The Spine Dictionary

The Spine Dictionary

A Comprehensive Guide to Spine Terminology

Christopher J. Centeno, MD
Executive Medical Director
Trauma Care, IPA
Boulder, Colorado

HANLEY & BELFUS, INC./Philadelphia

Publisher: HANLEY & BELFUS, INC.
Medical Publishers
210 South 13th Street
Philadelphia, PA 19107
215-546-7293; 800-962-1892
FAX 215-790-9330
Web site: http://www.hanleyandbelfus.com

Text Editor: Tara Pogoda, Cecelia Bayruns
Project Manager: Terri Velasquez
Editorial Board Manager: William Masisak

Note to the reader: Although the information in this book has been carefully reviewed for correctness of dosage and indications, neither the author nor the publisher can accept any legal responsibility for any errors or omissions that may be made. Neither the publisher nor the author make any warranty, expressed or implied, with respect to the material contained herein. Before prescribing any drug, the reader must review the manufacturer's current product information (package inserts) for accepted indications, absolute dosage recommendations, and other information pertinent to the safe and effective use of the product described. This is especially important when drugs are given in combination or as an adjunct to other forms of therapy.

Library of Congress Cataloging-in-Publication Data

Centeno, Christopher J., 1963-
The spine dictionary / Christopher J. Centeno.
p. cm.
ISBN 1-56053-270-X (alk. paper)
1. Spines—Dictionaries. 2. Spine—Diseases—Dictionaries.
3. Spine—Diseases—Treatment—Dictionaries. I. Title.
[DNLM: 1. Spine dictionaries. 2. Spinal Diseases—therapy dictionaries. 3. Spinal Injuries—therapy dictionaries. WE 13 C397s 1998]
RD768.C43 1998
616.7′3′003—dc21
DNLM/DLC
for Library of Congress 98-3975
CIP

THE SPINE DICTIONARY 1-56053-270-X

To my wife, who taught me how to be someone,
instead of something.

To my parents, whose sacrifices I
only now truly understand.

Editorial Board

Pamela Barker, P.T.
Back and Sports Injury Physical Therapy
Fort Collins, Colorado

Pete Emerson, P.T.
Director
Back and Sports Injury Physical Therapy
Director
Manual Physical Therapy Seminars of Colorado
Denver, Colorado

Matt Ferguson, M.S., P.T.
Challenge Sport and Spine Center Northwest
Westminster, Colorado

Cary Gold, P.T.
Cary Gold Physical Therapy
Boulder, Colorado

Ginny E. Johnson, M.S., P.T.
Back and Sports Injury Physical Therapy
Denver, Colorado

Candace R. Kenyon, M.S., P.T.
Challenge Sport and Spine Center Northwest
Westminster, Colorado

Patty Penell, M.S., P.T.
Back and Sports Injury Physical Therapy
Denver, Colorado

Pain Anesthesia

Scott Hompland, D.O.
Rehabilitation Associates of Colorado
Denver, Colorado

Chiropractic

David P. Gilkey, D.C., D.A.B.C.O., D.A.C.B.O.H., F.I.C.C.
Colorado Chiropractic Association
Denver, Colorado

Donald Kuppe, D.C.
Denver, Colorado

Craig E. Lincoln, D.C.
East Hampden Chiropractic
ChiroQualNet
Denver, Colorado

James C. Wagner, D.C.
Westminster Chiropractic
Westminster, Colorado

Insurance Industry

David McPherson
Progressive Insurance Companies
Denver, Colorado

Amy Newton
Colorado Compensation Insurance Authority
Denver, Colorado

Psychology

Kirk E. Peffer, Ph.D.
Behavioral Health Psychologists
Denver, Colorado

Nurse Case Management

Jill Adams, M.S.W., C.R.C., C.C.M.
Advanced Rehabilitation Management
Arvada, Colorado

Donna M. Cruz, L.P.N.
Sloans Lake Managed Care
Denver, Colorado

Nora Palmer Fox, R.N., C.C.M.
Fogel, Keating, and Wagner Law Firm
Englewood, Colorado

Deborah J. Grawet, B.S.N., R.N.
QMC3
Denver, Colorado

Linda Morris, R.N., C.C.M.
Bonnie Ruth and Associates
Denver, Colorado

Kathleen Solheim, R.N.
QMC3
Denver, Colorado

Fran Tafuro, R.N., CRRN, CIRS, C.C.M.
Centenial Rehabilitation Associates
Denver, Colorado

Marney Vaananen, R.N., B.Sc., N.Ed.
Lakewood, Colorado

Headache/Neurology

Judy Lane, M.D.
Head Pain Center
Englewood, Colorado

Legal

Angela R. Ecton
Norton Frickey and Associates
Lakewood, Colorado

Pharmacy

Gary W. King, R.Ph.
Infusion Treatment Centers
Englewood, Colorado

Alternative Medicine

Carol Flynn, C.M.T.
Fort Collins, Colorado

Preface

This book started as a small vocabulary list. After a while, I became obsessed with the idea of creating a truly comprehensive spine dictionary, a book that would include ideas that had never before been brought together on the same pages. The goal was to collect every single word that had ever been spoken about the spine. In reality, I still have a distance to go, but that will have to wait for subsequent editions.

There are many languages of the spine. Orthopedic surgeons, neurosurgeons, physical therapists, and chiropractors all speak different languages. Some terminology is so different that often professionals can barely communicate. This book was written to break down those barriers.

My career goal is to create a "unified field theory" of spine rehabilitation. The only way to accomplish this is to understand all dialects of "spine language" so that the best of many diverse concepts can be unified into one treatment technique.

Christopher J. Centeno, M.D.

Acknowledgments

I would like to acknowledge Joseph Centeno for all his hard work. Without his help this book would not be a reality. I also want to acknowledge Terri Velasquez for her work in pulling this book together.

I would like to thank James Wagner, David Gilkey, and Don Freuden for all their hard work educating me in the field of chiropractic. Without their help, this work would have very few chiropractic terms. Terry Yochum assisted with the radiology terms. His text was a fantastic resource.

I am grateful to Pete Emerson for his tireless attempts at educating me in the world of physical therapy. Pete has acted as my musculoskeletal mentor throughout this process and is a dear friend. I would like to thank Matt Ferguson for his help with lending me copies of his "boot-leg" books to use and for getting me excited about physical therapy in the first year of my practice. I would like to thank all the therapists at Back and Sports Injury for putting up with me for far too many afternoons. Candace Kenyon and Cary Gold have also taught me a great deal.

I would like to thank Kevin Reilly for his help with exercise physiology, Henry Roth and Howard Entin for giving me my start some time ago, and Nora Palmer Fox, Marney Vaananen, and Angela Ecton for going above and beyond the call of duty with some excellent medical editing.

SYMBOLS AND NUMBERS

+: A chiropractic notation which corresponds to less than appropriate movement in a vertebral segment. This can be placed after a Gonstead listing such as PRS+.

++: A chiropractic notation which refers to a vertebral segment which has appropriate or good movement. This can be used after a Gonstead listing such as PRS++.

+++: A chiropractic notation which refers to a segment which is over-adjusted. This can be used after a Gonstead listing such as PRS+++.

−: A chiropractic notation used for no joint movement. This can be used after a Gonstead listing. For instance, PRS−.

#: A symbol for pound or pounds. For instance, "15#" would be equivalent to "15 pounds."

↑: A chiropractic notation used to denote a vertebra which is posterior.

↓: A chiropractic notation used to denote a vertebra which is anterior.

→: A chiropractic notation used to denote a vertebra which is right facing.

←: A chiropractic notation used to denote a vertebra which is left facing.

↖: A chiropractic notation used to denote a vertebra which is posterior and left facing.

↗: A chiropractic notation used to denote a vertebra which is posterior and right facing.

↘: A chiropractic notation used to denote a vertebra which is anterior and right facing.

↙: A chiropractic notation used to denote a vertebra which is anterior and left facing.

✓: A physical therapy notation for flexion.

0: A grade of passive joint mobility which is defined as ankylosed (no movement).

1: A grade of passive joint mobility which is defined as considerable limitation to movement. There is, however, some small amount of movement.

2: A grade of passive joint mobility which is defined as a slight limitation to movement. This is a hypomobile joint.

2.5/500: A pharmacy abbreviation for 2.5 mg of hydrocodone and 500 mg of acetaminophen. This is equivalent to a Lortab 2.5.

3: A grade of passive joint mobility which is defined as normal joint movement.

4: A grade of passive joint mobility which is defined as a slight increase in joint movement. This is considered to be a hypermobile joint.

4/5: A notation in manual muscle testing which denotes a grade 4 manual muscle test. This would be the ability to move a joint and muscle through its range of motion against resistance. See 4 out of 5.

4 out of 5: A notation in manual muscle testing which denotes a grade 4 manual muscle test. See 4/5.

5: A grade of passive joint mobility which is defined as a considerable increase in joint mobility.

5/5: A grade 5 manual muscle test which implies normal muscle strength. See 5 out of 5.

5/500: A pharmacy abbreviation for 5 mg of hydrocodone and 500 mg of acetaminophen. This is equivalent to a Lortab 5.0, a Vicodin tablet, or a Lorcet-HD.

5 out of 5: A grade 5 manual muscle test which implies normal muscle strength. See 5/5.

6: A grade of passive joint mobility which is defined as pathologically unstable.

7.5/500: A pharmacy abbreviation for 7.5 mg of hydrocodone and 500 mg of acetaminophen. This is equivalent to a Lortab 7.5.

7.5/650: A pharmacological abbreviation referring to Lorcet Plus. This is 7.5 mg.

90/90 Hamstring Test: A test for hamstring length in which the patient is supine with the hip and knee in 90° of flexion. The knee is then extended and hamstring tightness is measured in degrees of extension lag.

360 Fusion: A surgical technique in which posterior instrumentation is combined with an anterior discectomy and fusion. Both anterior and posterior surgical approaches are used under the same general anesthesia.

10/650: A pharmacological abbreviation referring to the generic form of Lorcet. This refers to 10 mg of hydrocodone and 650 mg of acetaminophen.

A

A: An abbreviation for *anterior*. See Anterior.

AA Joint: An abbreviation for *atlantoaxial joint*. Referring to the C1–C2 articulation. See Atlantoaxial Joint.

AAO: American Academy of Osteopathy.

AAOS: American Academy of Orthopedic Surgeons.

AAPMR: American Academy of Physical Medicine and Rehabilitation.

A&W: An abbreviation for *alive and well*.

Abasia: A neurologic term referring to the inability to ambulate.

abd: An abbreviation for *abduction*.

Abd hallucis: An abbreviation for *abductor hallucis*.

Abdominal Curl-up: An abdominal strengthening exercise. The patient starts in the hook-lying position and is asked to slowly raise the head, bringing the shoulder blades off the floor. The focus should be on lifting the shoulder blades and not flexing the neck.

Abdominal Mechanism: A theory made popular by Gratavetsky whereby the abdominal musculature is used to increase intra-abdominal pressure and allow the lumbar spine to "float" on the abdominal contents. This is one reason behind strengthening the abdominals in low back rehabilitation.

Abdominal Support: A soft low back brace without metal stays with a Velcro enclosure anteriorly. The theory behind this type of bracing is that this increases interabdominal pressure and off loads some of the weight of the trunk. This then decreases some of the strain on the erector spinae musculature (back muscles) during lifting. See Abdominal Mechanism.

Abd Poll Brev: An abbreviation for *abductor pollicis brevis*.

Abduction External Rotation Test: A test for thoracic outlet syndrome. See Roos Test.

Aberrant Intersegmental Motion: Abnormal movement between two vertebral segments. This terminology is often used to refer to the subluxation complex.

ABNL: An abbreviation for *abnormal*.

Abnormal Spinal Segmental Motion: A chiropractic term which refers to an abnormality of spinal biomechanics involving a loss of normal movement of a vertebral motion. See Somatic Dysfunction, Vertebral Subluxation Complex.

Abortive: A medication used to treat headache which decreases pain once the headache has started.

ABOS: American Board of Orthopedic Surgery.

Abrupt Check: A type of end feel described by Cyriax which is caused by muscle spasm secondary to joint-related disorders.

Absolute Stenosis: Central canal stenosis involving a normal central canal with superimposed stenosis (commonly degenerative changes). This is in contrast to relative stenosis, which involves a congenitally small canal with superimposed stenosis. See Central Canal Stenosis.

ACA: American Chiropractic Association or Australian Chiropractors Association.

ACC: Association of Chiropractic Colleges.

Acceleration–Deceleration Injury: A sprain/strain syndrome of the cervical spine caused by a hyperextension–hyperflexion injury. See Flexion–Extension Injury, Whiplash Injury.

Accessory Atlantoaxial Ligament: The alar ligaments are wing-like structures which extend outward from the dens. The inferior wings are sometimes called the accessory atlantoaxial ligaments. These ligaments check atlantoaxial rotation from side to side. The right accessory atlantoaxial ligament checks AA rotation to the left. For example, when testing, the patient's cervical spine is brought into maximal flexion to "lock down" the lower cervical spine. The head is then rotated to the right or to the left. The end feel of rotation is the integrity of the accessory atlantoaxial ligament on the opposite side. See Alar Ligaments.

Accessory Movement: Movement that is necessary for normal range of motion but cannot be performed under voluntary control of the muscles. See Joint Play.

Accessory Occipital Vertebra: When the most distal portion of the occiput fails to fuse embryologically. An occipital vertebra can be found as a complete vertebral ring, accessory atlantal arches, or accessory pericondylar mass. These lesions can occur unilaterally or bilaterally and are often associated with narrowing and crowding of the foramen magnum as well as with other malformations of the bony and neural structures.

Accessory Process: An irregular bony prominence on the posterior surface of the transverse process near its attachment to the pedicles. These vary in size from a small bump to a more prominent mass of bone or a pointed projection of variable length.

Accessory SI Ligaments: The sacrotuberous, sacrospinous, and iliolumbar ligaments.

ACCO: American College of Chiropractic Orthopedists.

ACCR: American College of Chiropractic Radiologists.

Acetaminophen: An analgesic and antipyretic (reduces fever). Usual dosage is two 325-mg tablets every 8 hours. See Tylenol.

Acetaminophen and Codeine Phosphate: A narcotic pain reliever. See Tylenol No. 3.

Achilles' Reflex: An "ankle jerk" reflex. A physical exam maneuver in which the examiner taps on the Achilles' tendon to elicit a reflex response from the gastrocsoleus complex. Patients with an S1 radiculopathy *can* exhibit a decreased Achilles' reflex if there is motor involvement. An Achilles' reflex can also be decreased symmetrically with advanced age. This reflex represents a mono-synaptic arc and can be elicited electronically during an H-reflex study (part of a nerve conduction study). See Ankle Jerk, Achilles' Tendon Reflex.

Achilles' Tendon Reflex: An "ankle jerk" reflex. A physical exam maneuver in which the examiner taps on the Achilles' tendon to elicit a reflex response from the gastrocsoleus complex. See Achilles' Reflex, Ankle Jerk.

Achondroplasia: The most common form of congenital dwarfism. This is an autosomal condition. Spinal stenosis is commonly seen due to short pedicles and facets. This is most frequent in the thoracolumbar and lumbar regions. Multiple decompressive laminectomies are commonly performed to treat the spinal stenosis.

ACJ: An abbreviation for *acromioclavicular joint.*

Acquired Stenosis: Spinal stenosis due to degenerative disease. See Central Canal Stenosis.

ACR: American College of Rheumatology.

Acromegaly: A bony overgrowth that occurs from a persistently elevated growth hormone level. In the spine, widening of the vertebral bodies is commonly seen. This can narrow the spinal canal and cause spinal stenosis.

Acroparesthesia: A neurologic condition with symptoms of intense prickling, tingling, or numbness of the fingers and hands.

ACSM: American College of Sports Medicine.

Activator Technique: A chiropractic technique. See Activator Therapy.

Activator Therapy: A chiropractic technique that involves a small mechanical device which delivers a low-force "thump" to specific points in an attempt to rebalance the neuromuscular system through the spine. It can also be used in place of manipulation to small joints that would otherwise require very low force. This technique is used by more than half of all U.S. chiropractors. See Nonforce Technique.

Active Assistive Range of Motion: A type of active range of motion where assistance is provided by an outside force, either manually or mechanically.

Active Inhibition: A stretching maneuver which causes reflex inhibition of the muscle being stretched so that a greater stretch can be applied.

Active Mobility: Range of motion in the spine the patient can actively perform under his or her own power. See Active Range of Motion.

Active Range of Motion: Range of motion in the spine the patient can actively perform under his or her own power. For the lumbar spine, this would include flexion, extension, side bending, or rotation. See Active Mobility.

Active Trigger Point: An area of hyperirritability within a muscle or its associated fasciae that is tender and "shoots" or refers pain or other sensations to a distant site. An easy way to remember this is that, like a gun, this point is the trigger that shoots pain or other sensations to another location. It differs from a latent trigger point in that it is also tender. It may be associated with a local twitch response when stimulated. See Trigger Point.

Activities of Daily Living (ADL, Functional Activities): Those self-care functions that an individual must perform every day for normal hygiene. For instance, bathing, dressing, eating, toileting, and grooming. This also involves communication activities and home maintenance activities including cleaning and meal preparation.

Activity Restriction: Limiting the patient's physical movements, positions, and lifting after an injury for the purposes of healing.

Acupressure: The application of manual pressure to acupuncture meridians for the purpose of decreasing pain. See Acupuncture, Ischemic Compression.

Acupuncture: A Chinese treatment modality where needles are applied to specific points along "meridians" (channels of energy in the body). This is thought to have a neurophysiologic effect on decreasing pain. These same points can also be activated using pressure (acupressure) or various forms of electrical stimulation (electroacupuncture). See Alarm Points.

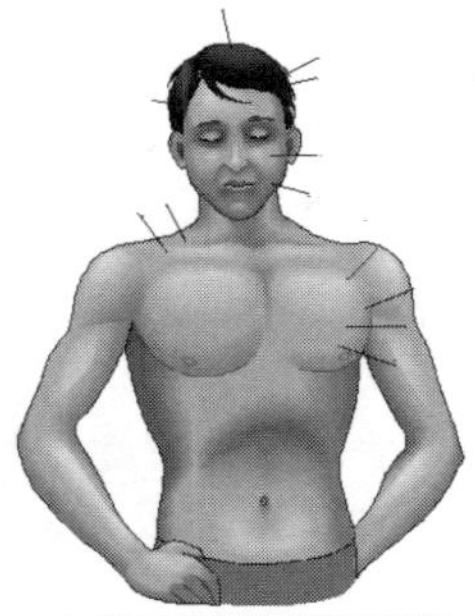

ACUPUNTURE

Acuscope: A proprietary name for a microcurrent electrical stimulation device. A function that reportedly allows the examiner to determine where to treat based on the electrical conductivity of the skin. This modality is used to block pain and decrease muscle spasm.

Acute: An injury of recent onset. The definition of *acute* varies considerably, however. To some, an injury is considered acute up to 2 weeks postinjury, to others it is up to 6 weeks postinjury. See Subacute, Chronic.

Acute Exacerbation: A sudden aggravation of symptoms or increase in severity of an already existing condition.

Acute Facet Syndrome: The acute facet syndrome may be more responsive to manual medicine than the chronic facet syndrome. See Facet Syndrome.

Acute Kyphosis Sign: A kyphotic angulation of the cervical spine which indicates severe damage to the posterior ligamentous structures. This injury can be caused by a hyperflexion force, and clinical instability should be ruled out.

Acute Low Back Strain: An injury to the musculature of the low back and sacral regions. See Lumbosacral Sprain/Strain.

Acute Sciatica: Dysfunction of a nerve root that can cause (1) radiating pain, numbness, or tingling in a specific pattern corresponding to that nerve root, or (2) muscle weakness in the muscles innervated by that nerve root. See Radiculopathy.

ADA: Americans with Disabilities Act.

Adalat: A calcium channel blocker used primarily for angina but is also used for patients with migraine headaches and reflex sympathetic dystrophy. See Procardia, Procardia XL, Adalat CC.

Adalat CC: A calcium channel blocker used for angina. See Procardia, Procardia XL, Adalat.

Adamkiewicz's Artery: The artery which supplies the anterior spinal artery and the thoracic and lumbar spinal cord. See Artery of Adamkiewicz.

Adaptive Changes: Changes in a spinal segment which occur secondary to another biomechanical problem in the spine. This usually involves loss of range of motion in a specific direction to compensate for the trauma at another area. Adaptive changes occur to restore the normal balance to the spine.

Adaptive Curve: A lateral curvature of the spine which is secondary to soft tissue imbalance and not to bony changes (structural). See Nonstructural Scoliosis, Nonstructural Curve, Adaptive Scoliosis, Adaptive Rotoscoliosis.

Adaptive Rotoscoliosis: A lateral curvature of the spine which is secondary to soft tissue imbalance but not to bony changes (structural). This term also implies a rotatory component to the lateral curve. See Nonstructural Scoliosis, Nonstructural Curve, Adaptive Scoliosis, Adaptive Curve.

Adaptive Scoliosis: A lateral curvature of the spine which is secondary to soft tissue imbalance and not to bony changes (structural). See Nonstructural Scoliosis, Nonstructural Curve, Adaptive Curve, Adaptive Rotoscoliosis.

add: An abbreviation for *adduction.*

Adhesive Arachnoiditis: An inflammatory reaction of the arachnoid membrane (one of the coverings of the spinal cord or brain) which causes scarring. See Perineural Fibrosis, Epidural Fibrosis.

Adhesive Capsulitis: Marked decreased range of motion, usually in one shoulder, of unknown etiology.

There are folds in the shoulder joint capsule which allow free movement and these become fused, thus limiting shoulder range of motion. Pain is usually noticed both in the shoulder joint area, as well as in the periscapular musculature. This can often be confused with primary thoracic pain. See Scaphohumeral Periarthritis, Frozen Shoulder.

ADI: The distance between the posterior margin of the anterior atlas and the anterior surface of the odontoid. See Atlanto-dental Interspace, Transverse Ligament of the Atlas, V Sign.

ADIO: An abbreviation for *above, down, inside, out.*

adj: An abbreviation for *adjustment.* See Adjustment, Manipulation.

Adjustment: The application of a force to a joint that takes it beyond its normal range of motion into its elastic range. See Manipulation.

Adjustment Disorder: A negative reaction to a known stressful situation. This usually results in symptoms far in excess of what would be considered a normal reaction to the stressful situation. Depression and/or anxiety are common features. See Adjustment Reaction.

Adjustment Reaction: A negative reaction to a known stressful situation. See Adjustment Disorder.

ADL: Those self-care functions that an individual must perform every day for normal hygiene. See Functional Activities, Activities of Daily Living.

Adolescent Scoliosis: A lateral spinal curvature that presents after puberty and before maturity.

Adson's Test: A physical exam test used to evaluate thoracic outlet syndrome at the first rib. See Costoclavicular Maneuver, Wright's Hyperabduction Maneuver.

Adult Scoliosis: Scoliosis which occurs after skeletal maturity. There are three major types: degenerative, posttraumatic, and developmental.

Adverse Mechanical Tension: The concept that the nervous system must be mobile to allow movement of the vertebral column and limbs. See Adverse Neural Tension.

Adverse Neural Tension: A concept first developed by Maitland and then developed further by Butler that the nervous system must be mobile to allow movement of the vertebral column and limbs. The nervous system interfaces with the surrounding connective tissue at a "mechanical interface." When the nervous system is not able to move and compensate for movements in the body, pain and nerve dysfunction can result. There are tests for specific nerves, and treatment is focused on mobilizing segments of the nervous system through stretches directed toward specific nervous system structures (epineurium) and "releasing" the mechanical interfaces through myofacial release. See Dural Mobilization, Mechanical Interface, Nerve Release, Neural Mobilization.

Adverse Neural Tension Test: Stressing specific nerves through maneuvers of the extremities or spine. Positive results can be a pulling sensation or radiating numbness in the distribution of that nerve. Both sides should be tested and compared. See Adverse Neural Tension, Brachial Plexus Tension Test, Tension Test.

Advil: A nonsteroidal anti-inflammatory drug which is in the propionic acid class. See Motrin, Ibuprofen.

Aerobic Capacity Assessment: This is usually included in a functional capacity evaluation. This is a submaximal screening of an individual's ability to sustain exertion at a given aerobic level. In other words, this is a measure of fitness. The measurement is usually expressed in METs.

Afferent (Afferent Input; Afferent Nerve Fiber): Sensory impulses which are carried toward the central nervous system and away from receptors in the periphery. See Afferent Nerve Fiber, Afferent Neuron, Afferent Input.

Afferent Neuron: Sensory impulses which are carried toward the central nervous system and away from receptors in the periphery. See Afferent, Afferent Nerve Fiber, Afferent Input.

AFO: An abbreviation for *ankle-foot orthosis.*

Agenesis of the Anterior Arch: A congenital defect of the anterior portion of the atlas which is extremely rare. Cervical flexion–extension views are recommended to rule out cervical instability.

Agenesis of the Posterior Arch: A congenital anomaly of the atlas which is usually detected on lateral cervical x-rays. There is lack of a bony posteroneural arch and often times a "megaspinous" process (an excessively large spinous process to C2). The integrity of the transverse ligament may be compromised; therefore, flexion–extension views should be performed looking at the ADI.

agg: An abbreviation for *aggravated* or *aggravation.*

Agonist: The muscle which is the prime mover. For instance, with respect to elbow flexion, the biceps would be the agonist and the triceps the antagonist. See Agonistic Muscles.

Agonist Contraction: A proprioceptive neuromuscular facilitation technique (PNF) used for inhibition (relaxation) of a muscle. The muscle opposite the tight muscle is contracted against resistance. This causes a reciprocal inhibition of the tight muscle and allows for better stretching of that muscle.

Agonistic Muscles: The muscle which is the prime mover. For instance, with respect to elbow flexion the biceps would be the agonist and the triceps the antagonist. See Agonist.

AH: An abbreviation for *abductor hallucis.*

Ah Shi Points: Acupuncture points that arise spontaneously and are not listed. They are said to occur in relation to particular joint problems or disease and are apparently suitable for needle or pressure treatment. They are thought to be very similar to the points described by Jones in the strain/counterstrain technique.

AIIS: Anterior inferior iliac spine.

AIIS Avulsion Fracture: An avulsion fracture of the anterior inferior iliac spine caused by the rectus femoris muscle. See Avulsion Fracture of the AIIS.

Air Contrast Myelography: A myelogram in which air is injected as the contrast agent to outline the nerve roots and dural sac. See Myelogram.

Airdyne: A brand name for an exercise bicycle that increases resistance as the pedaling speed increases.

AJ: An "ankle jerk" reflex. A physical exam maneuver in which the examiner taps on the Achilles' tendon to elicit a reflex response from the gastrocsoleus complex. See Ankle Jerk, Achilles' Reflex, Achilles' Tendon Reflex.

AK: (1) An abbreviation for *above knee*; (2) chiropractic diagnostic technique based on the idea that the neuromuscular system can be accessed through specific neuromuscular pressure points. See Applied Kinesiology.

Akabane Points: Acupuncture points which represent the terminal portions of the meridians. Sensitivity in these points is supposed to correspond to imbalance of the *chi* (life energy) in the meridian. See Acupuncture.

Ala of the Sacrum: The large lateral mass of the first sacral vertebral body. The iliacus muscle takes its origin from the most lateral portion of the tip of the sacral ala. See Sacrum, Sacral Ala.

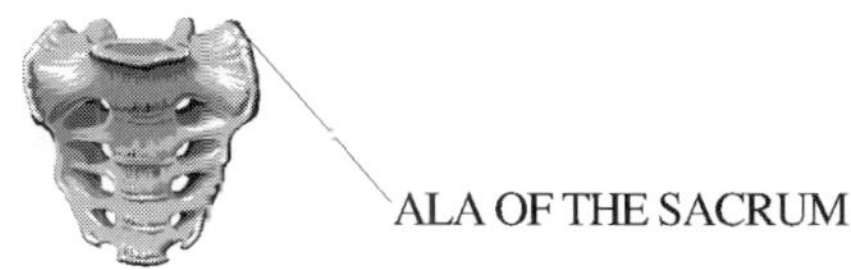

Alar Ligaments: A pair of wing-like, upper cervical ligaments that attach to the tip of the dens and to the medial surfaces of the occipital condyles. There is an upper and lower bundle on each side. Side bending to the right causes a C2 rotation to the left and involves the upper ligament on the left and the lower ligament on the right. The lower ligaments check AA rotation to the opposite side. AA rotation to the right thus ends with the end feel of the left lower alar. The upper bundles are sometimes referred to as the atlantal portion while the lower bundles are sometimes referred to as the accessory atlantoaxial ligaments. It has been postulated that the alar ligaments can be stretched or partially ruptured in a whiplash injury in which the head is rotated and flexed. See Apical Alar Ligaments, Check Ligaments.

Alar Ligament Test: A test for alar ligament integrity. The patient is in the sitting or supine position. The examiner palpates the C2 spinous process and then side bends the head. The spinous process of C2 should rotate to the opposite side of the side bending while the vertebrae rotate to the same side as the side bending. If a lag is present with a significant history of trauma or a significant impact whiplash, the ligament is suspect. There may be a history of blackouts or excessive muscle guarding in the upper cervical spine. It should also be noted that congenital absence of the alar ligaments does occur.

Alarm Points: Acupuncture points which are found only on the ventral surface of the body and associated with one of the 12 meridians and its functions. It is thought that tenderness elicited by palpation of an alarm point may indicate dysfunction of the organ related to that point. See Acupuncture.

Aleve: A nonsteroidal anti-inflammatory drug in the phenylpropionic acid class. See Anaprox, Naprosyn, Naproxen Sodium.

Alexander Technique: A movement system developed at the turn of the century by F. Matthias Alexander, a Shakespearean orator. Alexander developed a consistent problem when projecting his voice, and he began studying the relationship of head and neck posture to voice projection. The objectives are improvement in both posture and body mechanics. The system is based on the relationship of dysfunctional patterns in the head and neck to dysfunctional patterns throughout the body. Both verbal feedback and palpatory feedback are used to pattern new movements. The three stages of the Alexander technique include: (1) awareness of the habit, (2) inhibition of the habit, and (3) conscious control of the habit. See Movement Patterning.

ALIF: Anterior lumbar interbody fusion.

ALL: A ligament that runs the length of the lumbar spine anterior to the vertebral bodies and is one of the major ligaments involved in lumbar spine support during standing. See Anterior Longitudinal Ligament.

All Fours Opposite Arm and Leg Extension: A lumbar stabilization exercise. See Quadruped Opposite Arm and Leg Extension.

Allodynia: Pain that is due to a stimulus which does not normally cause pain. There is a lowered threshold of pain. See Hyperalgesia, Hyperpathia.

Allograft: A type of graft used for spinal fusion which is from a source other than the patient. The most common type of allograft is human cadaver bone. See Fusion.

Alordosis: Loss of the normal lordosis and straightening of the cervical or lumbar spine. This is most commonly seen in the cervical spine and known as "cervical straightening." This is seen after whiplash injuries and is thought to be caused by longus colli spasm.

Alprazolam: See Xanax.

ALS: A commonly fatal neurologic disorder with an unknown etiology. See Amyotrophic Lateral Sclerosis, Lou Gehrig Disease.

Altered Sagittal Curve: A term that usually refers to a decrease in cervical or lumbar lordosis (straightening of the spine).

Altered Weight Bearing: A radiographic term which refers to the shift of physiologic load from the anterior portion of the functional spinal unit (the disc) to the posterior portion (the facet). This is commonly seen in degenerative disc disease with the decrease in disc height being the main cause of the shift in load. The altered weight bearing can also occur in the opposite direction.

Ambien: A nonbenzodiazepine sleeping medication. The usual dose for adults is 10 mg before bedtime. A 5-mg tablet is also available. It is thought that this medication causes fewer problems with sleep disruption. See Zolpidem Tartrate.

Amipaque: A water-soluble x-ray contrast medium used commonly for myelography and CT myelography. See Metrizamide.

Amitriptyline HCl: A tricyclic antidepressant with sedative side effects. See Elavil, Amitriptyline Hydrocloride.

Amitriptyline HCl: A tricyclic antidepressant with sedative side effects. See Elavil, Amitriptyline HCl.

Amoss's Sign: A physical exam maneuver used to detect severe low back pain. A positive test is defined as difficulty rising from the supine position. The patient uses his upper extremities to lift himself and prevent flexion or any motion in the lumbar spine.

Amyotrophic Lateral Sclerosis: A commonly fatal neurologic disorder with an unknown etiology. This is characterized by deterioration of alpha motor neurons and progressive weakness and atrophy of the musculature. Muscle cramping is common and fasciculations are seen in the atrophied musculature. Death typically occurs within 2–7 years from the onset of symptoms and diagnosis. Symptoms can either appear slowly or be rapidly progressive. There is no known treatment. Diagnosis can be confirmed on EMG/nerve conduction study. The finding of fasciculations in the tongue usually secures the diagnosis. See ALS, Lou Gehrig Disease.

ANA: A laboratory blood test which screens for systemic lupus erythematosus (SLE). A positive ANA test is considered a titre greater than 1:40. However, if the patient is over 70 years of age, a titre of 1:40 may be insignificant. A positive ANA test should be followed up with more specific tests, such as an anti-DNA and precipitating antibodies such as RMP, Sm, Ro/SS-A. A negative ANA test usually means that the patient does not have SLE. However, there may be a significant false-positive rate (a positive test in a patient without the disease). See Antinuclear Factor, ANF.

Analgesia Rebound Headache: Headache pain noted with withdrawal from a pain medication such as Tylenol, aspirin, Advil, Fiorinal, and ergotamine. It is thought that taking an abortive headache medication more than 2 days a week can actually increase headache pain due to a rebound withdrawal effect.

Analgesic: A medication used for systemic or local pain relief.

Anal Wink: A physical exam maneuver which tests the integrity of the cauda equina and is often performed to rule out a cauda equina syndrome. This is a normal cord-mediated reflex that travels through the conus medularis. The test involves pricking the perianal region which causes a contraction or a "wink" of the external anal sphincter. In patients with cauda equina syndrome or lumbar stenosis the anal wink can be absent. Also, in patients with spinal cord injury the anal wink can be absent. See Sphincter Reflex.

Anaprox: A nonsteroidal anti-inflammatory drug in the phenylpropionic acid class. See Naprosyn, Naproxen Sodium, Aleve.

Anaprox DS: The 500-mg dose of Anaprox, which is considered double strength. See Naprosyn.

Anatomic Barrier: The absolute end of range of motion of a vertebral segment. If a vertebral segment is pushed beyond the anatomic barrier, damage to the joint capsule or surrounding soft tissues will occur.

Anatomic Leg Length Discrepancy: A leg length discrepancy due to a long or short femur or tibia. This can also be caused by coxa vera or coxa valga. See Anatomic Short Leg.

Anatomic Short Leg: A leg length discrepancy due to a long or short femur or tibia. This can also be caused by coxa vera or coxa valga. See Anatomic Leg Length Discrepancy.

Andersson Lesion: Instability at a vertebral segment seen in late-stage ankylosing spondylitis. There is a fracture at an ankylosed segment. This can be confused with an intervertebral disc infection or neuropathic arthropathy.

Android Pelvis: Referring to the characteristic male pelvic shape.

Anesthesia: The partial or total loss of sensation.

Anesthesia Dolorosa: Painful sensation in an area that is otherwise numb.

Aneurysmal Bone Cyst: A rare benign spinal tumor found most commonly in the lumbar region and in the posterior elements. There is a tendency to involve adjacent vertebra, and 3–4 vertebrae may be involved in sequence. Radiographs usually show an expansile, osteolytic cavity with strands of bone forming a bubbly appearance. The surrounding cortex is usually eggshell in appearance. Treatment can be through curettage or excision with reoccurrence in approximately one out of 10 cases.

ANF: A laboratory blood test which screens for systemic lupus erythematosus (SLE). See Antinuclear Factor, ANA.

Anghelescu's Sign: A test for tuberculosis spondylitis in the thoracic and lumbar spine. The patient lies supine on an examining table and attempts to extend the thoracic spine sufficiently to raise the upper back off of the table. The patient should be able to rest the weight of the body on the heels and shoulders. It is thought that this posture cannot be maintained in somebody with tuberculosis spondylitis. However, this would seem to be a very nonspecific test as anyone with significant thoracic or lumbar spine pathology other than tuberculosis may not be able to maintain this posture.

Angioma Racemosum Venosum: An AV fistula where the nidus is the nerve root sleeve dura. See Dural AV Fistula.

Angiothlipsis: A chiropractic term which refers to pressure on an artery in the intervertebral foramen caused by a bulging or herniated disc. Also, it is considered that foraminal stenosis can contribute to this problem.

Angle of Ferguson: A radiographic measurement of the angle between the superior end plate of L2 and the base of the sacrum. This is usually measured with a standing lateral x-ray film. See Lumbosacral Angle, Lumbosacral Lordotic Angle.

Angle of Louis: The angle between the manubrium and the body of the sternum. See Sternal Angle.

Angry Cat Stretch: A physical therapy exercise designed to stretch the erector spinae, posterior spinal ligaments, and gluteals. The patient starts in a quadruped position (on all fours) and is asked to tuck in the chin, tighten the stomach, and arch the back. This position is then held for a stretch.

Angular Kyphosis: A short-segment spinal curve with the apex pointing posteriorly. This is such a short segment that the curve appears to be more of an "angle." This angulation can cause irritation of the exiting nerve root. This deformity is usually due to fracture, inflammation, tumor, or laminectomy. It can also be congenital.

Ankle Jerk: Another way to say Achilles' tendon reflex. A physical exam maneuver in which the examiner taps on the Achilles' tendon to elicit a reflex response from the gastrocsoleus complex. See Achilles' Reflex, Achilles' Tendon Reflex.

Ankylosing Hyperostosis: A syndrome which involves diffuse ligamentous calcification and ossification seen in 5–10% of patients over 65 years of age. See Diffuse Idiopathic Skeletal Hyperostosis.

Ankylosing Spondylitis: An inflammatory disease of the spine which greatly restricts spinal movement. It is often associated with morning pain and occurs primarily in young adults. This is also known as "bamboo spine" because of its bamboo shoot–like appearance on x-rays. This "seronegative" (negative rheumatoid factor—not associated with rheumatoid arthritis) spondyloarthropathy (arthritis of the spine) involves inflammation, bony erosion, and ankylosis (spine joints that do not move). This disease process includes not only bony tissues, but also synovial joints and entheses (the points where ligaments, tendons, or joint capsules attach to bone). The SI joints, facet joints, and costovertebral joints are generally involved and may become ankylosed. There is involvement of the junction of the annulus fibrosus and the vertebral end plates (enthesiopathy). The cortical erosions and characteristic squaring of vertebral bodies lead to the classic "bamboo spine" on radiographs. End plate erosions are also seen. There can be involvement of the knees, and, peripherally, this is similar to rheumatoid arthritis. AS is associated with an HLA-B27 major histocompatibility complex. A positive HLA-B27 antigen is found in over 87.5% of American caucasians with AS, while only 8% of this group without AS have a positive HLA-B27. Prevalence is estimated at between 0.1 and 2%. The ratio of males to females is between 1 and 4 to 1. Patients usually complain of an insidious onset of low back pain and stiffness in the second and third decades. The location of pain varies from the trochanteric and gluteal regions to the thoracic spine. There may be some confusion of this symptom complex with sciatica because buttock pain with radiation to the legs is common. Symptoms are usually worse in the morning and improve with exercise. Nocturnal pain complaints are common. The disease is progressive, and patients assume a posture of lumbar flexion to transfer weight away from the inflamed facet joints. Pain from inflammation of the costovertebral joints inhibits chest expansion, and a decrease in pulmonary function is common. See AS, Marie-Strümpell Disease, Von Bechterew Disease, Rheumatoid Spondylitis, Pelvospondylitis Ossificans, HLA-B27, Romanus Lesion.

Ankylosis: An orthopedic term which describes a joint that no longer moves or has decreased motion. For instance, a spinal segment which has been fused is said to be ankylosed.

Annular Bulge: A disc bulge which is diffuse and usually due to degenerative changes. This is the first stage of disc degeneration.

Annular Rent: Another way to describe a radial tear in the annulus (outer covering of the disc) usually seen during discography, less commonly on MRI, or during surgery. It is thought that these tears are traumatic in origin. See Annular Tear, Radial Tear.

Annular Tear: A tear in the outer covering of the disc (the annulus) which is usually radial (from inside to outside or vice versa). Many low back injuries may include annular tears, especially those that heal slowly. This can lead to eventual disc disruption or herniation. See Annular Rent, Radial Tear, Internal Disc Disruption.

Anomalous Nerve Root: A congenital abnormality of the nerve roots. Approximately 15% of the population has anomalous lumbosacral nerve roots. The most frequent lumbar nerve root anomalies are two nerve roots that share the same dural sleeve and two nerve roots exiting the same foramen. One study found intradural connections between adjacent cervical nerve roots to be so common that they were regarded as normal variations.

Anomaly—Type 1: A nerve root anomaly with an aberrant course. See Type 1 Nerve Root Anomaly, Nerve Root Anomaly—Type 1.

Anomaly—Type 2: A nerve root anomaly where the number of roots in an intervertebral foramen is variable. See Type 2 Nerve Root Anomaly, Nerve Root Anomaly—Type 2.

Anomaly—Type 3: A nerve root anomaly in which there are extradural connections between roots, and a bundle of nerve fibers leaves one dural sleeve to enter an adjacent root. Also known as a conjoined nerve root. See Type 3 Nerve Root Anomaly, Nerve Root Anomaly—Type 3.

ANT: A concept first developed by Maitland and then developed further by Butler. The idea is that the nervous system must be mobile to allow movement of the vertebral column and limbs. See Adverse Neural Tension, Nerve Release.

Antagonist: The muscle opposite the prime mover. For instance, when you bend the elbow, the triceps is the antagonist and the biceps is the agonist.

Antagonistic Muscle: The muscle opposite the prime mover. See Antagonist.

Antalgic Tension Posture: The posture assumed to avoid tension on the sciatic nerve and nerve roots. The knee is flexed, the hip is flexed and abducted with slight external rotation. The cervical spine can be laterally flexed toward the side of the pain. The ankle can also be in slight plantar flexion. This is often associated with a lumbar radiculopathy.

Anteflexion: Forward flexion of the spine.

Antegrade Transport: The normal transport system from the cell body of a neuron along the axon distally. This occurs faster than retrograde transport. Neurotransmitters and nutrients are moved along the nerve and various toxic substances or ischemia can slow or block this transport. There are two types of antegrade transport, slow and fast. Fast antegrade transport occurs at approximately 400 mm per day and is involved in the transmission of neurotransmitters and transmitter vesicles. Slow antegrade transport occurs at 1–6 mm per day and is responsible for moving cytoskeletal material such as microtubules and neurofilaments.

Anterior: Located in the front, the opposite of posterior. See A.

Anterior Atlanto-dental Ligament: One of the upper cervical ligaments which runs between the anterior portion of the dens and the caudal portion of the anterior ring of C1. See Atlanto-dens Ligament.

Anterior Atlanto-occipital Membrane: A fibroelastic tissue that extends between the anterior margin of the foramen magnum and the upper border of the anterior arch of the atlas.

Anterior Cervical Cord Syndrome: An incomplete spinal cord lesion characterized by complete motor loss and loss of pain and temperature below the level of the injury. Proprioception, deep touch, and vibration remain intact. Direct trauma to the anterior spinal cord is a common etiology. Also, this syndrome is commonly seen after vascular repair of an aortic aneurysm. See Spinal Cord Syndrome.

Anterior Discectomy and Fusion: The removal of the intravertebral disc and placement of bone graft for fusion through an anterior approach. Instrumentation may be used.

Anterior Disc Herniation: An extrusion of the nucleus pulposus through the anterior annular fibers. This is in contrast to the more common posterolateral disc herniations. Since there are few neural structures anteriorly, this is usually *not* associated with radiculopathy or myelopathy. See Anterior HNP, Anterior Herniated Disc, HNP.

Anterior Elements: The opposite of the posterior elements. This refers to the vertebral body and disc.

Anterior Fusion: A surgical procedure which involves the replacement of some or all of the disc with a bony graft through an anterior approach. See Anterior Interbody Fusion, Transpedicular Fixation.

Anterior Herniated Disc: An extrusion of the nucleus pulposus through the anterior annular fibers. See Anterior HNP, Anterior Disc Herniation, HNP.

Anterior HNP: An extrusion of the nucleus pulposus through the anterior annular fibers. See Anterior Disc Herniation, Anterior Herniated Disc, HNP.

Anterior Horn: The portion of the spinal cord located ventrally which contains the anterior horn cells (cell bodies of the motor neurons). Injury to this area will cause motor weakness and atrophy without significant sensory loss. Diseases of this area include ALS.

Anterior Horn Cell: The cell body of a lower motor neuron which resides in the anterior portion of the spinal cord. This is a motor neuron (controls muscles).

Anterior Iliac Rotation: A movement dysfunction of the pelvis in which the ilium is noted to be anterior–inferior relative to the sacrum. See Anterior Ilium, Forward Ilium, Forward Innominate, Forward Innominate Rotation, Anteriorly Rotated Ilium, Anterior Innominate, Anteriorly Rotated Innominate.

Anterior Ilial Rotation: One of the many dysfunctions of the SI joint described in the osteopathic and manual physical therapy literature. The ASIS is noted to be anterior, inferior, and medial. The PSIS is anterior, lateral, and superior. In effect, the ilium has rotated forward on the sacrum. See Anterior Ilium.

Anterior Ilium: A movement dysfunction of the pelvis in which the ilium is noted to be anterior–inferior relative to the sacrum. The ASIS is noted to be inferior, anterior, and medial. The PSIS is noted to be superior, anterior, and lateral. Posterior rotation of the sacrum is decreased while anterior rotation of the sacrum is increased. It is thought that an anterior ilium can be compensatory for short leg or a structural scoliosis in the lumbar spine. See Forward Ilium, Forward Innominate, Forward Innominate Rotation, Anterior Iliac Rotation, Anteriorly Rotated Ilium, Anterior Innominate, Anteriorly Rotated Innominate, Anterior Ilium.

Anterior Inferior Iliac Spine Avulsion Fracture: An avulsion fracture of the anterior inferior iliac spine caused by the rectus femoris muscle. See Avulsion Fracture of the AIIS.

Anterior Innominate: A movement dysfunction of the pelvis in which the ilium is noted to be anterior/inferior relative to the sacrum. See Anterior Ilium, Forward Ilium, Forward Innominate, Forward Innominate Rotation, Anterior Iliac Rotation, Anteriorly Rotated Ilium, Anteriorly Rotated Innominate.

Anterior Innominate Shear: A manual medicine term which refers to a condition where the ilium is anterior in relation to the sacrum. See Anterior Shear.

Anterior Interbody Fusion: A surgical procedure which involves the replacement of some or all of the disc with a bony graft through an anterior approach. This is used commonly in the cervical spine to treat degenerative disc disease and HNP. This is also used in the lumbar spine when posterior attempts have failed, when the posterior elements are destroyed (facets), with a 360 fusion, or when the posterior approach is not possible. See Anterior Fusion.

Anterior Longitudinal Ligament: A ligament that runs the length of the lumbar spine anterior to the vertebral bodies and is one of the major ligaments involved in lumbar spine support during standing. See ALL.

Anteriorly Rotated Ilium: A movement dysfunction of the pelvis in which the ilium is noted to be anterior–inferior relative to the sacrum. See Anterior Innominate, Anterior Ilium, Forward Ilium, Forward Innominate, Forward Innominate Rotation, Anterior Iliac Rotation, Anteriorly Rotated Innominate, Right Anterior Innominate.

Anteriorly Rotated Innominate: A movement dysfunction of the pelvis in which the ilium is noted to be anterior–inferior relative to the sacrum. See Anterior Innominate, Anterior Ilium, Forward Ilium, Forward Innominate, Forward Innominate Rotation, Anterior Iliac Rotation, Anteriorly Rotated Ilium.

Anterior Nutation: A term derived from the Latin term meaning "nodding." In the lumbar spine, nutation usually refers to the ilium or the sacrum. See Nutation.

Anterior Pelvic Tilt: An anterior rotation of the pelvis in which the ASIS comes forward and the sacrum moves backward. This condition commonly occurs when the lumbar spine is hyperextended (excessive lordosis). This can place excessive loading on the facets and causes the abdominal muscles to be lengthened and weak and the erector spinae muscles to be shortened and tight.

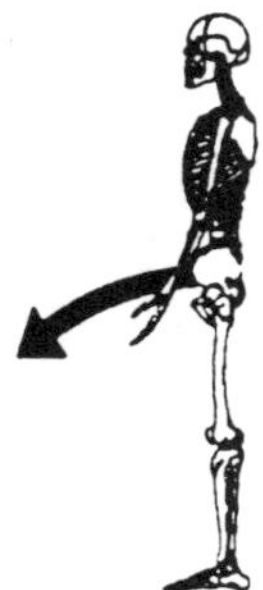

ANTERIOR PELVIC TILT

Anterior Posterior Diameter of the Pelvis: A measurement of the diameter of the pelvic inlet usually measured on lateral radiographs. This is the distance between the lower margin of the symphysis pubis and the tip of the sacrum. See AP Diameter of the Pelvis, Sacropubic Diameter.

Anterior Pubic Bone: A manual medicine term which refers to a condition where the ilium is anterior in relation to the sacrum. The pubic tubercle on that side is felt to be anterior on palpation. The ilium is noted to move more freely in an anterior direction than a posterior direction. See Anterior Shear.

Anterior Pubic Ligament: One of the supporting ligaments of the pubic symphysis.

Anterior Sacral Foramina: Foramina or openings which occur bilaterally and segmentally on the anterior sacrum through which pass the anterior branches of the sacral nerve roots. See Sacral Foramina.

Anterior Sacral Nutation: An osteopathic or manual physical therapy term used to denote a sacral position such that the base is anterior and inferior and the apex posterior and superior. See Bilateral Flexed Sacrum.

Anterior Sacroiliac Ligament: A thickening of the anterior joint capsule of the SI joint. This ligament is stressed with posterior pressure on the iliac wings.

Anterior Sacrum: An osteopathic or manual physical therapy term which refers to a sacrum with the sacral base anterior relative to the ilium on one side. The sacrum is noted to be side bent about a diagonal axis to the opposite side. See Unilaterally Flexed Sacrum.

Anterior Sacrum Left: An osteopathic or manual physical therapy term which refers to a sacrum with the sacral base anterior relative to the ilium on one side. The sacrum is noted to be side bent about a diagonal axis to the opposite side. Therefore, *anterior sacrum left* refers to a sacrum which is rotated right and side bent left; movement would then be restricted in the opposite directions, rotation left and side bending right. See Anterior Sacrum.

Anterior Sacrum Right: An osteopathic or manual physical therapy term which refers to a sacrum with the sacral base anterior relative to the ilium on one side. The sacrum is noted to be side bent about a diagonal axis to the opposite side. Therefore, *anterior sacrum right* refers to a sacrum which is rotated left and side bent right; movement would then be restricted in the opposite directions, rotation right and side bending left. See Anterior Sacrum.

Anterior Scalene Syndrome: Compression of the neurovascular bundle as it passes between the anterior and middle scalene muscles. This is synonymous with thoracic outlet syndrome as this is one of the more common areas of entrapment. See Scalene Anticus Syndrome, Thoracic Outlet Syndrome.

Anterior Shear: A manual medicine term which refers to a condition where the ilium is anterior in relation to the sacrum. The pubic tubercle on that side is felt to be anterior on palpation bilaterally. The ilium is noted to move more freely in an anterior direction than in a posterior direction. See Anterior Pubic Bone.

Anterior SI Ligaments: The weak supporting ligaments of the SI joint which lie anteriorly. These are defined as a thickening of the SI joint capsule.

Anterior Subluxation: A chiropractic term which refers to a vertebral body which is fixed in extension relative to the vertebral body above and below. Palpation of the spinous processes reveals that the spinous process of the involved vertebra is farther anterior.

Anterior Superior Iliac Spine: A common landmark for manual medicine diagnosis. This is a bony protuberance palpated on the anterior portion of the iliac bone. Abbreviated ASIS.

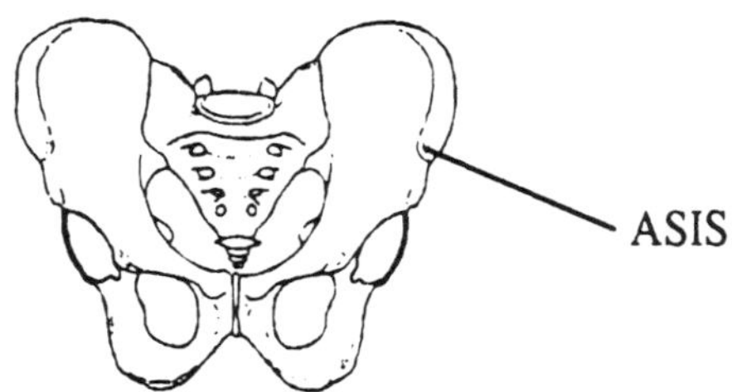

Anterior Torsion: An osteopathic or manual physical therapy term which describes a sacral torsion along an oblique sacral axis (from one sacral base to the opposite ILA). See Forward Sacral Torsion.

Anterior Translated Sacrum: An osteopathic term which refers to a sacrum that has moved forward relative to the ilia. See Translated Sacrum–Anterior.

Anterior Wedge Fracture: A fracture of the vertebral body characterized by anterior collapse of this structure. This most commonly occurs in the C5–T1 region. This fracture is usually clinically insignificant and complete recovery is common. Pain may persist for several months. The most common mechanism of injury is hyperflexion combined with axial loading. This is the number one nonfatal fracture of the cervical spine.

Anterolisthesis: A term which defines a vertebral segment which is moved forward relative to the segment above and below.

Anteroposterior View: An x-ray view in which the patient faces away from the x-ray film cartridge and toward the x-ray beam. The beam passes from anterior to posterior. See AP View, AP.

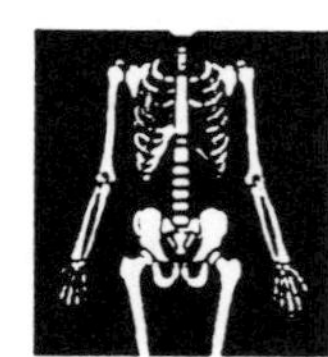

ANTEROPOSTERIOR X-RAY VIEW
AP VIEW

Anteversion of the Hip: A condition where the angle of torsion of the hip is greater than 150°. A simpler way to state this is that the acetabulum is facing farther forward than normal. This may cause a toed-in gait. There is a dramatic increase in internal rotation of the hips and a decrease in external rotation on physical exam. The lumbar lordosis may be increased. If the condition is unilateral, SI joint dysfunction or low back pain is common secondary to pronation causing a short leg and leg length discrepancy. Knee pain is also common with patellofemoral malalignment. Common treatment includes strengthening of the external rotators, mobilization to increase external rotation, orthotics, McConnel taping for the patellofemoral syndrome, correction of the SI joint dysfunction, correction of the leg length discrepancy, surgical correction, and others. See Anteverted Hip.

Anteverted Hip: A condition where the angle of torsion of the hip is greater than 150°. See Anteversion of the Hip.

Anthropoid Pelvis: A pelvic shape characteristic of primates. The pelvic inlet is widest in the AP direction with the transverse diameter being narrower.

Antinuclear Factor: A laboratory blood test which screens for systemic lupus erythematosus (SLE). See ANA, ANF.

Antivert: An antihistamine used most commonly for diseases affecting the vestibular system and causing dizziness. It is also used in the management of nausea and vomiting and dizziness associated with motion sickness. This medication does have anticholinergic side effects, such as dry mouth. The usual dosage for the control of vertigo is 25–100 mg in divided doses. This is usually given as 25 mg three times a day. See Meclizine.

Antrocollis: An abnormal flexion posture of the cervical spine. This is often associated with cervical dystonia.

AO: Abbreviation for the German name, Arbeitsgemeinschaft Osteosynthesefragen, a nonprofit European research group dedicated to the study and design of internal fixation. This is also a brand name of internal fixation devices.

AOA: American Orthopedic Association or American Osteopathic Association.

AO Joint: Atlanto-occipital joint, which is a joint between the skull and the atlas (C1). See Occipital-Atlantal Joint.

AOP: An abbreviation for AO plate. See AO group.

AO Plates: Plates designed by the AO group. See AO, AOP.

AO Screws: Screws designed by the AO group. See AO.

AO System: Fixation systems designed by the AO group. See AO.

Aortic Aneurysm: A ballooning out of the abdominal aorta, aortic arch, descending thoracic aorta, and, rarely, the ascending aorta that is due to atherosclerosis. This is a cause of low back pain and mid back pain, and caution should be taken in ruling out this diagnosis in unexplained back pain. Almost all aneurysms occur in the 60–80-year age group (95%). The male to female ratio is 4:1. This lesion can be seen radiographically if there is calcification within the aorta. The lesion is visible as a soft tissue density with a thin rim of continuous or discontinuous calcification. However, this calcification is present in only about 50% of the cases. Abdominal aortic aneurysm is suspected if the diameter of the aorta is greater than 3.8 cm. A measurement of greater than 5 cm is usually an indication for surgical intervention. Lesions greater than 6 cm are prone to rupture in over half of the cases. An ultrasound is recommended for confirming a diagnosis. Aortic arch aneurysms should be suspected in cases of trauma. They can develop slowly over years and remain clinically silent. Radiographically, they can enlarge the aortic silhouette superiorly and laterally and often displace the trachea and esophagus. Aneurysm of the descending aorta is best viewed on a lateral projection. Aneurysms of the ascending aorta are rare, but can be seen in patients with Marfan syndrome. Cystic medial necrosis of the ascending aorta can also lead to aneurysm.

AP: An x-ray view in which the patient faces away from the x-ray film cartridge and toward the x-ray beam. The beam passes from anterior to posterior. See Anteroposterior View, AP View.

APA: American Psychiatric Association or American Psychological Association.

AP and Lat: Anterior-posterior and lateral x-ray views.

AP Diameter of the Pelvis: A measurement of the diameter of the pelvic inlet usually measured on lateral radiographs. This is the distance between the lower margin of the symphysis pubis and the tip of the sacrum. See Anterior Posterior Diameter of the Pelvis, Sacropubic Diameter.

Apex of the Sacrum: The most inferior portion of the sacrum that articulates with the coccyx. See Sacral Apex.

Apical Alar Ligaments: The upper portion of the alar ligaments which check side bending and rotation of the upper cervical spine. See Alar Ligaments, Check Ligaments.

Apical Dentate Ligament: One of the dentate ligaments that attaches the superior portion of the dens to the anterior edge of the foramen magnum. See Apical Ligament.

Apical Ligament: One of the dentate ligaments that attaches the superior portion of the dens to the anterior edge of the foramen magnum. See Apical Dentate Ligament.

Apical Vertebrae: A term used in scoliotic spines to identify the vertebra that is the greatest distance from the midline. This would be the vertebra at the apex of the scoliosis and the most rotated vertebra.

Aplasia: The congenital absence of a structure. This is caused by a defect in development.

APOM View: A chiropractic x-ray series which involves lateral bending and left and right rotation of the C1 and C2 region. This is done to rule out ligamentous rupture or laxity involving the alar ligaments and/or accessory atlantoaxial ligaments.

Aponeurosis: Connective tissue in the shape of a flat sheet which attaches muscle to bone or bone to other tissues.

Aponeurositis: Inflammation in an aponeurosis.

Apophyseal Articulation: A synovial joint about the same size as the PIP joints (small joints at the end of the fingers). See Facet Joint.

Apophyseal Joints: A synovial joint about the same size as the PIP joints (small joints at the end of the fingers). See Facet Joint.

Apophysis Sign: A radiographic sign used to determine when vertebral growth is complete. See Risser's Sign.

Apparent Hypomobility: A decrease in normal joint movement which corrects with simple mobilization procedures. For instance, this would be the equivalent of the hypomobility in an SI joint seen on a squish test.

Apparent Leg Length: The functional length of a lower extremity measured from the umbilicus to the medial malleolus. The difference between this and actual leg length is that pelvic tilt or an SI joint dysfunction can alter the apparent leg length. This difference in leg length is not due to the bony length of the lower extremities. See Functional Leg Length, Structural Leg Length.

AP Pelvis: An x-ray view which shows both innominates (ilia), the sacrum, coccyx, SI joints, and proximal femurs. The x-ray beam passes from anterior to posterior.

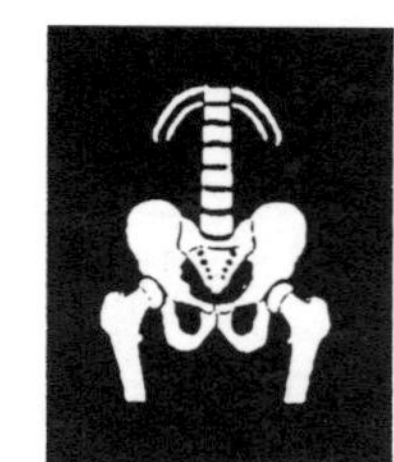

AP PELVIS

Applied Kinesiology: A chiropractic diagnostic technique based on the idea that the neuromuscular system can be accessed through specific neuromuscular pressure points. This is usually combined with manual muscle testing to determine which muscles are weak and need to be balanced. Some chiropractors use this technique as a way to plan their adjustments. This technique is used by approximately 37% of chiropractors in the U.S., according to the 1993 Job Analysis of Chiropractic. See A.K., Kinesiology.

Apportionment: The determination of the degree that various factors have contributed to a particular impairment. This is the amount of an injury that is due to a specific event. It must be determined that the factor in question could have caused the impairment or is "causally related." Take, for example, a patient who is involved in two motor vehicle accidents. Which injuries are due to the first accident and which to the second? If the patient had back pain only after the second accident, and the back pain was causally related, it would be apportioned 100% to the second accident. It should be noted that apportionment is a very inexact science and oftentimes there is no scientific way to determine apportionment.

Apraxia: The loss of motor coordination secondary to loss of higher (cortical) motor planning without loss of strength. An example would be a stroke patient who has normal strength in his right arm but does not have enough coordination to pick up a glass.

AP View: An x-ray view in which the patient faces away from the x-ray film cartridge and toward the x-ray beam. The beam passes from anterior to posterior. The anteroposterior x-ray view is included in many common x-ray series. The view of the cervical spine gives important information about the uncinate processes (bony ridges on the outer rim of the vertebra), facets, and overall bony alignment. Scoliosis is usually well appreciated on AP views. Information can also be gained in the lumbar spine about the posterior elements, pedicles, and transverse processes. See AP, Anteroposterior View.

ARA: American Rheumatism Association, the former name of the American College of Rheumatology. See ACR.

Arachnoid: A loose connective-tissue covering of the spinal cord which is below the dura mater and above the pia mater. This is a cobweb-like structure consisting of fine elastic fibrous tissue. It follows the contour of the dura mater and is separated from the dura by the subdural space and from the pia mater by the subarachnoid space.

Arachnoid Granulations: Tufts of arachnoid matter which protrude through the dura into the epidural space where they invaginate the walls of the epidural veins and drain the spinal cord and nerve root area of cerebrospinal fluid (CSF). The primary function of this system is to drain CSF and remove debris from the CSF into the vascular system. See Dural Cuff.

Arachnoiditis: Inflammation of the arachnoid membrane (one of the coverings of the spinal cord/brain) that can lead to fibrosis (scarring). This is one complication of epidural steroid injection, prior surgery, or myelography which is rare and usually self limited. However, chronic arachnoiditis can be a disabling condition.

Arachnoid Mater: A loose connective-tissue covering of the spinal cord which is below the dura mater and above the pia mater. See Arachnoid.

Arachnoid Membrane: A loose connective tissue covering of the spinal cord which is below the dura mater and above the pia mater. See Arachnoid.

Arachnoid Trabeculae: Small connective-tissue extensions between the arachnoid membrane and the pia mater. See Trabeculae.

Areflexic: Referring to the absence of deep tendon reflexes or other reflexes.

Arm Extension—Quadruped: A lumbar stabilization exercise. See Quadruped Arm Extension.

AROM Exercise: A physical therapy exercise designed to increase active range of motion. For instance, in the cervical spine, the patient is asked to actively move in all planes of cervical movement (forward flexion, backward bending, right/left rotation, right/left lateral bending) to increase range of motion. See Active Range of Motion.

Arm Pull: One of the many techniques of myofascial release which can be utilized to mobilize the fascia of the shoulder girdle.

Arm Raise Overhead—Hook-Lying: A lumbar stabilization exercise. See Hook-Lying Arm Raise Overhead.

Arteriovenous Malformation: A fistulous communication between intradural spinal arteries and a spinal vein. See AVM.

Artery of Adamkiewicz: The artery which supplies the anterior spinal artery and the thoracic and lumbar spinal cord. It enters through an intervertebral foramen on one side only (78% on the left side) between the T8 and L3 foramina. Injury to this artery can result in ischemia in the lumbar area of the cord. This is due to the poor vertebral anastomoses among the cervical, thoracic, and lumbar segments of the anterior spinal artery. Ischemia in the anterior spinal artery usually involves the anterior horn cells and produces a motor deficit. This artery takes off from T5 or above 15% of the time. See Adamkiewicz's Artery.

Arthralgia: Pain emanating from a joint.

Arthritis Deformans: A severely disabling and deforming destruction of the joints of the hands and feet seen in a minority of patients with psoriatic arthritis.

Arthrocentesis: The aspiration of a joint space through a needle, usually performed to remove fluid from a joint for diagnosis or treatment.

Arthrochondritis: Inflammation of the cartilaginous portion of a joint.

Arthrodesis: A bony surgical fusion possibly with internal fixation such as pins, plates, rodding systems, or bone grafts.

Arthrogram: The injection of radiographic dye into a joint followed by an x-ray. The outline of the joint can then be seen and inspected for irregularities. Also, SI and facet injections are usually accompanied by arthrograms.

Arthrokinetic Reflex: The muscles overlying a joint provide nerve supply to that joint. It is thought that a unique feedback mechanism between the joint and the overlying muscles receives the same innervation. The arthrokinetic reflex connects the articular mechanoreceptors to the overlying muscles of the joint so muscle tone can be regulated.

Arthroscopic Microdiscectomy: A surgical procedure performed arthroscopically (through a fiberoptic scope) for the removal of contained disc bulges. There is a minimum of dissection and damage to surrounding structures.

Arthrosis Temporomandibularis: Pain emanating from the temporomandibular joint. See TMJ Dysfunction, Temporomandibular Joint Arthrosis, TMJ Myofascial Pain, Temporomandibular Dysfunction, Mandibular Pain Dysfunction Syndrome.

Articular: Of or pertaining to a joint.

Articular Dysfunction: A chiropractic term which refers to an abnormality of spinal biomechanics involving a loss of normal movement of a vertebral motion segment. See Joint Blockage, Vertebral Subluxation Complex, Abnormal Spinal Segmental Motion, Somatic Dysfunction, Osteopathic Lesion.

Articular Dyskinesia: A joint that does not move freely in all directions due to a muscular imbalance in the muscles surrounding the joint.

Articular Fixation: A joint that does not move freely in all directions. See Fixation, Subluxation.

Articular Pillar: The bony portion of the C3–C7 vertebra which occurs at the junction of the pedicles and lamina and supports the superior and inferior articular facets. This projects laterally and is a bony landmark for many manual medicine diagnostic maneuvers as well as for Jones points.

Articular Pillar Fracture: A fracture of the articular pillars of the cervical spine. This is one of the most frequently missed fractures of the cervical spine because these structures are not well visualized on standard x-ray views. The articular pillar is formed by the superior and inferior articular processes. Pillar fractures most commonly occur at C4–C7 with C6 being the most common level. This site is involved in approximately 40% of cases. The most common mechanism is MVA. See Pillar Fractures.

Articular Spondylolisthesis: A "slipping" of one vertebra onto another due to destructive, degenerative changes within the facet joints. See Degenerative Spondylolisthesis.

Articular Strain: Stressing of the joint capsule beyond its limits causing small tears within the capsule.

Articulatory Technique: A repeated oscillatory mobilization of low velocity and varying amplitudes. This is performed within the available range of motion and has a rhythmic quality.

Artifact: A radiologic term for an incidental finding not related to pathology. For instance, during a CT scan, any metal within the patient can produce an artifact which may obscure the true pathology from view. Another example would be an MRI image of a patient who moved too much during the MRI; when the final picture is fuzzy, it is called an artifact.

AS: A chiropractic term denoting an SI joint in which the PSIS has moved anteriorly and superiorly with the ilium fixed in extension in relation to the sacrum. The axis of rotation has thus shifted inferiorly and the superior portion of the joint remains mobile. See Sacroiliac Extension Fixation.

AS: An inflammatory disease of the spine which greatly restricts spinal movement and is often associated with morning pain, and primarily occurs in young adults. It is also known as "bamboo spine" because of its bamboo shoot–like appearance on x-rays. See Ankylosing Spondylitis, Marie-Strümpell's Disease, Von Bechterew Disease, Rheumatoid Spondylitis, Pelvospondylitis Ossificans.

Asensate: The lack of sensation to all stimuli.

ASEX: A chiropractic term which denotes an anterior, superior, and externally rotated ilium. See ASEX Ilium.

ASEX Ilium: A chiropractic term which denotes an anterior, superior, and externally rotated ilium. See ASEX.

AS Ilium: A chiropractic term used in SI joint dysfunction. The ilium is found to be anterior and superior relative to the sacrum. The landmarks used include the ASIS or PSIS.

ASIN: A chiropractic term which denotes an ASIS which is anterior, superior, and internally rotated. This would be equivalent to an osteopathic inflare combined with a posterior ilium. See ASIN Ilium.

ASIN Ilium: A chiropractic term which denotes an ASIS which is anterior, superior, and internally rotated. See ASIN.

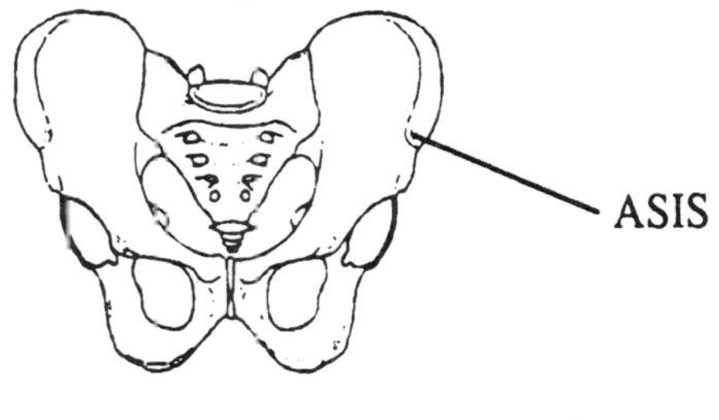

ASIS (Anterior Superior Iliac Spine): A common landmark for manual medicine diagnosis. This is a bony protuberance palpated on the anterior portion of the iliac bone.

ASIS

Asnis Screw: A cannulated screw used in orthopedic surgery.

Aspinall's Test: A physical exam maneuver for testing the integrity of the transverse ligament. The patient is in a supine position, and one examining hand is placed in the suboccipital region. Upward pressure is placed between the skull and C2 (on the atlas) while the other hand immobilizes the chin. Cord signs or excessive movement indicate transverse ligament laxity or rupture. Caution must be used when performing this test for obvious reasons. Transverse ligament dysfunction is relatively common in patients with Down syndrome (20%) and rheumatoid arthritis.

ASRF: Australian Spinal Research Foundation.

Associated Trigger Point: A focus of hyperirritability within a muscle or its surrounding fasciae that is due to compensatory overload, decrease in range of motion, or referred pain from another trigger point. Types of associated trigger points include satellite trigger points and secondary trigger points.

Aston Patterning: A system of movement education and deep tissue work to provide muscle balance and proper body mechanics. Emphasis is placed on the idea that accumulated stress is held in certain areas of the body and can be caused by compensation or muscle imbalances. These are called "functional holding patterns." There is also an element of deep tissue release and a focus on working with the body's natural asymmetries. See Movement Patterning.

asym: An abbreviation for *asymmetrical.*

Asymptomatic: Without symptoms.

At: An abbreviation for *atlas.*

Ataxic Gait: Walking which lacks coordination and is characterized by a wide base (the feet are farther apart). This gait is unsteady and can be caused by central nervous system diseases including cerebellar dysfunction. Also, spinal stenosis producing bilateral lower extremity weakness can cause an ataxic gait.

ATC: Athletic Trainer Certified.

Ativan: A benzodiazepine used for the management of anxiety disorders or for the short-term relief of symptoms of anxiety or anxiety associated with depressive symptoms. The use of this drug is contraindicated in patients with acute narrow-angle glaucoma. Physical addiction is possible, and withdrawal symptoms do occur. The usual adult dosage is 2–6 mg a day in divided doses. For anxiety, dosage is usually 1 mg two or three times a day. For insomnia, 2–4 mg are given at bedtime. Tablets are available in 0.5 mg, 1 mg, and 2 mg. See Lorazepam.

Atlantoaxial: Referring to the C1–C2 area.

Atlantoaxial Angle: A radiographic finding determined by lateral radiographs of the cervical spine. This is the angle formed between the first two cervical vertebrae.

Atlantoaxial Dislocation: Subluxation of C1 on C2. See Atlantoaxial Subluxation.

Atlantoaxial Impaction: Vertical subluxation of the odontoid into the foramen magnum. See Basilar Invagination, Vertical Subluxation, Vertical Settling, Cranial Settling.

Atlantoaxial Instability: Excess motion at C1–C2, usually due to trauma. The distance between the anterior border of the dens and the posterior border of C1 should not exceed 3 mm. The distance between the posterior margin of the dens and the anterior cortex of the posterior ring of C1 should not exceed 13 mm. Axial rotation to one side should not exceed 56°. See Atlanto-dental Interspace, ADI, Rheumatoid Arthritis.

Atlantoaxial Joint: Referring to the C1–C2 articulation. This joint supplies the head with about 50% of the rotation available in the cervical spine. The atlas (C1) rotates about the dens of the axis (C2). See AA Joint, Atlanto-odontoid Joint.

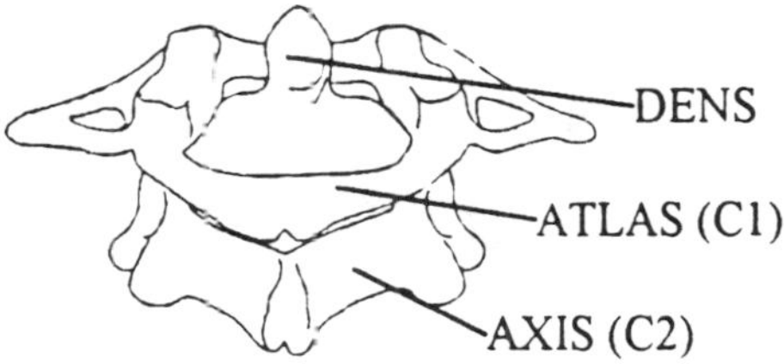

Atlantoaxial Joint Disruption—Bilateral Anterior: A condition in which the atlas has moved forward on the axis due to a fractured or dysplastic dens, and/or an attenuated or ruptured transverse ligament. This is usually caused by a traumatic blow, rheumatoid arthritis, or infectious processes. This is an unstable dislocation if the displacement is greater than 3 mm. Fusion is recommended for cases of transverse ligament disruption due to trauma. Immobilization is recommended if the transverse ligament laxity is due to infection. See Atlanto-dental Interspace, ADI, Bilateral Anterior Atlantoaxial Joint Disruption, Bilateral Anterior Transitory Displacement of C1 in relation to C2.

Atlantoaxial Rotatory Subluxation: A traumatic subluxation of the atlantoaxial articulation. This is a rotatory subluxation of the atlas in relation to both the occiput and C2. Patients usually present with torticollis and restricted neck range of motion. There is lateral mass asymmetry on open-mouth radiography. This can also be a difficult diagnosis to make and may require fluoroscopy or CT scanning. See Rotatory Subluxation of C1 on C2.

Atlantoaxial Subluxation: Subluxation of C1 on C2, often seen in severe rheumatoid arthritis. The synovial joint between the transverse ligament and the dens becomes involved, leading to eventual erosion of the transverse ligament. Common symptoms include occipital, retro-orbital, or temporal pain. Myelopathy can occur from compression of the spinal cord. Vertebral basilar insufficiency is also seen as the vertebral basilar arteries become kinked as they pass through the lateral arch of C1. This syndrome can also occur with the other inflammatory spondyloarthropathies: ankylosing spondylitis, psoriatic arthritis, Reiter's syndrome, and SLE. See Atlantoaxial Instability, Sharp-Pursor Test.

Atlanto–Dens Ligament: One of the upper cervical ligaments which runs between the anterior portion of the dens and the caudal portion of the anterior ring of C1. See Anterior Atlanto-dental Ligament.

Atlanto-dental: Referring to the C1–C2 area. See Atlantoaxial.

Atlanto-dental Interspace: A radiographic test for transverse ligament stability. A lateral flexion–extension view of the cervical spine is performed. The distance between the posterior margin of the anterior atlas and the anterior surface of the odontoid is measured. The distance is then measured again during a flexion view because this places the most stress on the transverse ligament of the atlas. The shape of the interspace usually alters in flexion and presents with a V configuration. In extension this becomes an inverted V. The minimum distance in adults is 1 mm and the maximum 3 mm. In children, the minimum is 1 mm and the maximum is 5 mm. The most frequent causes are trauma, Down syndrome, pharyngeal infections, occipitalization, the spondyloarthropathies, rheumatoid arthritis, and psoriatic arthritis. See ADI, Atlas-Odontoid Space, Atlas-Dens Interval, Predental Interspace, Predental Space.

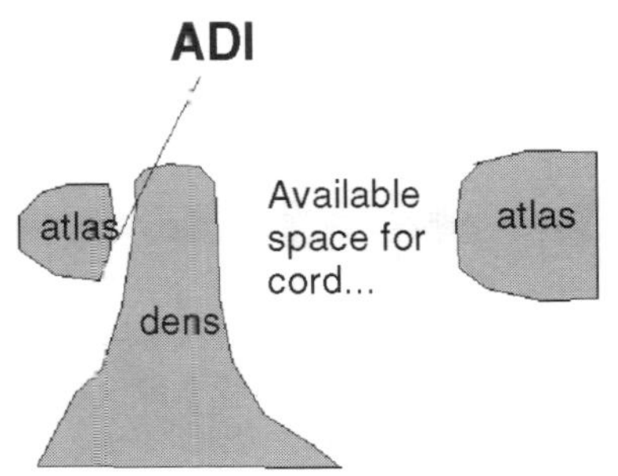

Atlanto-dental Interval: The distance between the posterior margin of the anterior atlas and the anterior surface of the odontoid. See Atlanto-dental Interspace

Atlanto-dental Joint: Referring to the C1–C2 articulation. See Atlantoaxial Joint, AA Joint.

Atlanto-occipital Dislocation: A dislocation of the upper cervical spine from the occiput. There is extensive ligamentous disruption allowing the skull to separate from the atlas. This is usually a fatal injury.

Atlanto-odontoid: Referring to the C1–C2 articulation. See AA Joint, Atlantoaxial Joint.

Atlas: The first cervical vertebra that supports the globe of the head, just as the mythical Titan Atlas supported the globe of the earth. This structure articulates with the skull above through the OA joints and with C2 below through the articulation formed with the odontoid process of the axis (C2).

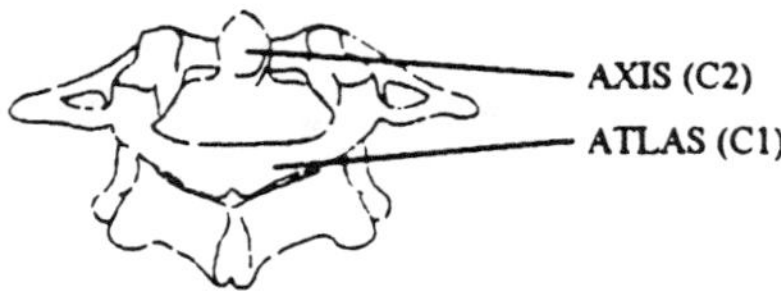

Atlas–Dens Interval: The distance between the posterior margin of the anterior atlas and the anterior surface of the odontoid. See Atlanto-dental Interspace.

Atlas–Odontoid Space: The distance between the posterior margin of the anterior atlas and the anterior surface of the odontoid. See Atlanto-dental Interspace.

atr: An abbreviation for *atrophy*.

Attenuated Nerve Root: A nerve root which is stretched over an object such as a herniated disc or bony structure. The implication is that this nerve root will likely have sustained some compression.

Atypical Sciatica: Radiation of pain, numbness, or tingling into one lower extremity which is not due to dysfunction of a nerve root or the sciatic nerve. The pain or numbness does not follow a dermatomal (sensory nerve root) distribution. There are many ligamentous, myofascial, or peripheral nerve referral patterns which can cause sciatic-like symptoms. See Mesodermal Pain, Sclerotomal Pain.

Autograft: A graft taken from the patient and used for fusion. For the spine, the most common site to take grafts is the iliac crest. See Autologous graft.

Autologous: A graft or tissue which is taken from the patient and moved from one location to another.

Autologous Blood: Blood used for transfusion which is taken from the patient prior to or during the surgical procedure.

Autologous Graft: A graft taken from the patient and used for fusion. For the spine, the most common site to take grafts is the iliac crest. See Autograft.

Automated Nucleotome: A device used for percutaneous discectomy. See Percutaneous Discectomy.

Automated Percutaneous Lumbar Discectomy: The removal of bulging disc material percutaneously through a large-bore needle inserted into the disc space. See Percutaneous Discectomy.

Automobile–Pedestrian Accident: A collision between an automobile and a pedestrian. See Auto–Ped Accident.

Autonomic Dysreflexia: A syndrome seen in paraplegics with spinal cord lesions at or above T6. This is most commonly due to a distended bladder which has not been emptied. The symptom complex is characterized by excessive sweating, pilomotor responses (goose flesh), headaches, hypertension, and in severe cases of bradycardia (slowing of the heart rate). This syndrome can represent a medical emergency and can be fatal.

Autonomic Ganglia: The portion of the nervous system that controls the glands, organs, and smooth muscle. See Autonomic Nervous System.

Autonomic Nervous System: The portion of the nervous system that controls the glands, organs, and smooth muscle. There are two divisions of the autonomic nervous system, sympathetic and parasympathetic. The sympathetic chain runs along the vertebral bodies on each side and consists of many ganglia. The postganglionic fibers are distributed to the body, and preganglionic fibers originate in the brain or spinal cord and lie in the lateral gray columns of the cord. These exit over the same cranial nerves and ventral roots as motor fibers, but synapse in the autonomic ganglia. The autonomic nervous system in the extremities is not known to have afferent nerve input. See Autonomic Ganglia.

Auto–Ped Accident: A collision between an automobile and a pedestrian. See Automobile–Pedestrian Accident.

Avascular Necrosis of the Femoral Head: A loss of blood supply to the femoral head which leads to destruction and necrosis of the bone. The femoral head, when displaced, is often rendered avascular secondary to trauma. Thus, fractures of the neck of the femur and dislocations of the head can cause avascular necrosis of the femoral head. Vascular occlusion as a consequence of immobilization and excessive steroid usage can also cause this disorder. The medial and lateral femoral circumflex arteries are vulnerable as they circle around the head of the femur, and this may explain the high incidence seen in femoral neck fractures. It is more common in the elderly because femoral neck fractures are more common in that age group. Clinically, there is an unexplained aching in the hip joint. X-rays may not show signs of this disease until it is advanced and the femoral head has begun to show signs of flattening and is irregularly shaped. See Femoral Avascular Necrosis.

AV Fistula: A fistulous communication between intradural spinal arteries and a spinal vein. See AVM.

AVM: A fistulous communication between intradural spinal arteries and a spinal vein. See Arteriovenous Malformation.

AVM—Direct: A fistulous communication between intradural spinal arteries and a spinal vein. See Direct AVM.

AVM—Type 1: A type of arteriovenous malformation which is commonly located on the dorsal spinal cord surface. It comprises a single-coiled vessel which accounts for approximately 80–85% of all AVMs. See Type 1 AVM.

AVM—Type 2: A glomus-type intradural, arteriovenous malformation which together with type 3 AVMs comprise approximately 15–20% of all spinal AVMs. There is often a fistula which connects the AVM to the dura. There is usually a tightly packed mass of blood vessels confined to a short segment of the spinal cord. This type of AVM typically occurs in the anterior half of the spinal cord and is supplied by the medullary arteries. It is possible to see acute clinical deterioration secondary to subarachnoid hemorrhage. See Type 2 AVM.

AVM—Type 3: An intradural arteriovenous malformation which is considered "juvenile." Together with a type 2 AVM this comprises approximately 15–20% of all spinal AVMs. Fistulas that connect this AVM intradurally often occur. The blood supply is derived from the medullary arteries via the anterior and posterior spinal arteries. There is almost always cord tissue within the interstitium between the vasculature. The nidus commonly involves bone and nonneural soft tissues including the paraspinal musculature and connective tissue. See Type 3 AVM.

Avulsion Fracture: The separation fracture and separation of a small piece of bone which is pulled away from its attachment by a ligament or tendon.

Avulsion Fracture of the AIIS: An avulsion fracture of the anterior inferior iliac spine caused by the rectus femoris muscle. A small bony fragment is pulled away from the AIIS and appears on x-ray displaced downward from the AIIS. Flexion of the hip is severely limited secondary to pain. This fracture most commonly occurs in rugby, soccer, and football. See AIIS Avulsion Fracture, Anterior Inferior Iliac Spine Avulsion Fracture.

Avulsion Fracture of the Ischial Tuberosity: Avulsion of the apophysis of the ischial tuberosity as a result of a large contraction of the hamstrings. This usually heals with bony overgrowth on the ischial tuberosity. This type of fracture is commonly seen in hurdlers, cheerleaders, and in horseback riders from chronic bony stress. See Ischial Tuberosity Avulsion Fracture, Rider's Bone, Hurdler's Fracture.

Avulsion Fracture of the Symphysis Pubis: An avulsion of the superior or inferior pubic rami near the pubic symphysis caused by the adductor major. This injury is commonly seen in soccer players. See Symphysis Pubis Avulsion Fracture.

Ax: An abbreviation for *axis.*

Ax-A: A chiropractic abbreviation for *axis anterior.*

Axial Cervical Distraction: The application of vertical, downward pressure on the spine. This can be placed on the head or other areas to determine if pain is elicited. If centralized pain is appreciated, this is called axial pain. See Traction.

Axial Extension Stretch: A physical therapy stretch designed to stretch the suboccipital musculature. See Chin Tuck.

Axial Loading Test: The application of vertical, downward pressure on the spine. This can be placed on the head or other areas to determine if pain is elicited. If centralized pain is appreciated, this is called axial pain. See Vertical Cervical Compression Test.

Axial Low Back Pain: Pain in the center portion of the low back.

Axial Neck Pain: Pain in the center portion of the posterior neck.

Axial Pain: Pain emanating from the spine or "axial skeleton." This pain is centrally located and thought to be due to the intervertebral disc. See Discogenic Pain.

Axial Rotation: Rotation about the y-axis to one side or the other. In the cervical spine, this can be accomplished at the atlantoaxial joint or in the lower cervical spine. In the thoracic and lumbar spine, this happens through the collective rotation of one vertebra on the other.

Axis: The second cervical vertebra or C2. The head and C1 rotate around the dens of the axis. About half of all neck rotation occurs at C1–C2.

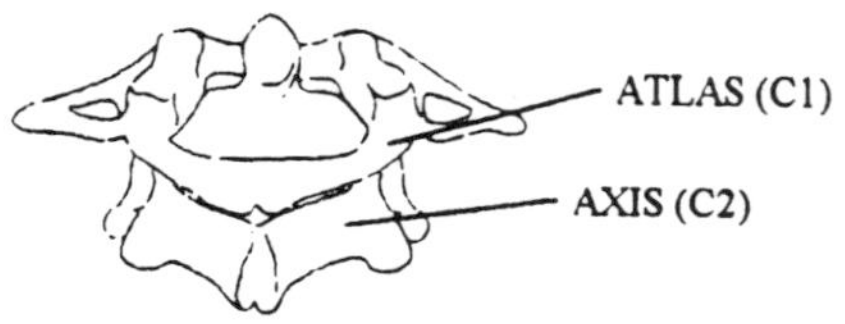

Ax-L: A chiropractic abbreviation for *axis left.*

Axontomesis: Damage to a nerve which results in loss of axons in which the epineurium and myelin sheath remain intact. Wallerian degeneration occurs distally and regeneration and spontaneous recovery is possible.

Axoplasmic Flow: The flow of protoplasm in the axons. This is how the nerve cell transports nutrients and wastes within the cell.

Axoplasmic Fluid Damming: This is a block in axoplasmic flow. See Axoplasmic Flow.

Ax-P: A chiropractic abbreviation for *axis posterior.*

Ax-R: A chiropractic abbreviation for *axis right.*

B

B: An abbreviation for *bilateral* or *burning pain.*

B-200: A proprietary name for a computerized low back testing machine. This measures strength in all three axes isoinertially. Angular displacement, velocity, torque, work, and power for each axis is recorded simultaneously. It can also be used for strength training.

B4: An abbreviation for *before.*

BA: A chiropractic abbreviation for *base anterior*. This denotes a sacral base that is found to be forward.

Baastrup's Disease: An inflammatory reaction seen in the lumbar and interspinous ligaments with degenerative joint disease characterized by bridging osteophytes between the spinous processes. See Kissing Osteophytes, Michotte Disease.

Babinski Sign: A physical exam maneuver performed to detect an upper motor neuron dysfunction (brain injury, spinal cord injury above the lower lumbar area). This is part of a primitive flexion reflex that is normal in infants but abnormal in patients older than 12–16 months. A blunt object such as a stick or the end of a reflex hammer is drawn across the foot starting from the heel moving toward the fifth toe and then across towards the big toe. A normal response is flexion and adduction of the toes and is described as a downgoing toe. An abnormal response is an up-going toe or dorsiflexion of the great toe with fanning of the other toes. An abnormal response indicates dysfunction in the motor area of the brain or the corticospinal tracts. See Up-going Toe.

Back Brace—Warm and Form: A soft low back brace with a thermoplastic insert which can be custom-molded to the lumbar spine and then placed within a special insert posteriorly. See Warm and Form Low Back Brace.

Back School: A class or course in body mechanics, proper lifting techniques, and back care.

Backward Bending: Extension of the spine. See Bending—Backward.

Backward Bent Sacrum: An osteopathic or manual physical therapy term which denotes a sacral base which is superior and posterior. See Bilateral Sacral Extension.

Backward Extension View: The extension portion of a flexion–extension series. See Flexion–Extension Views.

Backward Ilium: A movement dysfunction of the pelvis in which the ilium has "moved" posterior on the sacrum. See Posterior Ilium.

Backward Innominate: A movement dysfunction of the pelvis in which the ilium has "moved" posterior on the sacrum. See Posterior Ilium.

Backward Sacral Torsion: An osteopathic or manual physical therapy term which describes a sacral torsion found in lumbar backward bending. The sacral sulcuses are of equal depth on both sides with forward flexion, but on backward bending, one sacral sulcus is more prominent. One ILA is noted to be posterior and inferior. This can be caused by a biomechanical abnormality at L5 and can be described as right-on-left or left-on-right. The sacral sulcuses can also be used as landmarks. See Left-Facing Sacrum, Posterior Torsion.

Baclofen: A muscle relaxant and antispasticity drug used most commonly in patients with spasticity due to spinal cord injuries. Abrupt drug withdrawal can cause hallucinations and seizures, therefore, this drug is weaned before being discontinued. It is cleared through the renal system, so it should be given with caution in patients with renal impairment. This drug does not appear to be effective in patients with spasticity due to CVAs or centrally mediated spasticity. There are contraindications in pregnant patients. One of the side effects is sedation. The usual dosage is between 40 and 80 mg daily. Dosages usually start at 5 mg three times a day for 3 days, 10 mg three times a day for 3 days, 15 mg three times a day for 3 days, then 20 mg three times a day for 3 days. Tablets are available in 10 mg and 20 mg. See Lioresal.

Baer's Sacroiliac Point: A tender point over the sacroiliac area anteriorly. This is thought to indicate a nonspecific back injury or SI joint syndrome. The patient is supine and the point is situated 2 inches from the umbilicus in a line between umbilicus and the ASIS.

Bailey-Badgley Arthrodesis: A technique for anterior cervical fusion in which a rectangular "window" is cut in the anterior vertebral body. Through this opening a discectomy is performed. However, unlike the Cloward technique, removal of structures causing compression is not performed. It is thought the posterior and posterior lateral osteophytes will be reabsorbed once stabilization has been achieved. A cancellous bone graft and onlay graft is inserted.

Bakody Sign: A physical exam test for nerve root sydrome. The patient is asked to abduct and externally rotate the ipsilateral shoulder by moving the hand toward the head and then placing the hand on top of the head. If this position relieves radicular pain complaints, then it is considered a positive sign for a nerve root syndrome. See Shoulder Abduction Test, Cervical Foraminal Compression Test.

Ballottement Test: A physical exam maneuver which evaluates the atlanto-occipital joint. The patient is in a supine position while the examiner's thumbs and index fingers grasp the top of the head while the palm supports the occiput. The examiner induces traction of the head while palpating joint play.

Baltimore Testing Equipment: A brand name for an upper extremity isokinetic testing device. See BTE.

Bamboo Spine: A radiographic term associated with ankylosing spondylitis in which the spine on an AP view looks like a bamboo shaft. There is extensive calcification of the outer fibers of the annulus and the formation of marginal syndesmophytes which fuse one vertebra to another. See Poker Spine.

Banding: A palpable band of muscle fibers usually associated with a trigger point. See Taut Band, Trigger Point.

Bank Bone: Bone which is preserved through rapid freezing and then dehydrating in a vacuum. See Allograft, Freeze-dried Bone.

Barre-Lieou Sign: A physical exam test for vertebral atery compression. The patient is asked to rotate the head maximally from side to side. This is performed slowly at first and then accelerated until tolerance is reached. Vertebral artery compression is thought to be indicated by vertigo, blurry vision, nausea, syncope, or nystagmus. However, this is a nonspecific test because patients with benign positional vertigo or inner ear dysfunctions will also likely report dizziness or similar symptoms. Another test has been reported which combines rotation and lateral bending to the opposite side. The patient is supine and the same symptoms indicate a positive test.

Barre-Lieou Syndrome: Dizziness, headaches, blurry vision, tinnitus, vertigo, and nausea seen after a whiplash injury and thought to be caused by several mechanisms. See Syndrome of Barre-Lieou.

Barrel-shaped Vertebra: A radiographic sign seen in ankylosing spondylitis. The vertebral bodies become convex instead of the normal concave. This is due to corner erosions and subligamentous ossification. The vertebral bodies take on the appearance of a barrel.

Barrier: The limit of unimpeded motion. For instance, the anatomic barrier in manipulation is that point at which movement beyond will cause tissue damage.

Barr's Triad: A triad of signs which includes lumbar scoliosis, loss of disc height, and absence of the normal lumbar lordosis.

Bartschi-Rochain Syndrome: A relatively uncommon syndrome characterized by dizziness, light-headedness, vertigo, vasomotor face disturbances, retro-orbital pain, disturbances of vision, and other symptoms. See Syndrome of Barre-Lieou.

Base of the Sacrum: The superior-most portion of the sacrum that is the inferior portion of the L5–S1 disc space. See Sacral Base.

Basilar Impression: An abnormality of a skull base resulting in a protrusion of the upper cervical spine into the foramen magnum. Upper cervical cord or brain stem compression may occur. Common causes include atlas occipitalization (atlas fused with the skull), softening of the skull base such as with Paget's disease and osteomalacia, and platybasia. Occasionally, rheumatoid arthritis can be an etiology. See Primary Basilar Impression, Secondary Basilar Impression.

Basilar Invagination: An abnormality of a skull base resulting in a protrusion of the upper cervical spine into the foramen magnum. See Basilar Impression, Pseudobasilar Invagination, Vertical Settling.

Basilar Ischemia: Dizziness, headaches, blurry vision, tinnitus, vertigo, and nausea seen after a whiplash injury and thought to be caused by several mechanisms. See Syndrome of Barre-Lieou.

Batson's Plexus: The network of venous plexus surrounding the vertebral column that is just anterior to the posterior longitudinal ligament. These veins pierce through a thin fibrous membrane to enter the vertebral body and also cross the disc space. It is thought that this venous system plays a part in the spread of tumor and infection. See Vertebral Vein System.

Bear Hug Fracture: A fractured rib caused by the compressive force of a hug. See Passion Fracture.

Bechterew's Sitting Test: An obscure physical exam test which, if positive, is reported to suggest a disc lesion in the lumbar spine or a nerve root irritation. The patient is in the seated position and attempts to extend each leg one at a time. The examiner then resists hip flexion with downward pressure on the thigh. The test is reported to be positive if this maneuver increases backache or sciatic pain or if this maneuver is impossible. The patient then attempts to extend both legs simultaneously. With disc involvement, extending both legs will usually increase spinal and sciatic discomfort. However, this test is nonspecific in that biomechanical abnormalities such as psoas tightness could also cause pain in the lumbar spine. Also, many patients may not be able to extend both lower extremities simultaneously, which may just represent weak hip flexors and/or abdominals.

Bed Rest: Almost complete inactivity. The patient is usually instructed to "go to bed" for several days. Of late, the trend seems to be moving toward less bed rest (approximately 2 days at most). Prolonged bed rest has adverse side effects on multiple organ systems including the musculoskeletal system.

Beevor's Sign: A clinical examination finding indicating paraplegia which causes an asymmetrical paralysis of the rectus abdominis. The umbilicus is observed while the patient attempts a sit-up maneuver. Movement of the umbilicus in a superior direction is a positive test.

Bench Test: A physical exam maneuver to test for disc disease versus back strain. The patient kneels on a chair and attempts to touch the floor with outstretched hands. It is reported that, with disc disease, the patient is able to perform this test without difficulty. With a back strain, pain will be increased. See Chicago Test.

Bending—Backward: Extension of the spine. See Backward Bending.

Bending—Forward: Flexion of the spine. See Forward Bending.

Benign Positional Vertigo: Vertigo (a sensation that the room is spinning) that occurs only with a change in head position. This usually occurs while rolling over in bed, looking up, turning the head, or rising from a chair. Orthostatic hypotension needs to be ruled out. The vertigo lasts for less than 30 seconds and the response diminishes when the change in position is repeated many times. There can be associated rotary nystagmus without other brain stem signs on examination. Common treatments include repeated head position in the offending direction in an attempt to extinguish the response, positional maneuvers to allow free bodies to clear the inner ear, antivertigo medications, and surgical correction of a perilymph fistula. See Vertigo.

Bent Leg Lift—Hook-Lying: A lumbar stabilization exercise. See Hook-Lying Bent Leg Lift.

BEST Technique: Bio-energetic Synchronization Technique. A treatment technique which is controversial in the chiropractic community.

BID: A true subluxation of the bilateral facet joints due to a severe hyperflexion injury of the cervical spine. See Bilateral Interfacetal Dislocation.

b.i.d.: An abbreviation for *twice a day*.

Bikele's Sign: One of the more obscure tests for thoracic outlet syndrome. The patient is seated and is asked to abduct the shoulder to 90° while externally rotating the shoulder. The arm is then fully extended at the elbow and the patient attempts to reach behind. A positive test for this maneuver is a reproduction of radicular or thoracic outlet syndrome complaints.

Bilateral Anterior Atlantoaxial Joint Disruption: When the atlas has moved forward on the axis due to a fractured or dysplastic dens, and an attenuated or ruptured transverse ligament. See Atlantoaxial Joint Disruption—Bilateral Anterior, Bilateral Anterior Transitory Displacement of C1 in Relation to C2.

Bilateral Anterior Ilium: A pelvic dysfunction in which both ilia are noted to be rotated anteriorly on the sacrum.

Bilateral Anterior Transitory Displacement of C1 in Relation to C2: When the atlas has moved forward on the axis due to a fractured or dysplastic dens, and an attenuated or ruptured transverse ligament. See Bilateral Anterior Atlantoaxial Joint Disruption, Atlantoaxial Joint Disruption—Bilateral Anterior.

Bilateral Facet Dislocation: A cervical spine injury involving extensive ligamentous destruction including tearing of the interspinous, intertransverse, capsular ligaments, ligamentum flavum, and some portion of the annulus. The inferior facet of the superior vertebrae moves anteriorly on the superior facet of the inferior vertebrae. A flexion mechanism is considered the etiology, but other mechanisms have been proposed. This is also described as "jump facets." Instrumentation fusion is usually suggested. See Facet Dislocation—Bilateral.

Bilateral Flexed Sacrum: An osteopathic or manual physical therapy term used to denote a sacral position such that the base is anterior and inferior and the apex posterior and superior. There is a positive seated flexion test bilaterally. The patient will have difficulty with lumbar flexion. This dysfunction is commonly seen with an increased lordosis. See Bilateral Sacral Flexion, Sacral Flexion—Bilateral, Forward Bent Sacrum.

Bilateral Interfacetal Dislocation: A true subluxation of the bilateral facet joints due to a severe hyperflexion injury of the cervical spine. This is most commonly found in the C4–C7 region and does not involve fracture of the facets, but rather extensive ligamentous damage. On lateral x-ray, the superior facets are seen to lie anterior to the inferior facets. Chip fractures of the tip of the facets are often seen with this type of dislocation. This is an unstable lesion with a high incidence of cervical cord injuries. This is usually treated with cervical fusion. See BID.

Bilateral Isometric Hip Flexion: A lumbar stabilization exercise in which the patient is in a supine position with knees bent and feet on the floor. The patient is asked to tighten the stomach and raise both knees to meet outstretched arms. The arms are kept straight while pushing against the knees and stabilizing the spine. See Hip Flexion—Bilateral Isometric.

Bilateral Leg Lowering Test: A physical exam maneuver which, if positive, reportedly indicates mechanical lumbosacral involvement. The patient is lying supine with both legs fully extended. The patient's legs are lifted to approximately 90° of flexion at the hip. From this position, the patient then lowers both legs simultaneously from a 90° to a 45° angle. The test is reported positive if the legs drop or if lower back pain is elicited.

Bilaterally Extended Sacrum: An osteopathic or manual physical therapy term used to denote a sacral position such that the sacral base is anterior and inferior and the apex is posterior and superior. See Flexion Dysfunction of the Sacrum, Sacral Base Anterior.

SACRAL BASE MOVES MORE FREELY IN AN ANTERIOR DIRECTION THAN IN A POSTERIOR DIRECTION

BILATERALLY EXTENDED SACRUM

Bilaterally Flexed Sacrum: An osteopathic or manual physical therapy term used to denote a sacral position such that the sacral base is extended or posterior and the apex is anterior. The sacral base then moves more freely in a posterior direction and is restricted in anterior motion. Lumbar flexion is less restricted than lumbar extension. See Extension Dysfunction of the Sacrum, Sacral Base Posterior.

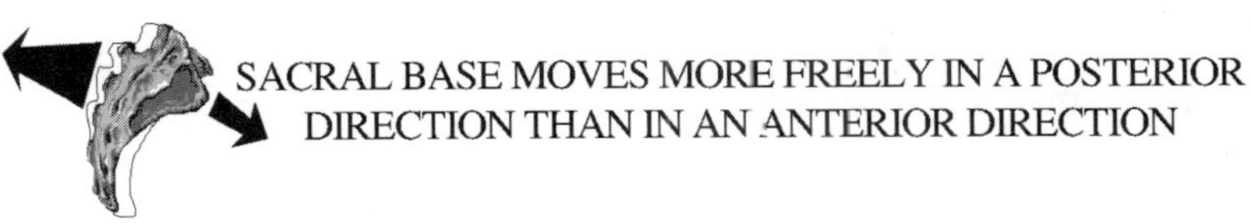

BILATERALLY FLEXED SACRUM

Bilateral Posterior Ilium: A pelvic dysfunction in which both ilia are noted to be rotated posteriorly on the sacrum.

Bilateral Sacral Extension: An osteopathic or manual physical therapy term denoting a sacral base which is superior and posterior. The sacral base is prominent posteriorly, and the ilia is less prominent. This is the reaction of the sacrum to lumbar flexion, thus lumbar extension is limited. See Posterior Sacral Nutation, Backward Bent Sacrum, Nutated Sacrum.

Bilateral Sacral Flexion: An osteopathic or manual physical therapy term used to denote a sacral position such that the base is anterior and inferior and the apex posterior and superior. See Bilateral Flexed Sacrum.

Bilateral Straight-Leg Raising Test: A physical examination maneuver. See Double Leg Raise Test.

Bilateral Weight Distribution: A technique in which the patient is asked to stand on weight scales or load cells positioned under each foot. The idea is that asymmetric posture in weight bearing might contribute to the development of degenerative joint disease, sacroiliac problems, chronic lumbar strain, and other conditions.

Bindegwebb's Massage: A massage technique developed in the 1920s by Dicke and Ebner. See Connective Tissue Massage.

Bioenergetic Synchronization Technique. A treatment technique which is controversial in the chiropractic community. See BEST Technique.

Biomechanical LBP: Low back pain. See Biomechanical Low Back Pain.

Biomechanical Low Back Pain: Low back pain caused by muscular strain or ligamentous damage that shunts work to structures, which become overloaded and painful. See Biomechanical LBP.

Bitemporal: This refers to a type of headache which occurs on both sides of the head.

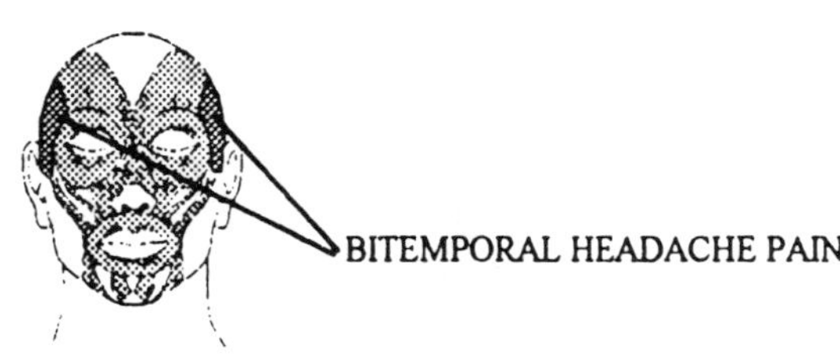

Biventor Line: A radiographic sign for basilar impression. See Digastric Line.

Blind Vertebra: A radiographic term which refers to bilateral pedicle destruction usually through neoplasm. On the AP view, the "eyes," which represent the normal pedicles, are absent bilaterally.

Block Stenosis: A type of severe central canal stenosis in which the flow of cerebrospinal fluid is blocked around the spinal cord. This is usually a radiographic diagnosis made on myelogram or CT myelogram.

Block Vertebrae: The congenital fusion of two adjacent vertebrae. This is clinically insignificant because there is no motion at this level. The neural foramina may be smaller, larger, or normal size at this level. See Congenital Block Vertebrae.

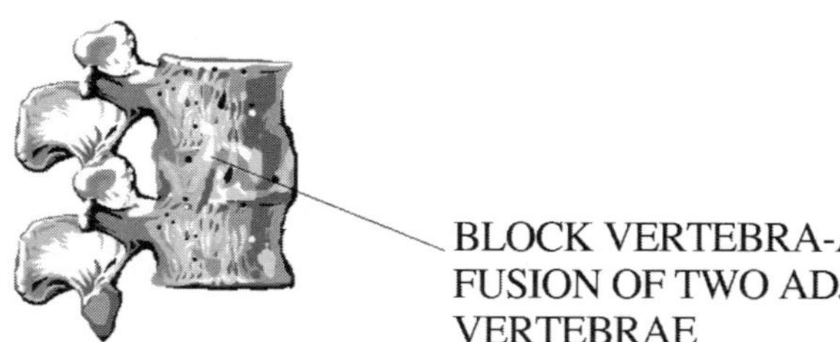

BMD: An abbreviation for *bone mineral density.*

Body Cast: A cast that encompasses the trunk and extends from the clavicles to the iliac crests. This is often used for postoperative stabilization status post-fusion.

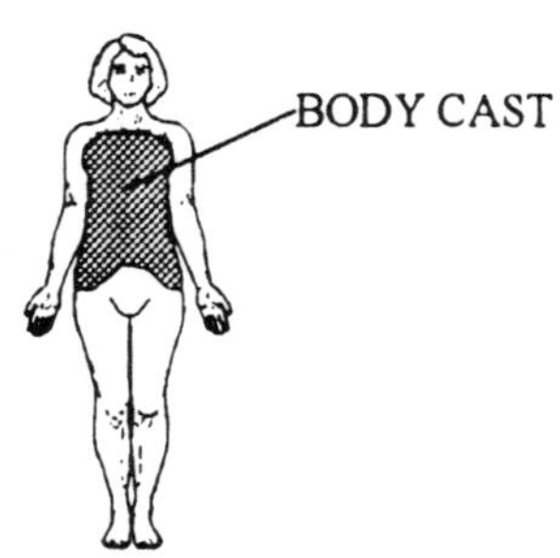

Body Cast with a Leg In: A thoracic, lumbar, sacral orthosis with a unilateral thigh attachment. See TL-SOT.

Body Drop: A chiropractic manipulative technique. See Body Drop Adjustment.

Body Drop Adjustment: A chiropractic manipulative technique used to deliver more force through the arms during a manipulation. The body is dropped suddenly by bending the knees such that the body weight is transmitted through the upper extremities. The elbows are locked straight.

Body Drop Manipulation: A chiropractic manipulative technique. See Body Drop Adjustment.

Body Jacket: A cast that encompasses the trunk. See Body Cast.

Body LP: A chiropractic listing that refers to a vertebral body that faces left and is positioned posteriorly.

Body LPI: A chiropractic listing which refers to a vertebral body which is left facing, posterior, and with its left transverse process inferior.

Body LPS: A chiropractic listing which refers to a vertebral body which is left facing, posterior, and with its left transverse process posterior.

Body Mechanics: The study of the biomechanics or movements of the dynamic human body. With respect to the spine, body mechanics are often considered in a person's work situation—such as the correct way to lift or twist.

Body RP: A chiropractic listing which refers to a vertebral body which faces right and is positioned posteriorly.

Body RPI: A chiropractic listing which refers to a vertebral body which is right facing, posterior, and with its right transverse process inferior.

Body RPS: A chiropractic listing which refers to a vertebral body which is right facing, posterior, and with its right transverse process superior.

bog: An abbreviation for *bogginess of tissue.*

Bogginess: A descriptive term which refers to a tissue which is spongy due to the accumulation of excess fluid. See Boggy.

Boggy: A descriptive term which refers to a tissue which is spongy due to the accumulation of excess fluid. See Bogginess.

Bone Graft: The use of bone in spinal fusion, which can be either *autograft* (from the patient) or *allograft* (cadaver bone). Autografts can be taken from many places in the body including the iliac crest, fibula, ribs, and tibia. Allografts are usually freeze-dried bone taken from a cadaver. Bone grafts can be placed in many locations in the spine to promote fusion, including the disc space, lateral to the transverse processes, and posteriorly. See Fusion.

Bone Island: A sclerotic density seen on radiographs which is asymptomatic and usually not clinically significant. See Enostosis.

Bone Scan—Limited: A bone scan of only one region of the body. See Limited Bone Scan.

Bone Spur: An overgrowth of bone in response to injury. See Osteophyte.

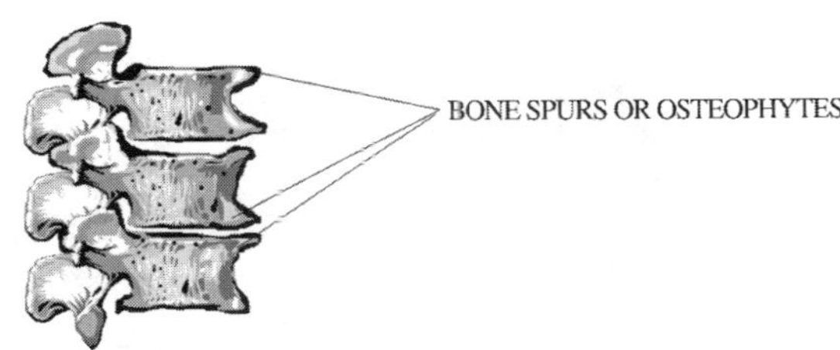

Bone to Bone: A type of end feel described by Cyriax. Elbow extension is one example. See Bony End Feel.

Bone Window: A CT scan image which shows bony structures more clearly than soft tissue structures. This also refers to the settings which allow the CT scanner to show bone in more detail.

Bony Alignment: Referring to manual medicine findings, such as the alignment of the ilium on the sacrum or the alignment of one specific segment of the spine to another.

Bony Compression: Pressure placed on the spinal cord or nerve roots through bony hypertrophy (enlargement). See Foraminal Stenosis, Central Canal Stenosis, Lateral Recess Stenosis.

Bony End Feel: An abrupt halt to the movement. An example of bony end feel is the abrupt halt experienced with elbow extension. See End Feel.

Bony Overlap: A radiographic term which refers to the neural foramen. In this instance, severe degeneration or acute trauma has allowed one vertebra to move forward on another, thus reducing the overall size of the intervertebral foramen.

Borg Scale: A measurement of perceived exertion used during exercise tolerance testing. The scale is from 6 to 20, with 6 being the least exertion and 20 being the most. Patients are asked to rate their own level of exertion, and this is compared to their actual exercise tolerance.

BOTOX: A proprietary name for purified botulinum toxin type A. This is an injectable substance which blocks neuromuscular conduction by inhibiting the release of acetylcholine. This is used in patients with intractable torticollis. See Botulinum Toxin Type A, Torticollis.

Botulinum Toxin Injections: The injection of purified botulinum toxin into the muscle belly of a dystonic muscle in order to block neuromuscular transmission and to "release" the muscle. This is commonly used in the treatment of torticollis. See BOTOX.

Botulinum Toxin Type A: A proprietary name for purified botulinum toxin type A. See BOTOX.

Bougery Ligament: A ligament connecting the base of the transverse process to the mamillary process below. See Ligament of Bougery.

Bow Sign: A density seen on x-ray that gives the appearance of a bow with the convex surface facing downward. This indicates severe spondylolisthesis and is seen as a result of the overlap of vertebral bodies.

Bowstring Sign: A physical examination maneuver used to test for radiculopathy. The patient begins in the supine position with both legs extended. The examiner places the patient's affected leg on top of one of the examiner's shoulders. The examiner then exerts firm pressure near the insertion of the hamstring musculature. If this is painful, firm pressure is applied to the popliteal fossa. Pain in the lumbar region or radiculopathy is a positive sign for nerve root compression. This sign has also been described in a different way. In this instance, the examiner carries out a straight leg raising test. If pain is produced in the back of the leg, the knee is slightly flexed to approximately 20°. The examiner then exerts pressure in the popliteal region to re-establish the radicular symptoms.

Bowstring Test: A physical examination maneuver. See Bowstring Sign, Cram Bowstring Test.

Box Lift and Carry: A portion of a functional capacity evaluation which tests the patient's ability to lift boxes of various weights and carry them various distances. This is done to simulate work tasks and give an estimate of lift/carry abilities.

BP: A chiropractic abbreviation for *base posterior*. This denotes a sacral base that is found posteriorly.

BPTT: A physical exam test. See Brachial Plexus Tension Test.

Brachial Neuritis: Compression of the neurovascular bundle (irritation of usually nerves) in the shoulder girdle area between the first rib and clavicle, by a cervical rib, at the second and third ribs, between the anterior and middle scalenes, or underneath the pectoralis minor and clavipectoral fascia. See Thoracic Outlet Syndrome.

Brachial Plexus: A complex network of nervous tissue located in the neck and axilla formed from the C5–T1 nerve roots. This acts as the "switchboard" for the nerves that go on to enter the upper extremity. The first section is divided into three trunks: superior, middle, and inferior. These trunks separate into anterior and posterior divisions with the next level being called "cords." These cords give off indi-

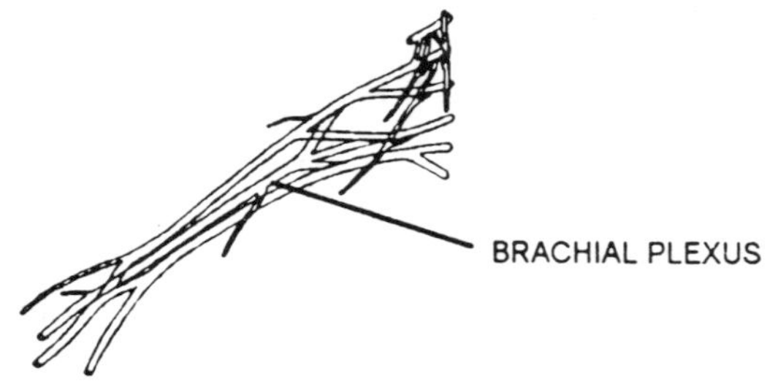

vidual peripheral nerves that supply the upper extremity. These include the axillary, radial, median, musculocutaneous, and ulnar nerves.

Brachial Plexus Neuropathy: Another term for thoracic outlet syndrome or for an acute traumatic lesion of the brachial plexus, usually involving neuropraxia (stinger) or complete disruption (axonotmesis). This is also referred to as brachial plexopathy and may be unassociated with trauma in idiopathic cases.

Brachial Plexus Tension Test: A physical exam test for thoracic outlet syndrome or any significant nerve irritation throughout the course of the nerve. The patient is seated and is asked to fully abduct the shoulders to the end point of joint play. The elbows are extended, and the examiner supports the patient's arms in this position. The patient then externally rotates the shoulders to the onset of discomfort. The elbows are then flexed with the shoulders being supported in this position. Reproduction of neurologic symptoms suggests a positive test. This terminology has also been used to describe an upper limb tension test. See ULTT, Adverse Neural Tension Test, BPTT.

Brachial Radiculitis: Compression of the neurovascular bundle (usually irritation of nerves) in the shoulder girdle area between the first rib and clavicle, by a cervical rib, at the second and third ribs, between the anterior and middle scalenes, or underneath the pectoralis minor and clavipectoral fascia. See Thoracic Outlet Syndrome.

Brachial Radiculopathy: Another term for cervical radiculopathy. See Cervical Radiculopathy.

Brachioradialis Reflex: A physical exam maneuver that tests the integrity of the C6 nerve root. A reflex hammer is used to strike the styloid process of the radius with the arm midway between pronation and supination. The corresponding muscle jerk in the brachioradialis is measured as the wrist extends and radial deviates. The deep tendon reflex can be rated 1+, 2+, or 3+. See Periosteoradial Reflex, Supinator Reflex.

Brachypelvic: A pelvis in which the transverse diameter is larger than the anterior-posterior diameter.

Braggard's Sign: Dorsiflexion of the ankle with a straight leg raising maneuver often combined with internal rotation at the hip (both maneuvers increase stretch on the sciatic nerve and nerve roots). If dorsiflexion markedly increases the patient's radiating pain pattern, this is considered a positive test due to root or neural irritation. Also, some would argue that an increase in low back pain with dorsiflexion of the foot is a positive test. See Slump Test.

Bridge Position: See Bridging.

Bridging: A physical therapy term which describes starting in a hook-lying position and then lifting the buttocks off the table so that the hip comes to a neutral position. This is one of the maneuvers performed in a lumbar stabilization program. This is also used to "clear" the pelvis in manual medicine testing. See Bridge Position.

Bridging Osteophytes: Bone spurs which seem to bridge across the disc space. It is thought that this type of osteophyte is formed by the body in an attempt to stabilize an unstable spinal motion segment. See Claw Osteophyte.

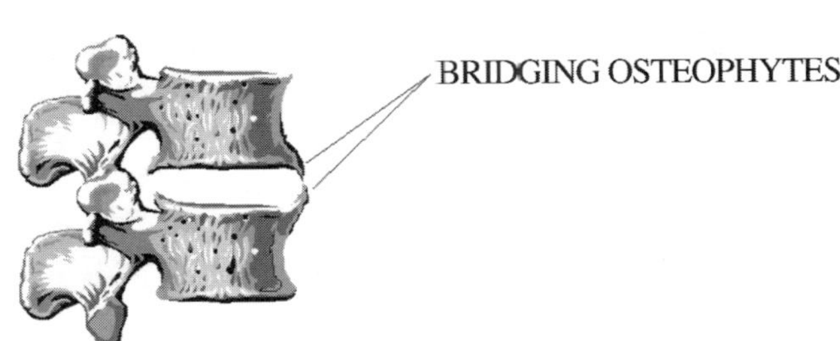

Bridging—Single Leg: A lumbar stabilization exercise. See Single Leg Bridging.

Brooks and Jenkins Surgical Technique: A type of atlantoaxial fusion in which two full-thickness iliac crest bone grafts are placed in the vertebral column between the arch of the atlas and the lamina of the axis bilaterally. Wiring is used to secure the grafts in place. This apparently provides superior postoperative stability when compared with the Gallie method. See Brooks Method.

Brooks Method: A type of atlantoaxial fusion. See Brooks and Jenkins Surgical Technique.

Brown-Sequard Syndrome: An incomplete form of spinal cord injury usually seen after a penetrating knife wound or gunshot wound. This involves injury to only half of the spinal cord and is characterized by loss of pain and temperature sensation on the side opposite the side of the injury and loss of motor function, vibratory sensation, and proprioception on the same side as the injury. See Hemicord Syndrome, Spinal Cord Syndrome.

Bru: An abbreviation for *bruised.*

Bruxism: Grinding of the teeth. Bruxism usually occurs at night while sleeping, but it can occur during the day. This can be a perpetuating factor of TMJ dysfunction. Common treatments: TMJ splints (occlusal splints), long-acting benzodiazepines, low-dose tricyclic antidepressants with CNS depressant side effects, myotherapy or deep tissue work, spray and stretch to eliminate myofascial trigger points, rehabilitation directed at the associated cervical musculature, and various electrical modalities.

BSE: An abbreviation for *bilaterally symmetrical deep tendon reflexes.*

BT: An abbreviation for *bitemporal.*

BTE: A brand name for an upper extremity isokinetic testing device. The device has multiple attachments to simulate work tasks. Coefficients of variation can be determined to rule out malingering or symptom magnification. See Baltimore Testing Equipment.

BTW: An abbreviation for *back to work.*

Bubble Inclinometer: A joint measuring device which uses an air fluid level in a circular configuration to quantify joint range of motion. This instrument can be easily zeroed. See Inclinometer.

Bucket Handle Fracture: A fracture through the superior pubic ramus and ischial pubic junction. The fracture line occurs on the side opposite an oblique impact. There is an associated fracture/dislocation of the SI joint on the side of impact. This is most commonly due to a motor vehicle accident or auto/ped accident.

Bucket Handle Restriction: An abnormality in the normal mechanics of the lower rib cage. This can be noted in inhalation (the rib does not elevate fully) or in exhalation (the rib does not depress fully). See Bucket Handle Rib Motion, Pump Handle Restriction, Inhalation Restriction, Inhalation Rib.

Bucket Handle Rib Motion: The movement of the lower ribs during respiration. With inhalation, the lateral aspect of the rib elevates and with exhalation it depresses. This results in an increase in the transverse diameter of the thorax with inspiration. Osteopaths and manual physical therapists refer to a bucket handle restriction when an abnormal movement is palpated. See Bucket Handle Restriction.

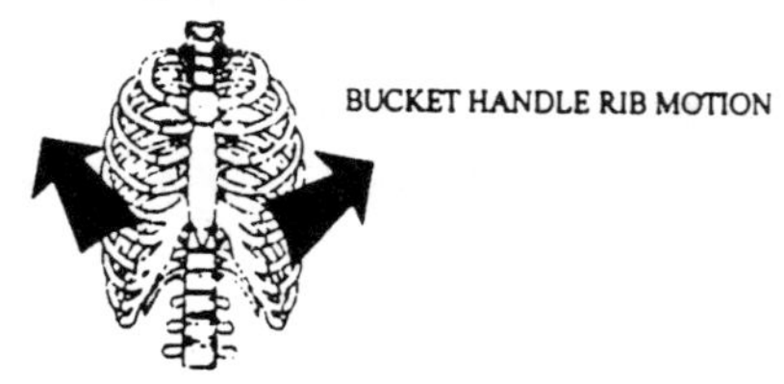

Bulbocavernosus Reflex: A spinal cord reflex mediated through the sacral portion of the spinal cord. The glans penis is squeezed while the anal sphincter is monitored with the opposite hand. A positive reflex is involuntary contraction of the anal sphincter. This test is helpful for determining the integrity of the sacral cord and can also be useful in determining when patients are out of "spinal shock."

Bulging Disc: A bulging of the outer covering of the disc which is diffuse and secondary to a loss in disc height. This differs from a disc protrusion in that a disc protrusion is

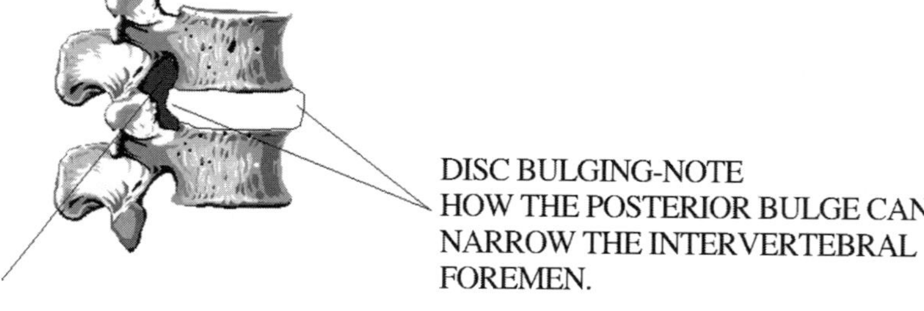

more focal and less diffuse. However, in both cases there is no herniation of the disc material outside of the confines of the annulus.

Bupivacaine: An amino amide anesthetic which has a significantly prolonged duration of action relative to traditional amino amides. This is used in concentrations of 0.125%, 0.25%, 0.5%, and 0.75% for local infiltration, peripheral nerve blocks, and epidural and spinal anesthesia. Average duration of anesthesia is 3–10 hours. When used in peripheral nerve blocks, duration of action is 10–12 hours. There is a differential blockade of sensory and motor fibers with sensory fibers clearly affected more heavily than motor fibers. There is some cardiotoxicity if bupivacaine is injected intravenously. Onset of action is usually within 5 minutes. See Marcaine, Sensorcaine.

Burner: A neuropraxic lesion of the brachial plexus which is self-limited. See Stinger.

Burns' Bench Sign: The patient is asked to sit on a low stool and bend forward and touch the palms of the hands to the floor. Since flexion in this particular position is mostly attained at the hip joints, this maneuver should not markedly increase his or her low back pain. If low back pain is markedly increased, then symptom magnification may be suspected.

Burns' Bench Test: A physical exam maneuver in which the patient kneels on a chair and attempts to touch the floor with outstretched hands. It is reported that, with disc disease, the patient is able to perform this test without difficulty. With a back strain, pain will be increased. See Chicago Test.

Bursa Atlanto-dentalis: The bursa between the transverse ligament of the atlas and the dens of the axis.

Burst Fracture: A comminuted fracture of the vertebral body, usually associated with bone fragments in the spinal canal. The obvious danger is that the bone fragments will compress or damage the spinal cord. Both the superior and inferior end plates are usually fractured. The etiology is usually significant trauma and instability is commonly present. See Crush Cleavage Fracture, Thoracolumbar Burst Fracture.

Bursting Fracture of the Atlas: A comminuted fracture of the ring of the atlas. See Jefferson's Fracture.

BuSpar: An antianxiety drug not related to the benzodiazepines. This drug is less sedating than other drugs used for treating anxiety. The mechanism of action is unknown. Unlike the benzodiazepines, there is no muscle relaxant effects. Significant side effects have been noted in approximately 10% of patients in premarketing clinical trials. The more common side effects were CNS disturbances, dizziness, insomnia, nervousness, drowsiness, and GI disturbances. There appears to be no potential for abuse or physical addiction. The usual adult dosage is 5 mg three times a day. In an interval of two to three days, the dosage can be increased 5 mg per day as needed. The maximum daily dosage is 60 mg, and dosages of 10 mg three times a day are not uncommon. See Buspirone.

Buspirone: An antianxiety drug not related to the benzodiazepines. See BuSpar.

Butterfly Vertebra: An x-ray finding in which the vertebra appears to have a biconcave or butterfly shape. There is notching of the end plates by the nucleus pulposus and the central part of the vertebral body is narrowed. This congenital abnormality occurs most frequently in the thoracic and lumbar spine. It is usually not clinically significant.

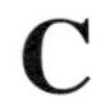

C

C: An abbreviation for *cervical.*

C0–C1: A notation which refers to the occipital-atlantal joint or OA joint.

C1–C2: A notation which refers to the atlantoaxial joint or AA joint.

C1-Odontoid Distance: A radiographic finding seen on a lateral x-ray views of the upper cervical spine. It is noted to be the distance between the anterior odontoid and the posteroinferior tubercle of C1. A distance of more than 2.5 mm in women or 3.0 mm in men is indicative of atlantoaxial subluxation. See ADI, Atlanto-dental Interspace.

C1L: A chiropractic notation which denotes a cervical segment with its transverse process or lamina on that side posterior. See C [Number] L.

C1R: A chiropractic notation which refers to a transverse process or lamina in the cervical spine denoted by the number given which is posterior. See C [Numbers 1–7] R.

C [number]: A notation which refers to the occipital condyles as they articulate with the axis. For example, C0–C1 denotes the occipito-atlantal joint.

C [number] L: A chiropractic notation which denotes a cervical segment with its transverse process or lamina on that side posterior. For example, C4L means that the transverse process or lamina of the fourth cervical vertebra was posterior or that the segment was left facing.

C [numbers 1–7] R. A chiropractic notation which refers to a transverse process or lamina in the cervical spine denoted by the number given which is posterior. For example: C3R would mean that the transverse process or lamina of C3 on the right is posterior or that the C3 segment is right facing.

CA: Chiropractic Assistant.

Café-au-Lait Spots: Irregular areas of pigmented skin which are light yellowish brown with smooth margins. These can occur normally, or can be indicators of neurofibromatosis. The criteria for the diagnosis of neurofibromatosis is six or more café-au-lait spots larger than 1.5 cm in diameter. Café-au-lait spots associated with neurofibromatosis have smoother margins. Less commonly, similar macules can be associated with polyostotic fibrous dysplasia, Albright's disease, or Caffey's disease.

Cafergot: A drug used as an abortive for migraine headaches which contains 1 mg of ergotamine and 100 mg of caffeine. The usual adult dosage is two tablets at the start of a headache, and one additional tablet every half hour if needed for full relief. The total dose for any one headache should not exceed six tablets. See Ergotamine.

Calcification of the Intervertebral Disc: An ICD-9 code used most commonly when calcification is seen either in the disc space or annulus. This represents degenerative disc disease. See Degenerative Disc Disease.

Calcifying Bursitis: The deposition of hydroxyapatite crystals in multiple locations. See Hydroxyapatite Deposition Disease.

Calcifying Tendinitis: The deposition of hydroxyapatite crystals in multiple locations. See Hydroxyapatite Deposition Disease.

Calcium Pyrophosphate Deposition Disease: An arthritic condition which presents like osteoarthritis and involves tissue deposition of calcium pyrophosphate dihydrate crystals. Involvement of the spine is uncommon and involves the lumbar and cervical spine. There is symmetrical joint involvement and a rapidly progressive degenerative joint disease. On x-ray, chondrocalcinosis (calcification of the cartilage) is seen. See Calcium Pyrophosphate Dihydrate Deposition Disease, CPDDD.

Calcium Pyrophosphate Dihydrate Deposition Disease: An arthritic condition. See Calcium Pyrophosphate Deposition Disease.

Calf Muscle: A muscle that makes up the bulk of the calf and is responsible for dorsiflexion of the foot. See Gastrocnemius, Gastroc.

Caliper Rib Movement: The movement of the lower rib cage during respiration, such that the ribs move anterior in inhalation.

Canal–Body Index: A radiographic method for determining if lumbar spinal stenosis is present. AP and lateral lumbar x-rays are taken. The interpediculate distance is calculated (the smallest distance between the pedicles), and the sagittal canal measurement is measured using Eisenstein's method. The width of the vertebral body on the AP film is measured at the midpoint. The sagittal body dimension is also measured laterally at the midpoint. The canal-body ratio is the sum of the interpediculate dimension multiplied by the sagittal canal dimension divided by the sum of the transverse body dimension multiplied by the sagittal body dimension. In essence, the first two measurements multiplied together are divided by the second two measurements multiplied together. Normal lumbar canal–body ratios are as follows: at L3 a minimum of 1:2.0–1:6.0, at L4 a minimum of 1:3.0–1:6.0, at L5 a minimum of 1:3.2–1:6.5. The higher the ratio, the smaller the spinal canal. See Eisenstein's Method, Spinal Index.

Canal–Body Ratio: A measurement of the size of the cervical spinal canal. The width of vertebral body is measured at its center. The width of the spinal canal is also measured from the midpoint of the posterior cortex of the vertebral body to the closest point on the spinolaminar line. The measurement of the canal is compared with the measurement of the vertebral body and is expressed as a ratio. This method is thought to compensate for differences in measurement technique. See Ratio Method.

Canal Stenosis: A narrowing of the canal for the spinal cord. See Central Canal Stenosis.

Canal Volume: The three-dimensional space available within the spinal canal. In patients with decreased canal volume, there is an increased likelihood of the symptoms of spinal stenosis. See Spinal Stenosis.

Cancellous Bone Graft: Bone graft which is made up of cancellous bone (spongy, lattice work) and usually used to promote fusion. This is in contrast to a cortical bone graft, which is used primarily for fixation and has much less potential to promote bony fusion.

Cancellous Screw: Screws used for internal fixation which have larger threads than cortical screws to provide better stability in soft or cancellous bone.

Cancer: An abnormal growth which can be local or can spread to other locations. Four tumors (breast, thyroid, lung, prostate) commonly spread or metastasize to the spine.

TUMORS WHICH CAN METASTASIZE TO THE SPINE:

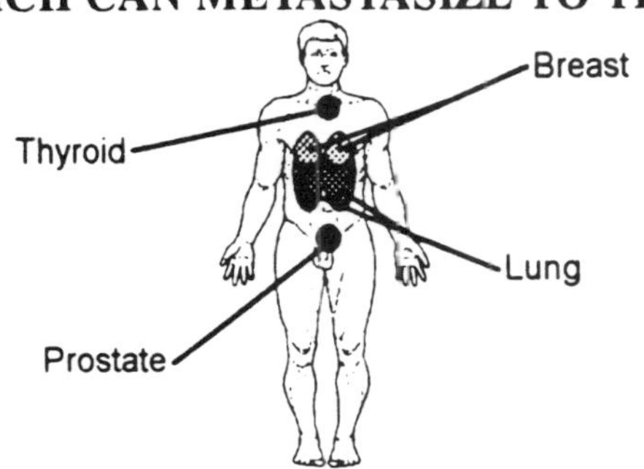

Candle Flame Hyperostosis: An osteophyte which is a calcification of the anterior longitudinal ligament (ALL) climbing upward. This is seen in diffuse idiopathic skeletal hyperostosis. See ALL.

Cannulated Screw: A threaded screw which has a hollow center and can be placed over a guide wire.

Capsular Adhesions: A term that refers to scarring of the facet joint capsules, which can restrict movement. See Facet Capsular Adhesions.

Capsular Pattern: Restriction of joint movement present when a joint capsule is tight. Each joint has a different capsular pattern. For instance, when the hip capsule is tight, it tends to lose internal rotation and abduction. This is in contrast to the capsular pattern of the shoulder, which results in a loss of external rotation and abduction. See Noncapsular Pattern.

Capsular SI Ligaments: The ventral SI ligaments, interosseous ligaments, the dorsal SI ligaments, and the lumbar sacral ligaments.

Carbamazepine: An anticonvulsant. See Tegretol.

Carisoprodol: A muscle relaxant which has sedative properties. See Soma.

Carisoprodol–Aspirin Tablets: A muscle relaxant which has sedative properties. See Soma Compound.

C-arm: This is a more maneuverable form of fluoroscopy. See Fluoroscopy.

Carotid Triangle: A portion of the anterior neck commonly used in surgical approaches bordered by the posterior belly of the digastric and stylohyoid muscles, the omohyoid muscle, and the sternocleidomastoid.

Carotid Tubercle: The tubercle on the anterior transverse process of C6. See Chassaignac's Tubercle.

Carrot Stick Fracture: A fracture through the ankylosed intervertebral disc in ankylosing spondylitis.

Cataflam: A nonsteroidal anti-inflammatory drug of the benzeneacetic acid class. This is the same drug as Voltaren, but is an immediate release version whereas Voltaren is a delayed-release version. As with all nonsteroidals, GI or hepatic side effects are possible. Renal side effects are also possible. There are drug interactions with aspirin, anticoagulants, digoxin, methotrexate, cyclosporine, lithium, oral hypoglycemics, and diuretics. The recommended starting dosage is 50 mg three times a day. A loading dose of 100 mg may be helpful. Only 50 mg tablets are available. See Diclofenac Potassium, Voltaren.

Catapres: A brand of clonidine, a centrally acting antihypertensive agent which is sometimes used in the treatment of reflex sympathetic dystrophy. This is an alpha-2 blocking agent which works in the brain stem to reduce the sympathetic outflow from the central nervous system. Clonidine should be used with caution in patients with severe coronary insufficiency, recent myocardial infarction, CVA, or chronic renal failure. Use with tricyclic antidepressants may reduce the effect of clonidine. Clonidine may also enhance the CNS depressant effects of alcohol, barbiturates, or other sedatives. Amitriptyline, in combination with clonidine, enhances the manifestation of corneal lesions in rats. Dry mouth and drowsiness are common side effects. The usual starting dosage is 0.1 mg twice a day. The dosage may be titrated up from that to achieve desired effect. However, hypotension obviously will increase with increased dosages. See Clonidine.

Catapres-TTS: A clonidine transdermal delivery system. There are three types of patches. The TTS-1 delivers 0.1 mg per day for 1 week, the TTS-2 delivers 0.2 mg per day for 1 week, and the TTS-3 delivers 0.3 mg per day for 1 week. See Clonidine.

CAT Scan: The use of x-rays taken at different angles and processed through a computer to produce a cross-sectional image. See CT Scan.

Caudad: The opposite of cephalad. In an inferior direction or toward the tail.

Cauda Equina: The "horse's tail" of the spinal cord. This is the lower-most portion of the spinal cord after the conus medularis. The cord splits into numerous nerve roots that give the appearance of a horse's tail.

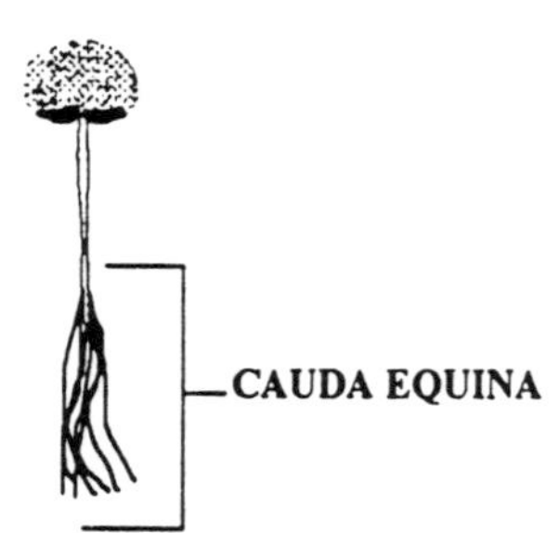

Cauda Equina Syndrome: Abnormal pressure on the bottom-most portion of the spinal cord, which can be caused by either bony stenosis or a large herniated disc. This can be associated with bowel and bladder incontinence, perianal anesthesia, and sphincter paralysis and is considered a surgical emergency requiring decompressive laminectomy. See Lumbar Disc Disorder with Myelopathy, Pseudo-Intermittent Claudication.

Caudal: Toward the tail, downward.

Caudal Anesthesia: Anesthesia given through a caudal epidural route introduced through the sacral hiatus and sacral canal.

Caudal Block: Epidural injection. See Caudal Epidural, Epidural Steroid Injection.

Caudal Epidural: An epidural injection through the sacral hiatus. The sacral hiatus is a defect in the lower part of the posterior wall of the sacrum formed by the failure of the lamina of S5, and usually a part of S4, to fuse medially. This is covered by a thick fibrous posterior sacrococcygeal ligament, and penetration of this ligament yields direct access to the epidural space in the sacral canal. It should be noted that the sacral epidural venous plexus usually ends at S4, but may extend throughout the canal. There is risk not only of damaging the venous plexus, but also of penetrating the dura; however, the dura usually ends at approximately S2. The needle is usually directed toward the sacral hiatus at an angle of about 30°. Once bone is reached on the opposite side of the hiatus, the needle is directed parallel to the sacral canal. It should be noted that any fluid injected can exit the anterior sacral foramina. The complication rate of dural puncture is rare, approximately 1% or slightly greater. A misplaced needle may enter the fourth sacral foramen, the sacral ligament, or into the sacral marrow. It has also been reported that even with fluoroscopy, there is a significant chance of incorrect needle placement. See Caudal Block, Epidural Steroid Injection, ESI.

Caudally: In an inferior direction or toward the tail. See Caudad.

Causalgia: (1) A burning pain that may result from a peripheral nerve injury or a radiculopathy. This is commonly associated with skin changes that involve skin atrophy and can include hair loss. (2) A clinical syndrome characterized by the presence of pain out of proportion to the severity of the injury. See Reflex Sympathetic Dystrophy.

CBT: Certified Biofeedback Therapist.

CC: An abbreviation for *cervical chair* or *chief complaint.*

CCA: Canadian Chiropractic Association.

CCE: Council on Chiropractic Education.

CCM: Certified Case Manager.

C-collar: A cervical orthosis. See Cervical Collar.

CCR: Consortium for Chiropractic Research.

CD: Cotrel-Dubousset instrumentation.

Central Canal Stenosis: A decrease in the size of the canal containing the spinal cord. This can be caused by pseudohypertrophy of the ligamentum flavum, facet joint hypertrophy, disc degeneration, or spondylosis. This is usually associated with radiating pain and numbness down both legs or weakness in both legs. Cervical stenosis can cause symptoms in all four extremities. These symptoms worsen with standing and are improved by sitting. This condition may require a decompressive laminectomy with or without fusion as surgical treatment. Conservative

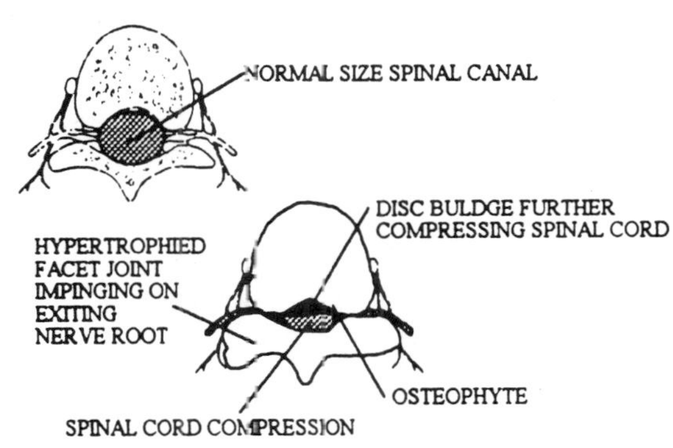

treatment tends to be only somewhat successful and can include a lumbar stabilization program. See Stenosis, Canal Stenosis, Bony Compression, Myelopathy.

Central Disc Herniation: A herniation of the nucleus pulposus that occurs in the midline instead of the usual posterior lateral direction. See Central HNP, Paramedian Herniated Disc.

Central Herniated Disc: A herniation of the nucleus pulposus that occurs in the midline instead of the usual posterior lateral direction. See Central HNP, Paramedian Herniated Disc.

Central HNP: A herniation of the nucleus pulposus that occurs in the midline instead of the usual posterior lateral direction. The disc usually herniates around the posterior longitudinal ligament (thus the posterior lateral configuration). However, here, the disc herniates through the posterior longitudinal ligament and thus more centrally. In the thoracic spine, this can lead to paraplegia owing to the small size of the spinal canal in that area. In the cervical and lumbar spines, this can lead to cord compression and sometimes myelopathy. See Paramedian Herniated Disc.

Centralization: A McKenzie physical therapy term used to describe a patient's pain pattern. When putting the patient through a series of movements, radiating low back pain recedes to the low back. This is often used in the phrase "centralization of pain."

Central Spinal Cord Syndrome: A syndrome usually following hyperextension injuries of the cervical spine without fracture or dislocation that results in a motor deficit in the upper limbs and a segmental level of impaired sensation. The sensation deficit is unique in that sensation to pain and temperature are lost, but sensation to touch is intact. Many theories have been proposed including edema and swelling in the central portion of the cord. This can occur in motor vehicle accident injuries in patients who have pre-existing cervical spondylosis who undergo a hyperextension injury without fracture or dislocation. Surgical intervention is usually not recommended. The cervical spine should be evaluated for clinical stability. See Spinal Cord Syndrome.

Centric Occlusion: The position of the jaw with the teeth maximally contacted.

Cephalad: The opposite of caudad denoting toward the head or superior.

Cephalgia: Headache.

Cephalic: The opposite of caudad. Superior or toward the head.

Cerebrospinal Fluid: The fluid which bathes the brain and spinal cord. This fluid circulates in the arachnoid space. See CSF.

Cervical: Of or referring to the neck. The cervical spine has 7 vertebrae, which allow head movement.

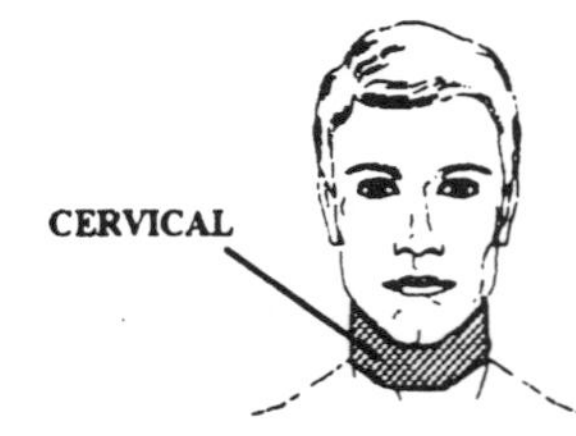

Cervical Acceleration–Deceleration Syndrome: A sprain/strain syndrome of the cervical spine caused by a hyperextension–hyperflexion injury. See Acceleration–Deceleration Injury, Whiplash Injury.

Cervical Brachial Syndrome: Compression of the neurovascular bundle (usually irritation of nerves) in the shoulder girdle area between the first rib and clavicle, by a cervical rib, at the second and third ribs, between the anterior and middle scalenes, or underneath the pectoralis minor and clavipectoral fascia. See Thoracic Outlet Syndrome.

Cervical Break: A chiropractic adjusting technique for the neck. The thrust does not rotate the neck; rather, the thrust is applied across the neck. See Lateral Break.

Cervical Clock: A home exercise in which the patient is supine with the hips and knees bent and the feet positioned comfortably with the head flat. A 6-inch clock face is visualized under the head with the 12 and 6 in line with the vertical axis of the head. The object of the exercise is to move the head and neck slowly in a controlled fashion through different movement patterns *without* bringing on discomfort at the extremes of range of motion. The top of the head can be brought back to the clock numbers 10 and 2 and the chin can nod toward the numbers 4 and 8. The head rotates without side bending to reach 3 and 9. The 11, 5 diagonals and 1, 7 diagonals can also be performed. The numbers can also be worked individually from 1 to 12 around the clock. See Neck Clock.

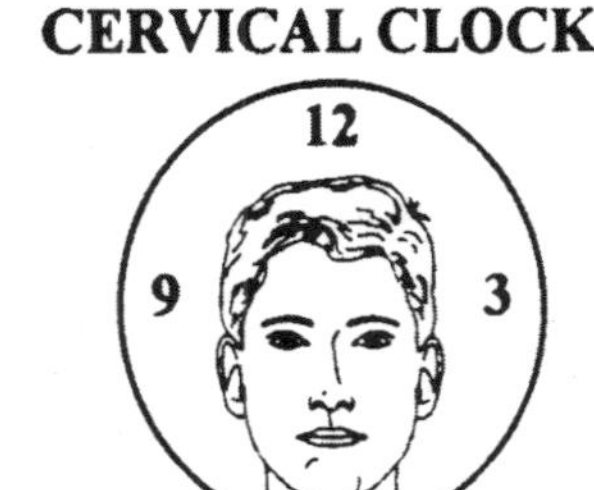

Cervical Collar: A cervical orthosis that wraps around the neck for support of the cervical spine, usually used following injury. There are several types of cervical collars. Perhaps the most common is the soft collar, which is made of foam rubber. There are also hard cervical collars, which are made of closed cell foam and tend to provide more support and further limit range of motion. See C-collar.

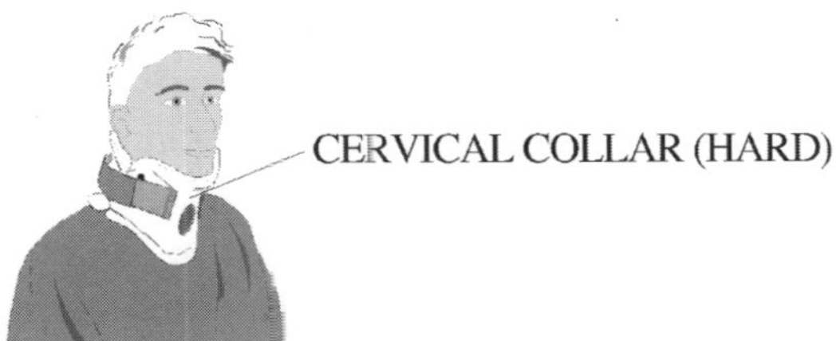

Cervical Compression Fracture: A crush fracture of a cervical vertebra. Cervical compression fractures are thought to be secondary to flexion injuries. This class of fracture includes a "teardrop fracture." A teardrop fracture occurs with more force than a simple vertebral compression fracture. Diagnosis is usually made on lateral radiographs but can be difficult to make secondary to the normal wedging of the cervical vertebral bodies. CT scan may be required. Clinical instability should be ruled out. Common treatments include cervical immobilization for fractures without neurologic deficit, axial traction, or laminectomy/fusion for severe teardrop fractures or fractures with neurologic deficit. See Compression Fracture—Cervical.

Cervical Compression Test: A physical exam maneuver that causes compression of the foramina and is positive if it reproduces radicular symptoms. The head can be compressed axially, and the test can be sensitized by rotation to the right and side bending. Extension can also sensitize the maneuver.

Cervical Cord Syndrome: A clinical syndrome. See Spinal Cord Syndrome.

Cervical Curve: A term that refers to a scoliosis in the cervical spine. The apex of the curve is between C1 and C6.

Cervical Disc Disorder with Myelopathy: An ICD-9 code diagnosis which usually refers to a large cervical HNP or central canal stenosis on the cervical spine. See Spinal Stenosis, Myelopathy.

Cervical Distraction Test: A physical exam maneuver which involves manual traction on the cervical spine to decrease pressure on a suspect nerve root. The test is positive if radicular symptoms subside during the test or a "release" phenomena is noted. See Release Phenomena.

Cervical Dizziness: A relatively uncommon syndrome characterized by dizziness, light-headedness, vertigo, vasomotor face disturbances, retro-orbital pain, disturbances of vision, and other symptoms. See Syndrome of Barre-Lieou.

Cervical Dystonia: An abnormal neck posture due to repetitive, clonic (spasmodic), and tonic (sustained) head movement. Approximately one third of these patients have involvement of a contiguous body part such as the jaw or shoulder. Botulinum injections are commonly used as treatment. See Spasmodic Torticollis.

Cervical Foraminal Compression Test: A physical exam test for nerve root syndrome. The patient is asked to abduct and externally rotate the ipsilateral shoulder by placing the hand on top of the head. If this position relieves radicular pain complaints, then this is considered a positive sign for a nerve root syndrome. See Bakody Sign.

Cervicalgia: Cervical pain. See Cervicothoracic Sprain/Strain, Whiplash Syndrome.

Cervical Gravity Line: An x-ray technique which assesses the gravitational stresses on the cervicothoracic junction. A vertical line is drawn through the apex of the dens downward. The line should pass through the vertebral body of C7. If the line is anterior to the vertebral body, it is thought that there is excessive stress on the posterior elements at the cervicothoracic junction.

Cervical Myelopathy: A clinical syndrome that involves impingement of the cervical spinal cord. This can be due to direct compression from cervical spondylosis (bone spurs) or central canal stenosis (a closing off of the bony canal that houses the spinal cord), ischemia caused by compromise of the vascular supply to the cord, or repeated trauma in flexion and extension of the neck secondary to spondylosis or central canal stenosis. Neck pain is a prominent symptom, but radiculopathy is uncommon. However, there may be paresthesias (diffuse tingling) in different root distributions. The most common symptom is an alternation in gait. Weakness and wasting of the upper extremities may be seen, and bowel and bladder problems actually occur in the minority of patients. This is a slowly progressive disease process. An EMG can be helpful in the diagnosis as well as SSEP. Cervical spinal tumors should be ruled out with MRI. Decompressive laminectomy is recommended. Multiple sclerosis, ALS, neurosyphilis, and other causes of this symptom complex should be ruled out. See Myelopathy—Cervical.

Cervical Plexus: A collection of nerve fibers made up of the ventral rami from the first four cervical nerve roots.

Cervical Radiculopathy: Dysfunction of the cervical nerve roots secondary to either pressure or inflammation that causes weakness or numbness in the hand, arm, forearm, or shoulder. This can be caused by a cervical disc bulge, HNP (herniated disc), foraminal stenosis (a closing off of the bony window through which the nerve root exits), or a mass lesion (for example, a tumor) in the cervical spine. It should be noted that the cervical nerve roots exit at the bottom portion of the cervical foramen. Symptoms include numbness or tingling in one extremity in a specific dermatomal pattern, weakness in muscle groups corresponding to the affected nerve root, or cervical pain or pain in the upper back. Common treatments include injections of epidural steroids, traction, physical therapy including muscle energy technique, Jones strain–counterstrain, cervicothoracic stabilization techniques, strengthening, or modalities to reduce spasm and/or inflammation. Cervical discectomy with fusion and/or foraminotomy may be considered if there is prolonged disability or significant motor involvement. See Radiculopathy—Cervical.

Cervical Rib: An "extra" rib which occurs in the cervical spine (rather than the usual thoracic spine). A cervical rib is present in 0.5% of the population and is most commonly found in females. They are bilateral in about two thirds of cases. They are most common at C5–C7. This phenomenon has been associated with thoracic outlet syndrome. This is thought to occur secondary to neurovascular compression caused by the rib as the thoracic outlet decreases in size with shoulder protraction.

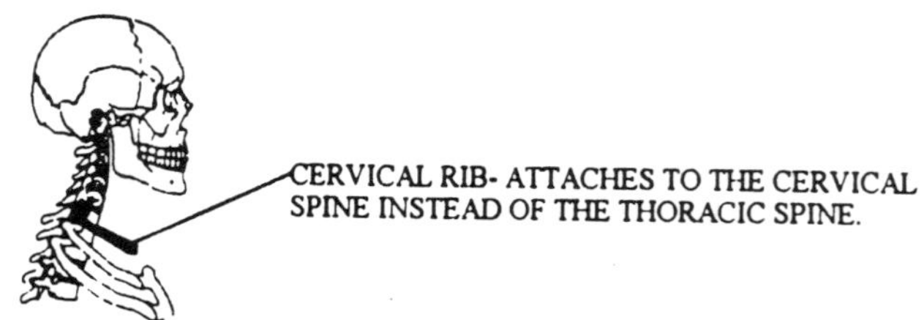

Cervical Spondylolisthesis: A rare disorder usually discovered incidentally during x-ray studies. The most common level is C6. This is more common in males. Fifty percent of patients have an associated spin-abifida occulta. Flexion extension x-rays are recommended to rule out clinical instability.

Cervical Spondylosis: A progressive degeneration of the intervertebral discs leading to bony spurring. This is so common that it is likely a part of normal aging. This is seen in 5–10% of patients between the ages of 20 and 30, 50% of patients at the age of 45, and more than 90% after age 60. This can lead to central canal stenosis or foraminal stenosis with myelopathy and radiculopathy. See Spondylosis—Cervical.

Cervicobrachial Syndrome: Compression of the neurovascular bundle (usually irritation of nerves) in the shoulder girdle area between the first rib and clavicle, by a cervical rib, at the second and third ribs, between the anterior and middle scalenes, or underneath the pectoralis minor and clavipectoral fascia. See Thoracic Outlet Syndrome.

Cervicocephalic Syndrome: A constellation of symptoms which includes headache, dizziness, and neck pain that is seen post whiplash. See Barre-Lieou Syndrome.

Cervicocranial: Referring to the C0–C2 area.

Cervicothoracic Block: The injection of a local anesthetic into the region surrounding the stellate ganglion in the cervical spine. See Stellate Ganglion Block.

Cervicothoracic Curve: A scoliosis with its apex at C7 or T1.

Cervicothoracic Disc: The C7–T1 disc.

Cervicothoracic Dysfunction: Decreased or abnormal mobility at the cervicothoracic junction (C7–T1). In this area, the much more mobile cervical spine connects to the less mobile thoracic spine. This is a common site of hypermobility after whiplash injuries. This area can also be hypomobile or directionally hyper- or hypomobile with abnormal movement or joint fixation.

Cervicothoracic Ganglion: A star-shaped collection of sympathetic cell bodies (ganglion) in the cervical spine. See Stellate Ganglion.

Cervicothoracic Junction: The C7–T1 area. This is the place where the more mobile cervical spine meets the less mobile thoracic spine.

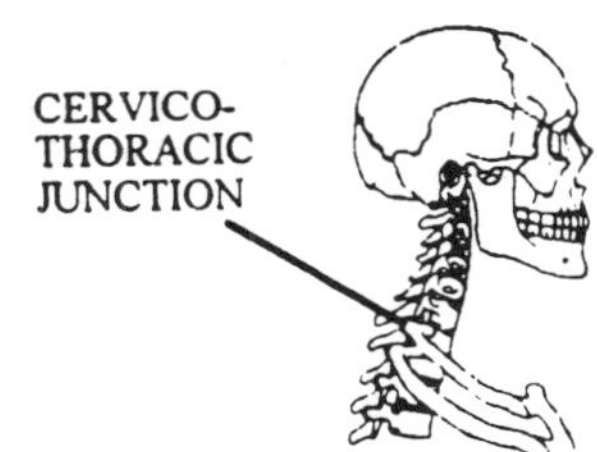

Cervicothoracic Sprain/Strain: A sprain/strain syndrome of the cervical spine caused by a hyperextension–hyperflexion injury. See Acceleration–Deceleration, Whiplash Injury.

CES: A microcurrent electrical stimulation device used to treat headache pain. The electrodes are usually placed over the temporal region of the head. See Cranial Electrical Stimulator.

CESI: An abbreviation for *cervical epidural steroid injection.*

Chair Back Brace: A lumbar support brace. See Macausland Brace.

Chakras: A traditional Indian medical concept which involves areas of focused energy within the body. There are seven chakras. They are located at the base of the spine, in the perineum, behind the navel, at the heart, at the throat, at the third eye (between the eyebrows), and in the crown.

Chamberlain's Line: A radiographic sign used to detect basilar impression. A lateral skull/lateral cervical view is used. A line is drawn from the posterior margin of the hard palate to the posterior aspect of the foramen magnum. The relationship of this line to the odontoid process is evaluated. In the majority of patients, the tip of the odontoid process should not project above this line. However, projection up to 3 mm above the line is still within normal limits. A measurement of 7 mm above the line is considered abnormal. See Palato-occipital Line, Pseudobasilar Invagination.

Chance Fracture: A horizontal fracture through both the vertebral body and the posterior elements produced by a hyperflexion injury. This most commonly occurs in the upper three lumbar vertebrae, and diagnosis is made radiographically. See Lap Seat Belt Fracture, Empty Vertebra Sign, Fulcrum Fracture, Lap Belt Injury, Seat Belt Fracture.

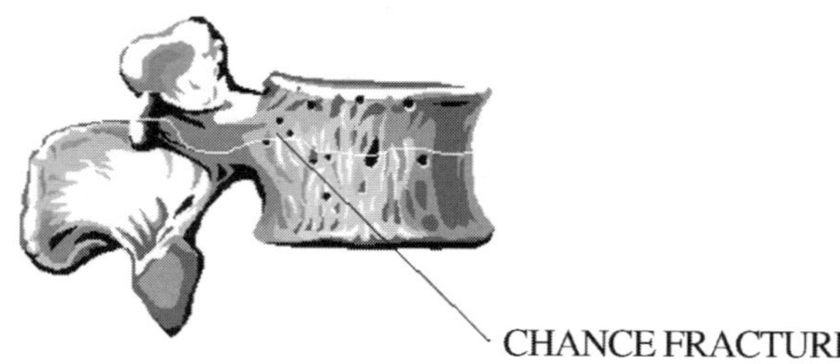

Chapman's Neurolymphatic Reflexes: An osteopathic term which refers to anterior and posterior reflex points associated with areas of tissue texture abnormality which correspond to specific visceral dysfunctions. See Chapman's Reflex.

Chapman's Reflex: An osteopathic term which refers to anterior and posterior reflex points associated with areas of tissue texture abnormality which correspond to specific visceral dysfunctions. See Chapman's Neurolymphatic Reflexes.

Chassaignac's Tubercle: The tubercle on the anterior transverse process of C6. See Carotid Tubercle.

Chatillion Gauge: A portable isokinetic dynamometer (force-measuring device). This is often used during job site analyses to determine the amount of push/pull forces required for a specific job. See Push/Pull Dynamometer.

Check Ligaments: The upper portion of the alar ligaments which check side bending and rotation of the upper cervical spine. See Apical Alar Ligaments, Alar Ligaments.

Chemical Radiculitis: An inflammatory reaction within a nerve root that occurs due to leakage of nucleus pulposus from the disk. Since the nucleus is rich in inflammatory substances, a significant inflammatory reaction can ensue. See HNP, Radiculopathy, Radiculitis.

Chemical Shift: A phenomenon that occurs in musculoskeletal MR imaging because of the differing chemical environments of the hydrogen nuclei. Hydrogen nuclei bound to fat molecules experience a different chemical environment than those bound to water molecules. There is a shielding effect such that the hydrogen bound to water precesses at a slightly different larmor frequency than those bound to fat. The difference in the larmor frequency is the chemical shift.

Chemonucleolysis: The injection of chymopapain or another proteolytic enzyme into the nucleus pulposus. The injection decreases disc height and water content and decreases intradiscal pressure. Chemonucleolysis is no longer common in this country secondary to allergic reactions, but at one time it was done to treat HNP. See Chymopapain.

Chest Expansion Test: A test commonly used to determine if there is rib and thoracic spine involvement in ankylosing spondylitis. The patient is seated with arms at sides. A tape measure is placed around the patient's chest at a specific point. The patient exhales deeply and the measurement is recorded. The patient then takes a maximum inhalation and a second measurement is taken. The normal difference between inspiration and expiration is reported to be 1.5–3 inches or 3.81–7.62 cm.

Chicago Test: A physical exam maneuver in which the patient kneels on a chair and attempts to touch the floor with outstretched hands. It is reported that with disc disease, the patient is able to perform this test without difficulty. With a back strain, pain will be increased. See Burns' Bench Test, Bench Test.

Chin-on-Chest Forward Flexion: A physical exam term used to describe normal cervical flexion and meaning the patient is able to bring his or her chin to the chest in cervical forward bending.

Chin Tuck: A physical therapy stretch designed to stretch the suboccipital musculature. The patient's chin is brought posterior in the same plane (straight back) until a stretch is felt at the base of the skull. See Suboccipital Stretch, Neck Retraction, Axial Extension Stretch.

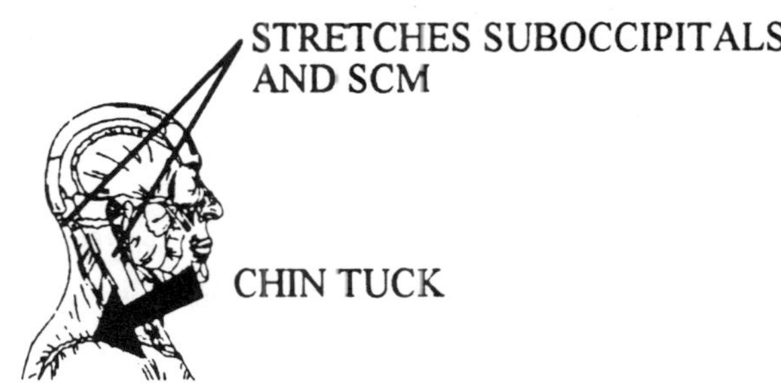

Chip Fracture: A fracture of the corner of a vertebral body. This can be "pulled off" by a sudden hyperflexion or hyperextension injury. Sudden hyperflexion or hyperextension that causes the two corners (inferior corner of the superior vertebrae and superior corner of the inferior vertebrae) to come together, which can cause a fracture. A teardrop fracture should be ruled out and flexion/extension views should be performed to rule out instability. See Limbus Vertebra.

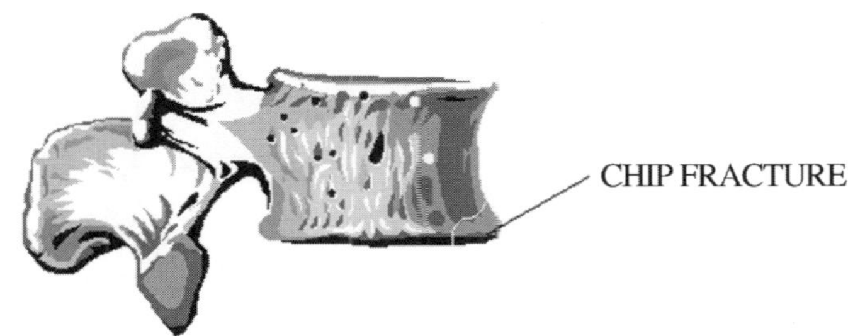

Chiro: An abbreviation for *chiropractor* or *chiropractic.*

Chiropractic: Referring to the chiropractic profession. See Chiropractor.

Chiropractic Biophysics: A chiropractic adjusting technique which uses high-velocity, high-acceleration, low-amplitude thrust.

Chiropractor: A medical provider who has completed an ACA-approved degree in chiropractic. A specialist in the use of hands-on treatment techniques such as manipulation.

Chondrocalcinosis: Calcification of cartilage on x-ray usually caused by calcium pyrophosphate deposition. This is also seen in rheumatoid arthritis, osteoarthritis, and gout.

Chondropathia Tuberosa: Inflammation of the costal cartilage (area between the ribs) due to trauma. This can also have an idiopathic etiology. See Costochondritis.

Chondrosarcoma: A malignant tumor which is found in the spine approximately 10% of the time. These tumors are usually resistant to radiotherapy and chemotherapy and are slow growing, often with local recurrences. When found in the spinal column, the prognosis is poor. Radiographically, there is a large area of bony destruction, an associated soft tissue mass, and flocculent calcifications. If no soft tissue mass is found, the lesion is usually lytic with sclerotic margins and with no mottling seen in the calcification. CT scanning and MRI are extremely helpful in diagnosis. Complete surgical excision is recommended, but may be difficult. Repeated local excisions of recurrent disease are sometimes necessary and, again, can be difficult.

Chordoma: A locally invasive malignant tumor primarily occurring in the spine which is relatively rare and usually found in patients in their 50s and 60s. Embryologically, it arises from the remnants of the primitive notochord found in the sacrococcygeal and the suboccipital regions and occasionally in the thoracic and lumbar regions. There is a slow, relentless local spread with the possibility of distant metastases. Symptoms are usually mild and progress slowly with these tumors reaching considerable size before metastasizing. Patients often complain of symptoms of constipation, urinary frequency, or nerve root compression before they present to their physician. A fixed and firm presacral mass can be palpated on rectal exam. Surgical excision with a wide margin is the only curative procedure, and biopsy is not recommended until appropriate staging studies have been evaluated. When local recurrence does occur, it portends a poor prognosis and dramatically reduces the cure rate. Radical surgical approaches are recommended to try to achieve excellent margins.

chr: An abbreviation for *chronic*.

Chronic: A long-standing injury. The definition of *chronic* varies considerably, however. A chronic injury is usually considered one that continues at least into the 3–6 month range.

Chronic Epstein-Barr Virus: A somewhat controversial diagnosis. See Chronic Fatigue Syndrome.

Chronic Fatigue Syndrome: A somewhat controversial diagnosis. The diagnostic criteria have been outlined as the following: (1) fatigue with no improvement on rest, (2) fatigue lasting for more than 6 months, and (3) activity level of 50% normal. Physical exam signs must be seen on two separate occasions, at least one month apart, and include the following: (1) an oral temperature of 99.7–101.5°F, (2) pharyngitis, and (3) enlarged tender lymph nodes (generalized). It is thought that this disorder is caused by the Epstein-Barr virus. See Chronic Epstein-Barr Virus, Myalgic Encephalomyelitis.

Chronic Pain: The definitions vary, but the most accepted seems to be significant disabling pain for more than 6 months that significantly alters activities of daily living and may or may not prevent return to work. See Chronic Pain Syndrome, CP.

Chronic Pain Management: The use of treatment techniques designed to palliate rather than cure chronic pain. This is used when the disorder causing the chronic pain is not readily treatable. It is thought that by decreasing the patient's pain complaints and by teaching self–pain management techniques, the patient will become more functional. See CPP.

Chronic Pain Program: The use of treatment techniques designed to palliate rather than cure chronic pain. See CPP, Chronic Pain Management.

Chronic Pain Syndrome: The definitions vary, but the most accepted seems to be significant disabling pain for more than 6 months that significantly alters activities of daily living and may prevent return to work. Most chronic pain syndrome patients have pathology, but this pain is often magnified by psychosocial issues. A chronic pain program may be helpful once attempts at abating the pain generator have been reasonably exhausted. Also, a chronic pain program may be necessary in some patients to allow them to participate in normal rehabilitation care before the search for the pain generator has been exhausted. See Pain Clinic, Somatoform Pain Disorder.

Chymopapain: A proteolytic enzyme. See Chemonucleosis.

Cigne de Shampoo: A physical exam maneuver which evaluates the parietal subcutaneous tissue. The palpating fingers are placed over the parietal region while the scalp is displaced from side to side in a sagittal plane. It is thought that this area corresponds to the C2–C3 motor unit and decreased displacement indicates C2–C3 dysfunction.

Circuit Weight Training: Resistance exercises that are carried out in a specific sequence using a variety of exercises for total body conditioning. Common circuit weight-training systems include Universal, Nautilus, or Eagle Systems. A rest period is usually taken between each set of exercise.

Circumlaminar Wires: A wiring system. See Harrington Rods, Segmental Wiring.

CJA: *Chiropractic Journal of Australia*.

Classic Migraine: A vascular headache with transient, visual, and other sensory or motor symptoms. See Migraine.

Clavicle Jump Test: A manual medicine test in which the patient abducts the shoulders bilaterally, and

Concentric Tear of the Annulus: A tear in the fibers of the annulus that is in the same direction as the fibers. These are not thought to be significant tears and likely represent normal aging and normal disc degeneration.

Concomitant Noncontiguous Spinal Fractures: Multiple fractures in nonadjoining areas due to trauma. For instance, 25% of transverse sacral fractures have an associated thoracolumbar burst fracture. See Concomitant Noncontinuous Thoracolumbar and Sacral Fractures.

Concomitant Noncontinuous Thoracolumbar and Sacral Fractures: Multiple fractures in nonadjoining areas due to trauma. For instance, 25% of transverse sacral fractures have an associated thoracolumbar burst fracture. See Concomitant Noncontiguous Spinal Fractures.

Concordant Pain Response: One possible pain response during discography. If the patient reports an exact or near-exact reproduction of usual pain, this is said to be a concordant pain response. Some question exists about how objective these findings are because they rely on patient report. See P2 Response, Discography, Pain Re-creation, Subjective Discography.

Conduction Block: The loss of conduction through a nerve, usually in one specific region. This can be due to direct compression, inflammation, loss of the myelin sheath (focal demyelination), or other causes. See Reversible Conduction Block.

Condylicus Tertius Syndrome: A syndrome involving a large abnormal dens which articulates with a third occipital condyle in the anterior rim of the foramen magnum. This can produce cord involvement because of narrowing of the foramen magnum and brain stem compression.

Coned-Down View: A close-up view of a specific area obtained by using a funnel-shaped attachment that controls x-ray scatter and concentrates the x-ray beam. This is commonly performed in the lumbar spine with a lateral of the L5–S1 area. See Cone View.

Cone View: A close-up view of a specific area obtained by using a funnel-shaped attachment that controls x-ray scatter and concentrates the x-ray beam. This is commonly performed in the lumbar spine with a lateral of the L5–S1 area. See Coned-Down View.

Congenital Block Vertebrae: The congenital fusion of two adjacent vertebrae. See Block Vertebrae.

Congenital Hypermobility: Excessive mobility found in multiple areas of the body. See Systemic Hypermobility.

Congenital Muscular Torticollis: A congenital condition which causes the head and neck to be side bent to the affected side and the chin to face the opposite direction. See Congenital Torticollis.

Congenital Scoliosis: A structural scoliosis caused by an anomalous or malformed vertebra. See Scoliosis, Scoliosis—Congenital.

Congenital Short Neck Syndrome: A syndrome of osseus malformations of the cervical spine most commonly associated with a "short" neck. See Klippel-Feil Syndrome.

Congenital Spinal Stenosis: A decrease in size of the spinal canal that is not related to trauma. This is a normal variant due to underdevelopment of the spinal canal and short pedicles. In congenital spinal stenosis, even minimal degenerative changes of the disc, facet, or ligamentum flavum can result in neurologic symptoms. Since there is less overall room in the spinal canal, any structure that moves into the spinal canal will impinge on the spinal cord or cauda equina. See Central Canal Stenosis.

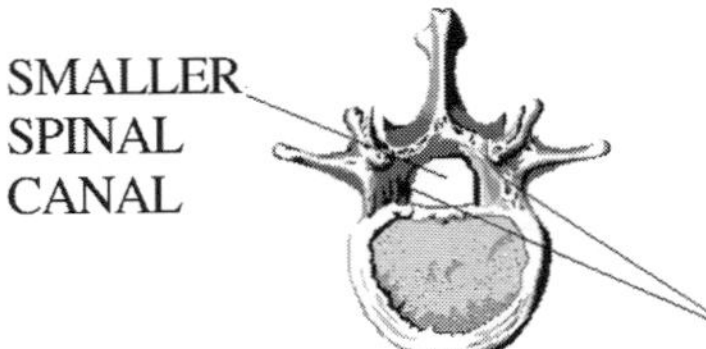

Congenital Torticollis: A congenital condition which causes the head and neck to bend to the affected side and the chin to face the opposite direction. This is caused by shortening and contracture of the sternocleidomastoid, usually at birth. Treatment usually involves aggressive stretching, traction, and positioning. Surgical intervention has been advocated for torticollis, which continues to occur into childhood. See Congenital Muscular Torticollis, Wryneck, Congenital Wryneck.

Congenital Wryneck: A congenital condition which causes the head and neck to bend to the affected side and the chin to face the opposite direction. See Congenital Torticollis.

Congestive Myelopathy: Myelopathy caused by venous congestion usually associated with a dural AV fistula or a direct spinal AV fistula.

Conjoined Nerve Roots: Nerve roots which are congenitally joined together. See Type 3 Nerve Root Anomaly.

Connective Tissue Disease: A group of disorders involving the connective tissue and can either be hereditary or autoimmune. Marfan and Ehlers-Danlos syndromes are examples of hereditary disorders. Autoimmune disorders include SLE, scleroderma, rheumatoid arthritis, and others.

Connective Tissue Massage: A massage technique developed in the 1920s by Dicke and Ebner. The CTM is systematic and protocol-oriented. Each stroke is performed three times with the right side always first. The low back and sacral areas are always treated first. CTM is used to influence connective tissue, increase circulation, and "release" nerve impulses along specific paths. CTM is often used for hypersensitive patients, i.e., reflex sympathetic dystrophy. See Bindegwebb's Massage.

Contact Point: The area on the patient where the hand of the manipulator makes contact to deliver the manipulation. Also, the area on the manipulator's hand where the contact is made.

Contained Herniation: When the nucleus of the disc ruptures through the inner annular fibers, but does not rupture through a majority of those fibers. See Disc Protrusion, Protruded Disc.

Contoured Anterior Spinal Fixation System: Instrumentation used for anterior interbody fusion which consists of a plate with multiple holes which is applied to the lateral aspect of the vertebral bodies to be fused. Screws are then placed through the contoured plate into the vertebral bodies.

Contract-Relax: A proprioceptive neuromuscular facilitation (PNF) muscle energy technique. The patient performs a contraction of the tight muscle isometrically against resistance (to relax the muscle) and then that muscle is stretched. This utilizes the concept of autogenic inhibition. See Hold-Relax.

Contract-Relax-Contract: A variation of the contract-relax technique during which the tight muscle is contracted, then relaxed, followed by a contraction of the muscle opposite the tight side. This technique combines the concepts of autogenic inhibition and reciprocal inhibition to lengthen a tight muscle. See Hold-Relax-Contract.

Contracture: This is usually meant to describe muscle, tendon, or ligament shortening. Chronic shortening of the musculature can lead to fibrosis. A contracture can be caused by a sustained position of muscle shortening or increased tone secondary to upper motor neuron dysfunction.

Contralateral: Pertaining to the opposite side.

Contrast Column: The column of dye seen on a myelogram. Indentations in this column are associated with a herniated disc, tumors, stenosis, and other mass lesions. See Column, Myelographic Column.

Contusion: Discoloration of the skin seen after trauma that is caused by rupture of the capillary bed.

Conus: The caudal end of the spinal cord located in the T12–L1 area. See Conus Medullaris.

Conus Medullaris: The caudal end of the spinal cord located in the T12–L1 area.

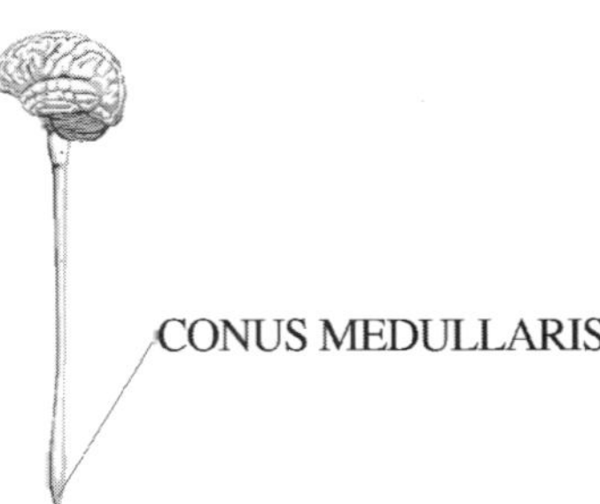

Conus Medullaris Syndrome: An ICD-9 diagnosis code which usually refers to a large centrally herniated lumbar disc causing pressure on the conus medullaris. See Lumbar Disc Disorder with Myelopathy.

Conversion Disorder: A pain disorder which involves pain or loss of bodily function without a physical cause. An emotional conflict seems to play a role in the etiology of this disorder. This differs from symptom magnification in that the most common manifestations involve paralysis, loss of sight, and movement disturbances. This is a psychiatric diagnosis and is relatively uncommon in chronic pain patients. See Conversion Hysteria, Hysterical Neurosis, Conversion Reaction.

Conversion Hysteria: A pain disorder which involves pain or loss of bodily function without a physical cause. See Conversion Disorder, Hysterical Neurosis, Conversion Reaction.

Conversion Reaction: A pain disorder which involves pain or loss of bodily function without a physical cause. See Conversion Disorder, Hysterical Neurosis, Conversion Hysteria.

Cordotomy: A surgical lesioning of the spinal cord. Usually, the anterolateral tracts are separated. This uncommon surgical technique is performed for treatment of severe chronic pain. One risk of this procedure is significant weakness of the leg contralateral to the lesion. After an extended period of time, the degree of pain relief may decrease.

Cord Traction Syndrome: A progressive neurologic deficit seen in patients with spina bifida and myelomeningocele. See Tethered Cord Syndrome.

Core Control: A rehabilitation program used to stabilize the lumbar spine through the pelvis; it involves neuromuscular retraining, flexibility, and strengthening. See Dynamic Lumbar Stabilization.

Core Stabilization: A rehabilitation program used to stabilize the lumbar spine through the pelvis; it involves neuromuscular retraining, flexibility, and strengthening. See Dynamic Lumbar Stabilization.

Corner Stretch: A stretching maneuver for the anterior chest and shoulder structures which includes the clavipectoral fascia, pectoralis minor, pectoralis major, subscapularis, subclavius, and other structures. This is usually given as a home stretch to correct a protracted shoulder, which may be causing postural misalignment or thoracic outlet syndrome. The patient is asked to place the forearm and hand on a wall near a corner and place the other hand on the other wall for support. The stretch is applied to the shoulder and anterior chest in various positions by asking the patient to push farther into the corner or push farther into the doorway. See Doorway Stretch.

Corset: A type of TLSO (brace that extends from under the shoulders to the pelvis) which is made of fabric and provides minimal support to the lumbar spine. This restricts flexion/extension and lateral bending to a small degree. Metal stays can be added posteriorly to provide further stability. Also, a thermoplastic insert can be added posteriorly and molded to the shape of the lumbar spine. See Warm and Form Low Back Brace, Lumbosacral Corset.

Cortical Bone Graft: A bone graft used for fusion composed of cortical bone and used primarily for fixation. Unlike a cancellous bone graft, this type of graft is not used to stimulate bone growth and bone fusion.

Cortical Screw: A screw drilled into cortical bone used for internal fixation.

Corticospinal Tract: Nerve fibers which originate from the motor cortex of the brain and travel in the dorsolateral portion of the spinal cord. See Pyramidal Tract.

Corticosteroid: A potent anti-inflammatory which can be supplied in tablet form, for intravenous, intramuscular, or intra-articular use. See Steroid.

Costal Cartilage: The cartilage that connects the ribs to the sternum anteriorly.

Costochondral Junction Syndrome: Inflammation of the costal cartilage (area between the ribs) which can be due to trauma or more likely is idiopathic. See Costochondritis.

Costochondritis: Inflammation of the costal cartilage (area between the ribs) which can be due to trauma or more likely is idiopathic. This is usually self-limited and symptoms include pain in the rib cage which is increased with coughing, sneezing, or motion. The second rib is most frequently involved. See Tietze's Syndrome, Chondropathia Tuberosa, Costochondral Junction Syndrome.

Costoclavicular Maneuver: A physical exam test used to evaluate thoracic outlet syndrome at the first rib. See Adson's Test, Wright's Hyperabduction Maneuver.

Costoclavicular Syndrome: Compression of the neurovascular bundle (usually irritation of nerves) in the shoulder girdle area between the first rib and clavicle, by a cervical rib, at the second and third ribs, between the anterior and middle scalenes, or underneath the pectoralis minor and clavipectoral fascia. See Thoracic Outlet Syndrome.

Costophrenic Angle: The angle between the ribs and diaphragm.

Costotransverse Arthrosis: Degenerative joint disease of the costovertebral joints.

Costotransversectomy: A surgical technique used to excise laterally herniated thoracic discs and to evacuate tuberculous abscesses in the thoracic spine. This technique provides good access to the lateral aspect of the vertebral bodies and to the posterior elements. This is commonly used when a more conventional anterior approach is not possible.

Costovertebral Angle: The angle between the twelfth rib and the T12 vertebral body. This also refers to the area overlying this articulation. See CVA.

Costovertebral Arthrosis: Degenerative changes within the rib facet. See Rib Facet.

COTA: Certified Occupational Therapy Assistant.

Cotrel Cast: A casting technique developed by Cotrel for the treatment of scoliosis which involves applying a body cast during spinal traction while a patient is suspended by derotation slings.

Cotrel-Dubousset Rods: Stainless steel rods with hooks that are placed posteriorly and are used for three-dimensional correction of scoliotic deformities. Distraction, compression, and derotation forces can be applied. A bony fusion usually is performed along the length of a rodding system. This system is commonly used to correct scoliotic deformities and spinal fractures. It is a dual rod system with vertically planed hooks and parallel rods. Most patients are not immobilized postoperatively. See Cotrel-Dubousset System.

Cotrel-Dubousset System: Stainless steel rods with hooks that are placed posteriorly and are used for three-dimensional correction of scoliotic deformities. Distraction, compression, and derotation forces can be applied. A bony fusion usually is performed along the length of a rodding system. This system is commonly used to correct scoliotic deformities and spinal fractures. It is a dual rod system with vertically planed hooks and parallel rods. Most patients are not immobilized postoperatively. See Cotrel-Dubousset Rods.

Cotrel Dynamic Traction: Traction that is applied before surgical intervention for scoliosis. This involves a head halter, pelvic harness, and foot stirrups which allow for stretching of the soft tissues for 7–10 days before surgery.

Cough Fracture: Bilateral nondisplaced fractures of the sixth to ninth ribs which can result from violent coughing.

Counternutated Sacrum: An osteopathic or manual physical therapy term which refers to a sacrum that is extended backwards. It is often seen in patients who have very little lumbar lordosis. These patients often complain of difficulty with backward bending because the sacrum moves into nutation with this movement. The ILAs are deeper on both sides.

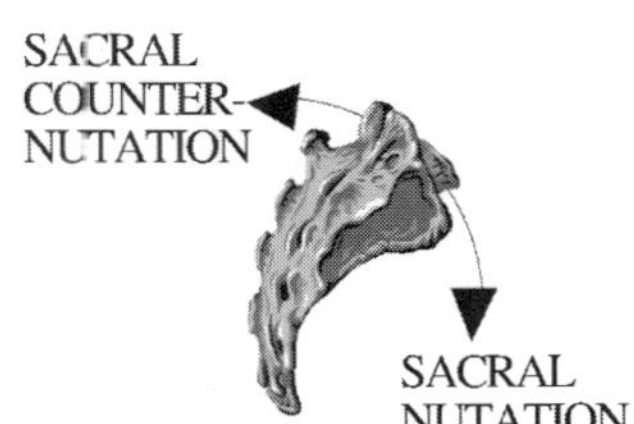

Counternutation: Since nutation means to nod, counternutation is moving in the opposite direction. In the spine, this usually refers to the ilium or sacrum, e.g., a sacrum which is extended or is bending backward. See Superior Nutation.

Counterstrain: A technique which is advocated for the treatment of acute and subacute muscular strain. See Strain-Counterstrain.

Coupling: A biomechanical phenomenon in the spine in which lateral bending is associated with rotation. This follows type I and type II mechanics. See Type 1 Motion, Type 2 Motion, Coupling Pattern.

Coupling Pattern: A biomechanical principle of the spine in which rotation is coupled with side bending. For instance, when the spine is in neutral position, side bending and rotation occur in opposite directions. When the spine is in a flexed or extended position, side bending and rotation occur in the same direction. See Coupling.

Coxa Valga: A valgus deformity of the hip characterized by a neck-shaft angle greater than 130°. Causes include trauma, dislocation of the hip, spastic paralysis, developmental stresses, and the congenital form. There is relative lengthening of the limb, and this causes obliquity which places the hip on the affected side in relative adduction. The acetabulum can become elongated and oval secondary to a shift of weight bearing that is closer to the center of the head of the femur. Gait analysis reveals a gluteus medius limp. Treatment includes equalizing leg length and stretching for the adductors as well as strengthening for the abductors of the same side. Surgical treatment has also been used.

Coxa Vera: A varus deformity of the hip where the neck shaft angle is less than 125°. Causes include trauma, a slipped femoral epiphysis, arthritis, or rickets. A congenital form is also described. The congenital condition is often bilateral. This condition causes extra stress to be placed on the femoral neck biomechanically. This may lead to a greater predisposition for fracture of the femoral neck. Also, shear forces across the capital femoral epiphysis enhance the tendency for a slipped femoral epiphysis. There is a relative shortening of the limb which results in a pelvic obliquity with a dropped pelvis on the affected side. There is a positive Trendelenburg's sign on the affected side. Back pain or SI joint dysfunction is common. There may be restriction of abduction secondary to impingement of the greater trochanter against the ilium. There is abductor inefficiency and contracture. Treatment includes equalizing leg lengths, osteotomy, and strengthening the abductors.

Coxalgia: Pain emanating from the hip.

Coxalgic Gait: The gait pattern that arises from a painful hip joint. The painful hip is held in slight flexion, abduction, and external rotation. This is the position that causes the least tension along the inflamed synovial tissues. Walking speed is notably slower and individual steps are shorter and unequal. Longer steps are taken with the painful limb than with the uninvolved limb. There is a Trendelenburg lurch. See Trendelenburg Gait.

Cox Flexion-Distraction: A chiropractic technique which uses traction force to reduce disc bulging into the intervertebral foramen and/or spinal canal. This traction force is imparted through flexion, usually over a Cox table and is thought to work by developing negative pressure inside the disc. This technique is used by more than half of all U.S. chiropractors. See Cox Technique.

Cox Sign: A chiropractic physical examination maneuver in which the patient is supine with the legs fully extended. The examiner places one hand under the ankle of the leg being tested and one hand on the knee. A straight leg raising maneuver is then performed. The test is said to be positive if the pelvis rises from the table rather than the hip flexing. This sign is positive in patients with far lateral disc herniations into the intervertebral foramen.

Cox Technique: A technique of "flexion-distraction" which is thought to pull the bulging intervertebral disc and tissues away from the spinal cord and the spinal nerves. A special table is used that adds additional traction force by flexing the patient during traction. Both sustained and intermittent traction are applied. See Cox Flexion-Distraction, Flexion-Distraction.

CP: An abbreviation for *cervical pillow*, *cold pack*, or *chronic pain*.

CPDD: An arthritic condition which presents like osteoarthritis and involves tissue deposition of calcium pyrophosphate dihydrate crystals. See Calcium Pyrophosphate Deposition Disease.

CPO: Certified Prosthetist/Orthotist.

CPP: The use of treatment techniques designed to palliate rather than cure chronic pain. See Chronic Pain Program, Chronic Pain Management.

Cram Bowstring Test: A physical examination maneuver positive in patients with radiculopathy. See Bowstring Test.

Cram Test: A physical examination maneuver positive in patients with radiculopathy. See Bowstring Sign.

Cranial: Of or referring to the skull. Also, this is short for craniosacral therapy. See Craniosacral Therapy.

Cranial Base: Referring to the suboccipital area.

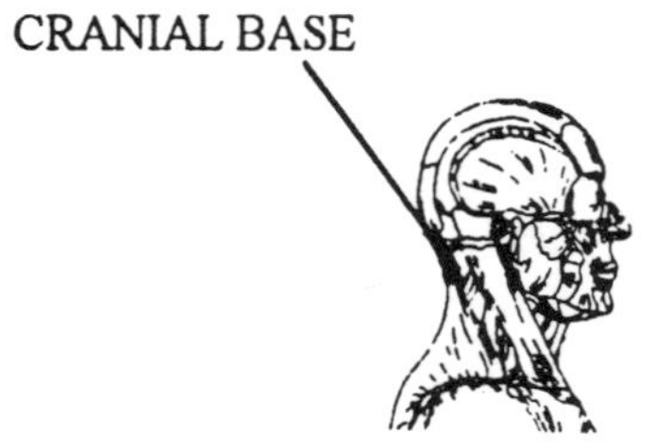

Cranial Base Release: A myofascial release technique which mobilizes the suboccipital musculature. This technique is used most often to treat headaches due to tightness in the suboccipital area. The therapist flexes his or her fingers at the MCPs forming a right angle to the palm with the fingers. The head is allowed to relax into the therapist's hand as the fingers are placed in the C1–2 area. Axial traction is often pulled on the skull, distracting the OA joints bilaterally. Occipital-atlantal extension is added with traction following the release technique. See Cranial Release.

Cranial Electrical Stimulator: A microcurrent electrical stimulation device used to treat headache pain. The electrodes are usually placed over the temporal region of the head. See CES.

Cranial Release: A myofascial release technique which mobilizes the suboccipital musculature. See Cranial Base Release.

Cranial Settling: An abnormality of a skull base resulting in a protrusion of the upper cervical spine into the foramen magnum. See Basilar Invagination.

Cranial Technique: A chiropractic technique similar to the osteopathic craniosacral technique. This focuses on correcting restriction and asymmetries of the cranial plates.

Craniocervical Junction: The articulation between the occipital condyle of the skull and the superior articular surface of the atlas. See Occipital-Atlantal Joint.

Craniosacral Extension: Motion that occurs during craniosacral rhythm when the sacrum nutates (flexes forward) and the sphenobasilar symphysis descends. See Extension—Craniosacral.

Craniosacral Flexion: Motion that occurs during craniosacral rhythm when the sacrum counternutates and the sphenobasilar symphysis ascends. See Flexion—Craniosacral.

Craniosacral Therapy: A healing system developed by William Sutherland, D.O., that is commonly used to treat headaches and TMJ. It is believed that the cranial plates are mobile and connected to the spinal cord and sacrum through the meninges. Some techniques concentrate on detecting cranial plates that are "out of place" and correcting these dysfunctions. While the mechanism of action is controversial, many patients seem to report relief of headaches with this technique. See CST.

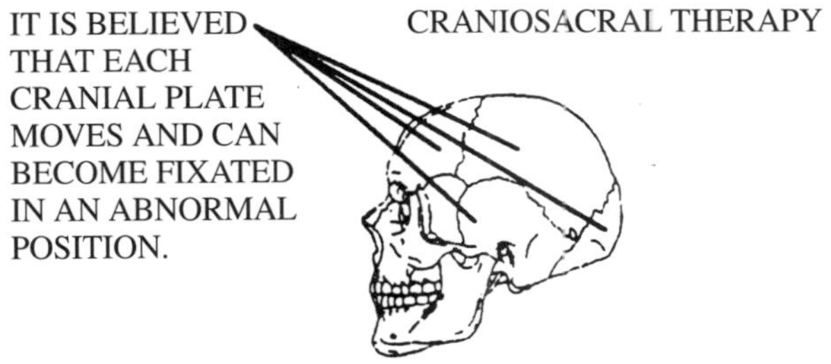

Craniovertebral Junction: A joint between the skull and the atlas (C1). See Occipital-Atlantal Joint, OA Joint.

Crawford Needle: A thin-walled needle used to deliver epidural anesthesia, which is often used for a paramedian approach. Using this system, a catheter can be threaded directly up to the epidural space if the needle is angled at approximately 45–60° upward. There is no curved tip. Since a Tuohy needle has a curved tip, a catheter can be threaded through this system with more ease.

C-reactive Protein: A laboratory blood test helpful in confirming the diagnosis of temporal arteritis, rheumatoid arthritis, polymyalgia rheumatica. This may also be elevated in patients with generalized inflammatory conditions or neoplastic disorders. This is used similar to an ESR test. See CRP.

Creep: Creep is what happens when you take a 5-pound weight and put it on a sponge soaked in molasses. Initially the weight will sink in a significant distance and then slowly continue to sink in over time. Similar phenomenon occurs in the lumbar spine. In flexed postures, the lumbar spine tends to "creep" into flexion. The tissues can be "reset" by standing and bending backwards into extension. It is known that degenerated discs creep more than healthy hydrated discs.

crep: An abbreviation for *crepitus*. See Crepitus.

Crepitus: Cracking noises heard or felt when moving a joint.

C-rod: Posterior segmental fixation with a wire that encircles the lamina in combination with a metal rod. The wire enters the spinal canal and has inherent risks by doing so, but forms a sturdy attachment.

Crossed Straight-Leg Raising Test: A physical exam maneuver in which one leg is raised with the patient in the supine position. This is similar to the straight-leg raising test, but the opposite leg is tested. This test is positive if the patient reports numbness in a dermatomal pattern in the nontested leg. This is thought to be a more sensitive indicator of radiculopathy than straight-leg raising. See Prostrate Leg Raising Test, Sciatic Phenomenon.

Cross-over Sign: A physical exam maneuver in which one leg is raised with the patient in the supine position. See Crossed Straight-Leg Raising Test.

Cross Pisiform: A manual adjusting technique which involves placing one hand atop the other and using the pisiform as the contact point for manipulation. This is more commonly used in the thoracic spine and ribs.

CRP: A laboratory blood test helpful in confirming the diagnosis of temporal arteritis, rheumatoid arthritis, polymyalgia rheumatica. See C-reactive Protein.

Cruciate Ligament: An important ligament in the upper cervical spine which contains the transverse ligament. This structure is shaped like a cross with vertically running fibers and horizontally running fibers. The vertical fibers attach to the anterior edge of the foramen magnum and to the body of C2. The horizontal fibers are the strongest and make up the transverse ligament. These fibers attach to the two condyles of the atlas and are the main ligamentous attachment keeping the dens in place. Between the dens and the transverse ligament is a bursa. An anterior dislocation of C1 on C2 can occur with a complete rupture of the transverse ligament only.

Crush Cleavage Fracture: A thoracic or lumbar fracture that is similar to a burst fracture. It is analogous to a teardrop fracture of the cervical spine. The mechanism of injury is a high energy impact with an axial load and bending moment. The upper half of the vertebral body is crushed and the lower half contains a cleavage fracture in the sagittal plane. There are often bone fragments in the canal, and a neurologic deficit can be seen. Evaluation and management is similar to a burst fracture except that these fractures are more likely to be unstable. See Burst Fracture.

Crutchfield Tongs: A form of cervical traction with the treatment of fractures and fracture dislocations of the cervical spine. Traction is pulled through hinged metal tongs which are attached to the parietal portions of the skull bilaterally through screws.

Cryoanalgesia: The destruction of a peripheral nerve or nerve root with extreme cold with the aim of achieving long-lasting pain relief. This is commonly performed in chronic pain patients. The medial branch is usually destroyed. See Medial Branch Block, Dorsal Rhizotomy.

Cryotherapy: The use of ice applied to the surface of the body after injury. This is thought to cause an initial period of vasoconstriction and decreased blood flow superficially. This occurs until temperatures fall below approximately 15°, then there is a vasodilatation with increased blood flow probably secondary to failure of the contractile mechanisms of the blood vessels. Skin temperature falls rapidly and approaches an equilibrium temperature of about 12–13°C in about 10 minutes. Deep muscle temperatures likely only fall a degree or less in 10 minutes. Cooling of at least 20 minutes is necessary to achieve significant decreases in temperature in the deeper muscles. Cryotherapy is particularly useful after acute injuries and is usually indicated for the first 48 hours after injury. Ice can also be used in chronic pain after an exercise program to reduce inflammation. Indications include acute sprains, fractures, and strains. Icing commonly is done for 20 minutes per hour and up to 30 minutes per 2 hours. See Ice Packs.

CSF: The fluid which bathes the brain and spinal cord. See Cerebrospinal Fluid.

CSF Reserve: The amount of CSF that separates the spinal cord from the surrounding bony structures of the spinal canal. This term is also used to refer to the distance on sagittal MRI images between the dura and the anterior vertebral column. If CSF reserve is low, then central canal stenosis is implicated.

C-spine: An abbreviation for *cervical spine.*

CSPT: An abbreviation for *cervical support.*

CST: A healing system that is used clinically to treat headaches and TMJ. See Craniosacral Therapy.

CT: An abbreviation for *computed tomography* scan. X-rays are taken at different angles and processed through a computer to produce a cross-sectional image. See CAT Scan, CT Scan.

CT: An abbreviation for *cervicothoracic.*

CT Discogram: A discogram followed by a CAT scan. See Computed Tomographic Discography.

CT Myelogram: A myelogram followed by a CT scan. This technique gives excellent visualization of the nerve roots as they relate to the surrounding bony structures. This study is commonly used for surgical planning. See CT Scan, Myelogram.

CT Scan: The use of x-rays taken at different angles and processed through a computer to produce a cross-sectional image. Bone settings and soft tissue settings are used to give better resolution in bone and soft tissues, respectively. This technology can be used to diagnose HNP, but MRI is considered a more sensitive imaging technique for that purpose. Bony resolution is excellent because of the use of x-rays, and many people believe CT scan to be superior to MRI for that purpose. This can be combined with a myelogram for better resolution of nervous structures. Sagittal images can be obtained through computer reformatting. See CAT Scan, Computed Tomography.

Cuneiform Synovial Fold: A meniscus-like body which is thought to become trapped in the facet joint and cause acute facet locking. See Meniscoid.

Curettage: Removal of bone by scrapping with a curette. A curette is a spoon- or ring-shaped surgical instrument with sharp edges.

Curvature of the Spine, Acquired: An ICD-9 diagnosis for scoliosis. See Scoliosis.

Curve Measurement: A method for quantifying the degree of scoliosis in the spine on an AP radiograph. See Cobb's Angle.

Cutaneous Axon Reflex: An increase in skin temperature seen with antidromic stimulation of the dorsal root ganglion.

CVA: The angle between the twelfth rib and the T12 vertebral body. This also refers to the area overlying this articulation. See Costovertebral Angle.

cx: An abbreviation for *coccyx.*

CX: An abbreviation for *cervical.*

Cybex: A brand name of exercise equipment and computerized muscle testing equipment. This term most commonly refers to a computerized isokinetic dynamometer. This is a machine which measures the patient's strength against a lever, which moves at a fixed speed. The speed at which the lever is moved is measured in degrees per second. For instance, with the device moving 60° per second, the patient gives a maximal effort against the system, and this is recorded in kilograms versus joint angle.

Cyclobenzaprine: A muscle relaxant which acts at the brain stem level to decrease muscular activity without acting directly on muscle contraction. See Flexeril.

Cyriax Technique: A treatment technique created by Dr. James Cyriax, a British orthopaedic specialist. Dr. Cyriax is considered the founder of orthopedic medicine (nonoperative office orthopedics). The Cyriax method is used by many physical therapists and physicians and involves manipulation and mobilization of specific structures. The traditional Cyriax technique emphasizes injection therapy of both local anesthetics and corticosteroids. Much attention is paid to the dura as a pain-sensitive and pain-generating structure.

D

D: An abbreviation for *dorsal* or *dull pain.*

d: An abbreviation for *dull.*

D1 Disc: A notation used to evaluate disc height on lateral radiographs. This represents a widened disc space which may be due to increased fluid uptake within the disc after an acute disc injury.

D2 Disc: A notation which refers to disc space height on lateral radiographs. This represents the first stage of disc degeneration in which there is a small decrease in the posterior aspect of the disc space with a slight retrolisthesis of the vertebral body.

D3 Disc: A notation which pertains to disc space height on lateral radiographs. This is the second stage in disc degeneration in which there is increased "creep" of the disc which is reported to be associated with a greater tendency for malalignment of the functional spinal unit. There is decreased disc height posteriorly with very little change occurring in the anterior portion of the disc. See Creep.

D4 Disc: A notation which is used to evaluate disc space height on lateral radiographs. This is the third stage of disc degeneration in which the anterior portion of the disc becomes progressively more involved. The disc height is reduced to approximately two-thirds of the original height. The weight bearing is transferred to the facet joints. It is thought that this will lead to facet joint hypertrophy.

D5 Disc: A notation which is used to evaluate disc space height on lateral radiographs. The disc space is reduced to one-third of its original height. It is thought that the D5 disc occurs between 5 and 20 years after the initial injury.

D6 Disc: A notation which is used to evaluate disc space height on lateral radiographs. Almost complete obliteration of the disc space is present with extensive osteophyte formation.

DABCO: Diplomate of the American Board of Chiropractic Orthopedists.

DACBR: Diplomate of the American Chiropractic Board of Radiology.

DACR: Diplomate of the Academy of Chiropractic Radiologists.

DAD: Developmental anteroposterior diameter. This is the distance across the spinal canal from the posterior portion of the vertebral body to the lamina. This varies by level. See SAD, Spondylitic Anteroposterior Diameter.

Dagger Sign: A radiographic sign in ankylosing spondylitis. This is calcification of the interspinous or supraspinous ligament that shows a single vertical stripe connecting the lumbar spinous processes.

Daily Adjustable Progressive Resistance Exercise: A system designed to determine when to increase resistance and how much to increase resistance in an exercise program. See DAPRE Technique.

DAPRE Technique: A system designed to determine when to increase resistance and how much to increase resistance in an exercise program. Initial working weight is determined at six repetitions. The patient then performs 10 repetitions at one-half of the working weight, six repetitions at three-quarters of the working weight, as many repetitions as possible of the full working weight, then as many repetitions as possible with an adjusted working weight. The adjusted working weight is based on the number of repetitions of the full working weight performed during the third set. The number of repetitions done in the last set is used to determine the working weight for the next day. There are specific guidelines for adjustment of the working weight. This technique was developed by Knight. See Daily Adjustable Progressive Resistance Exercise.

Darvocet-N 100: A narcotic pain reliever used to control mild to moderate pain which contains 100 mg of propoxyphene and 650 mg of acetaminophen. This is indicated for the use of moderate pain. Physical addiction is possible. The usual dosage is one tablet every 4 hours as needed for pain.

Dashboard Fracture: A fracture of the posterior rim of the acetabulum which usually occurs after a blow to the knee with the knee in flexion and the hip abducted. See Posterior Rim Fracture.

Davis Series: A radiologic study of the cervical spine which involves six views: anterior, flexion, extension, lateral, right oblique, and left oblique.

DayPro: A nonsteroidal anti-inflammatory drug in the propanoic acid group. It has anti-inflammatory, analgesic, and antipyretic properties. It is an inhibitor along the arachidonic acid pathway of prostaglandin synthesis. It is contraindicated in patients with complete or partial syndrome of nasal polyps, angioedema, and bronchospastic reactivity to aspirin or other NSAIDs. GI side effects are possible. There are drug interactions with aspirin, oral anticoagulants, H2 receptor antagonists, beta blockers, antacids, acetaminophen, or conjugated estrogens. The usual starting dosage is 600–1,200 mg a day and doses larger than 1,200 mg a day should be reserved for patients who weigh more than 50 kg and have normal renal and hepatic function with low risk of peptic ulcer. The usual daily dosage is two 600-mg caplets once a day. See Oxaprozine.

DC: Doctor of Chiropractic.

DCS: An electronic device inserted near the spinal cord which provides competitive sensory stimulation to the dorsal columns of the spinal cord in order to interfere with pain transmission. See Dorsal Column Stimulator.

DDD: Degeneration of the intervertebral disc. See Degenerative Disc Disease, Microtrauma.

DDS: Doctor of Dental Surgery.

Debridement: The surgical removal of dead or damaged tissue or foreign matter from a wound.

Decadron Phosphate Injection: A synthetic adrenal corticosteroid used for intramuscular injection in chronic inflammatory or acute inflammatory injections where oral steroids or NSAIDs are not advisable. There is a rapid onset and short duration of action. There is an enhanced effect of corticosteroids in patients with hypothyroidism and those with cirrhosis. Euphoria, insomnia, mood swings, personality changes, severe depression, and frank psychotic manifestations are possible. Aspirin should be used cautiously in conjunction with corticosteroids in chronic disorders. When large doses are given, antacids should be administered between meals to help prevent peptic ulcer as there are GI side effects. The use of steroids intramuscularly in the same location greater than 2–3 times a year is not advisable owing to the risk of muscle necrosis and collagen weakening. Multiple systemic side effects have also been tied to steroids, and the PDR should be consulted for this list. See Dexamethasone Sodium Phosphate.

Decadron Tablets: A synthetic adrenocortical steroid used for either acute or chronic inflammatory conditions. This drug is contraindicated in patients with systemic fungal infections, concomitant infections, hypothyroidism, or cirrhosis. This is a more potent steroid than cortisone as 0.75 mg of this drug equals approximately 25 mg of cortisone. The usual dosage varies depending on the disorder. It is available in 0.25-mg, 0.5-mg, 0.75-mg, and 1.5-mg tablets. Withdrawal of corticosteroids may result in symptoms of corticosteroid withdrawal when stopped abruptly during prolonged therapy. See Dexamethasone.

Decompensated Scoliosis: When the angle of the compensatory scoliotic curve does not equal the angle of the major curve, the scoliosis is termed decompensated. What this means functionally is that the shoulders are not level and the compensatory scoliosis has not been able to counteract the major curve. There is usually a list or lateral shift of the trunk to one side. See Scoliosis, Scoliosis—Decompensated.

Decompression: A surgical term that refers to removal of pressure from a nerve root or from a spinal cord through laminectomy, laminotomy, or foraminotomy. For instance, a decompressive laminectomy denotes removal of the lamina for the purpose of releasing pressure on the spinal cord.

Decreased Interosseous Spacing: A chiropractic term which refers to a vertebral segment which has undergone degenerative changes in the disc such that there is decreased disc height. This causes vertebral segment to be closer to the segment below and farther from the segment above. This is equivalent to an inferior subluxation.

Deep Posterior Sacrococcygeal Ligament: The deep ligament covering the sacral hiatus that is penetrated during an epidural steroid injection.

Deep Tendon Reflex: A physical exam maneuver that checks the integrity of the "wiring" of the muscle being tested. The examiner strikes the tendon of the muscle with a reflex hammer to elicit a contraction of the muscle. The muscle can be hyperreflexic (3+ or 3/3) (overactive with a big contraction), normal (2+ or 2/3), or hyporeflexic (1+ or 1/3) (underactive with a poor muscle contraction). This response is compared with the opposite side, which is assumed to be normal. If the muscle is hyperreflexic, then an upper motor neuron lesion is suspected. (A problem with the wiring of the nervous system in the spinal cord above the level tested or in the brain. A stroke would be one example.) If the muscle is hyporeflexic, then a lower motor neuron lesion is suspected. (A problem with the wiring of the muscle between the spinal cord and that muscle. An example would be a spinal cord injury, a nerve root irritation or radiculopathy, or a peripheral nerve injury.) See DTR, Tendon Jerk, Tendon Reflex, Spinal Reflex.

Degenerated Disc: A disc which has suffered wear and tear which may be related to normal aging or additional trauma over a long period of time. There are usually small circumferential tears within the anulus fibrosus (outer covering of the disc), and the nucleus (inner gel-like material inside the disc) has lost its ability to hold onto water. On x-ray, spondylosis (bone spurs) is usually seen as decreased disc height. On MRI, there is decreased signal intensity on T2 images of the nucleus pulposus. Also, outer annular tears can sometimes be imaged on fast spin echo sequences. There can be bony hypertrophy of the facet joints due to increased loading posteriorly as the disc height decreases. There can be buckling of a calcified ligamentum flavum, known as pseudohypertrophy of the ligamentum flavum, which can cause central canal stenosis. See Degenerative Disc Disease, Spondylosis.

Degeneration of Cervical Intervertebral Disc: An ICD-9 diagnosis for cervical spondylosis or degenerative disc disease. Degenerative disc disease is most common in the cervical spine at C4–5 and C5–6 and may or may not be associated with pain when seen radiographically. This is a nonspecific diagnosis.

Degeneration of Intervertebral Disc, Site Unspecified: An ICD-9 diagnosis which is nonspecific and roughly equates with degenerative disc disease.

Degeneration of Lumbar or Lumbosacral Intervertebral Disc: An ICD-9 diagnosis for lumbar degenerative disc disease or spondylosis. This is a nonspecific diagnosis that is usually made radiographically. Radiographic evidence of degenerative disc disease may or may not be associated with pain.

Degeneration of Thoracic or Lumbar Intervertebral Disc: An ICD-9 code diagnosis which roughly equates with degenerative disc disease or spondylosis of those areas.

Degeneration of Thoracic or Thoracolumbar Intervertebral Disc: An ICD-9 diagnosis which roughly equates with spondylosis or degenerative disc disease.

Degenerative Changes: This is usually meant to imply degeneration of the intervertebral disc. The degenerative changes seen on x-ray are decreased disc height and bony spurring such as osteophytes. Degenerative changes on MRI would be decreased signal intensity on T2 weighted images of the nucleus, outer annular tears, Schmorl's nodes, and other evidence of degenerative disc disease.

Degenerative Disc Disease: Wear and tear of the intervertebral disc which may represent normal aging or may be due to long-standing trauma. This involves small tears in the annulus (outer covering of the disc) and lack of water content of the nucleus (the gel-like center of the disc). This degenerative cascade can lead to disc bulging, bone spurs, and loss of disc height, which can effect the nerve roots. See DDD, Disc Changes, Disc Degeneration, Spondylosis, Hemispherical Annular Degeneration, Intradiscal Scarring, Postural Syndrome, Multilevel Disc Desiccation, Segmental Instability.

Degenerative Instability: The loss of the ability of the spine under physiologic loads to maintain its pattern of normal movement due to disc degeneration. See Spinal Instability.

Degenerative Joint Disease: This specifically refers to degenerative facets. See Degenerative Joint Syndrome.

Degenerative Joint Syndrome: This specifically refers to degenerative facets. See Degenerative Joint Disease.

Degenerative Listhesis: A "slipping" of one vertebra on another due to destructive, degenerative changes within the facet joints. See Degenerative Spondylolisthesis.

Degenerative Proliferative Disease: Degenerative disc disease which leads to bony hypertrophy including osteophytes and enlargement of the facet joints. This process can cause bony stenosis both in the central canal causing myelopathy and/or in the intervertebral foramen causing foraminal stenosis and radiculopathy. See Spondylosis, Facet Hypertrophy.

Degenerative Scoliosis: A lateral curvature of the spine due to advanced degenerative disease. There is usually minimal structural vertebral deformity. Degenerative disc disease causes the destruction of the articular facets and deformity within the vertebral body that results in a structural scoliosis. See Scoliosis.

Degenerative Spinal Stenosis: Narrowing of the canal that contains the spinal cord. See Spinal Stenosis.

Degenerative Spondylolisthesis: A "slipping" of one vertebra on another due to destructive, degenerative changes within the facet joints. The facet joints normally help to prevent the superior vertebrae from falling forward with respect to the inferior vertebrae. However, once the facets become degenerated, they are no longer capable of preventing that slippage. This is graded in much the same way as the other forms of spondylolisthesis. This can also lead to central canal stenosis, foraminal stenosis, and other clinical syndromes. See Articular Spondylolisthesis, Spondylolisthesis, Type III Spondylolisthesis.

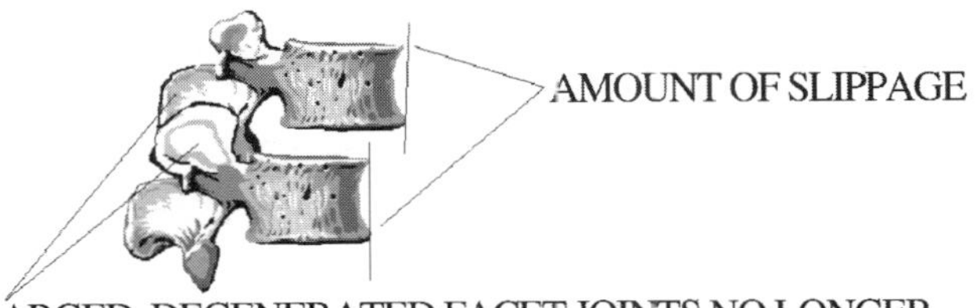

AMOUNT OF SLIPPAGE

ENLARGED, DEGENERATED FACET JOINTS NO LONGER PREVENT THE VERTEBRA ABOVE FROM SLIPPING FORWARD ON THE VERTEBRA BELOW.

Degenerative Symptoms: Physical complaints and pain due to degenerative disc disease. See Discogenic Pain.

Degrees of Freedom: The number of different types of motion in any vertebral segment. For instance, one degree of freedom is rotation around one axis. The spine is considered to have six degrees of freedom.

Dejerine's Sign: A test for dural irritation or compression. The patient is questioned as to reproduction of radicular symptoms with coughing, sneezing, or straining during defecation. A positive sign is the reproduction of radicular symptoms with any of these maneuvers. All of these maneuvers cause dural irritation by increasing intrathecal pressure. See Dejerine's Triad, Triad of Dejerine.

Dejerine's Test: A physical exam test in which the patient is supine and places the hands behind the head lifting the upper torso off the examining table. A positive test is reproduction of leg pain secondary to nerve root inflammation. See Soto Hall Test.

Dejerine's Triad: A test for dural irritation or compression. See Dejerine's Sign.

DeKleyn's Test: A test for vertebral artery insufficiency in which the patient extends the cervical spine while lying supine. The head is then rotated to one side. This is held for about 30 seconds and the patient is monitored for nystagmus or slurred speech. See Hall Pike Maneuver.

Delayed Union: The delayed fusion of two vertebral bodies following a surgical fusion.

DeLorme Technique: A technique for strength training that has been called heavy resistance exercise and progressive resistance exercise. The maximum weight a patient can lift at 10 repetitions is determined. The patient then carries out 10 repetitions at one half of that maximum, 10 repetitions at three quarters of that maximum, and 10 repetitions at that maximum weight. There is a brief rest period between sets. There is a built-in warm-up as the first two sets are submaximal. The maximum weight that the patient can lift is determined and increased weekly as strength increases. See Progressive Resistance Exercise, PRE, Oxford Technique.

Deltasone: A brand name of Prednisone. Deltasone is supplied in 2.5-mg, 5-mg, 10-mg, 20-mg, and 50-mg tablets. The usual dosage varies depending on indication. See Prednisone.

Deminoff's Sign: A physical examination maneuver in which the patient is in the supine position. The examiner then performs a straight-leg raising maneuver. The sign is positive if this action produces pain in the lumbar region while the leg is not more than 15° from the examination table. This sign is positive in patients with pain in the iliocostalis lumborum musculature.

Demyelination: A term used by electromyographers to describe a conduction block that results from loss of the myelin sheath around a peripheral nerve. This is usually diagnosed through the loss of nerve conduction velocity in a specific peripheral nerve.

Denervation: Loss of nerve supply to a muscle. This can be either partial or total. An example is radiculopathy secondary to direct pressure which causes axonal loss. An EMG will show characteristic fibrillation potentials and sharp waves in a muscle that has been denervated.

Dens: A tooth-like process which arises from the body of the axis. See Odontoid Process.

Dentate Ligaments: Ligaments which occur in pairs and support the spinal cord. They provide stability and protection to the spinal cord and are usually under significant tension. There are 20 dentate ligaments, the last of which occurs at the T12–L1 level. The dentate ligaments are found in the cervical and thoracic spine.

Denticulate Ligament: Ligaments which occur in pairs and support the spinal cord. See Dentate Ligaments.

Depo-Medrol: A long-acting injectable steroid. See Methylprednisolone.

Depressed End Plate Fracture: A radiographic sign sometimes seen with a compression fracture. There is significant depression of the end plate denoting an acute injury.

Depression, Major: An ICD-9 diagnosis involving depressed mood and/or loss of interest in life and/or loss of pleasure in normal, everyday activities for at least two weeks. Four of the following must be present: (1) an increase or decrease in appetite or a five percent or greater change in body weight in a one month period; (2) difficulty falling asleep or significant sleep changes; (3) psychomotor agitation—an increase in constant body movements or a decrease in body movements; (4) constant fatigue; (5) the thought of worthlessness or inappropriate guilt; (6) cognitive complaints such as problems with concentration or memory; and (7) suicidal thoughts or preoccupation with death. See Major Depression.

Derangement: A McKenzie physical therapy term that corresponds to a disc protrusion.

Derangement Syndrome: A McKenzie physical therapy term which describes derangement within the intervertebral disc causing either low back pain or radiating pain. There are seven types of derangements. Treatment involves movements which decrease or centralize pain, being able to maintain those movements during ADLs, recovery of the lost function, and preventing the derangement from recurring. See ADL, McKenzie Exercises.

Dermatomal Distribution: Radiating numbness, tingling, and/or pain which radiates into a specific dermatome. For instance, in the lower extremity, an L5 dermatomal distribution would be radiating numbness into the big toe.

Dermatomal Evoked Potential: A somatosensory evoked potential in which a dermatome is stimulated versus a peripheral nerve. See Dermatomal Somatosensory Evoked Potential.

Dermatomal Pain: Pain that radiates in the distribution of a specific nerve root. See Dermatome.

Dermatomal Somatosensory Evoked Potential: A somatosensory evoked potential in which a dermatome is stimulated versus a peripheral nerve. This technique is often used to monitor the integrity of the spinal nerve roots during spinal surgery. See SSEP, Somatosensory Evoked Potential, Dermatomal Evoked Potential, DSEP, DSCP.

Dermatome: The sensory distribution of a specific nerve root. For instance, the C6 dermatome is the area on the hand surrounding the thumb which carries sensation back from that area to the central nervous system. Several different dermatomal maps have been constructed and there is some variation between individuals. See Radicular Pain.

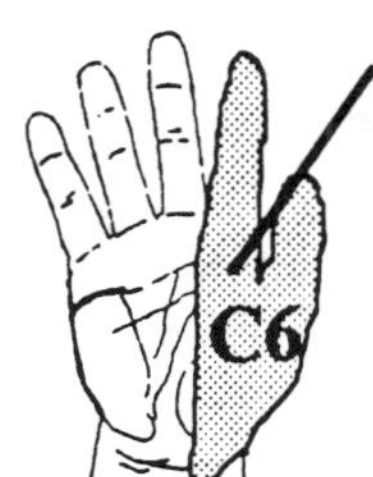

THE AREA OF THE HAND SUPPLIED BY THE SIXTH CERVICAL NERVE ROOT KNOWN AS THE C6 DERMATOME.

Designation Movement Diagram: A method for determining segmental instability that was described by Buetti and Bauml in 1954. A line is drawn along the posterior border of each vertebral body on flexion/extension radiographs. The angle between that line and a line drawn on the posterior border of the vertebral body above is measured. These angles are then compared to average values of segmental movement based on 28 healthy adults.

Destabilizing Laminectomy: A surgical procedure used to treat lateral stenosis by removing a large portion of the facet. This is defined as removal of over 50% of the joint. This procedure tends to make that segment unstable and is usually followed by fusion to regain stability at that level. See Laminectomy.

Destot's Sign: A large hematoma seen subcutaneously in the region of the inguinal ligament or in the scrotum after pelvic fractures.

dev: An abbreviation for *deviation.*

Developmental: An adjective which means congenital. This is a defect in the spine (or other area) which occurred during the patient's "development."

Developmental Anteroposterior Diameter: The distance across the spinal canal from the posterior portion of the vertebral body to the lamina. This varies by level. See DAD, SAD, Spondylitic Anteroposterior Diameter.

DEXA: One of the newer techniques for measuring osteoporosis in the spine. See Dual Energy X-ray Absorptiometry.

Dexamethasone: A synthetic adrenocortical steroid used for either acute or chronic inflammatory conditions. See Decadron Tablets.

Dexamethasone Sodium Phosphate: A synthetic adrenal corticosteroid used for intramuscular injection in chronic inflammatory or acute inflammatory disorders where oral steroids or NSAIDs are not advisable. See Decadron Phosphate Injection.

Dextro-convex: A radiology term used to describe scoliosis. The apex of the curve points toward the right.

Dextro-scoliosis: A scoliotic curve with the convexity pointing to the right.

Deyerle's Sign: A physical examination maneuver in which the patient is seated and extends the affected leg to the point in which pain is reproduced. The knee is then slightly flexed with strong pressure applied in the popliteal fossa. If radicular symptoms are reproduced, the test is said to be positive. This is very similar to a bowstring test but is performed in the seated position. See Bowstring Test.

DHE: A potent medication used to abort migraine headache. It is supplied in many different forms and may be useful in the resolution of analgesia rebound headache. See Dihydroergotamine.

Diagonal: A physical therapy exercise used to strengthen the obliques. See Diagonal Curl-up.

Diagonal Curl-up: A physical therapy exercise used to strengthen the obliques. The patient starts in the hook lying position with arms folded across the chest. The pelvis is tilted to flatten the lumbar curve. The patient is then asked to lift the shoulder blades from the floor while rotating to one side. See Diagonal.

Diaphragmatic Release: A myofascial release technique for the diaphragm. Diaphragmatic releases are common in combination with treatment for rib dysfunction and thoracic spine biomechanical abnormalities. It is thought that the diaphragm is also closely associated with the quadratus lumborum musculature. There is a gentle superficial technique release described, as well as a deeper more aggressive release technique. See Diaphragm Release.

Diaphragm Release: A myofascial release technique for the diaphragm. See Diaphragmatic Release.

Diastasis: With respect to the spine, this usually refers to a pubic symphysis that has been separated. A diastasis is dislocation or separation of two bones that are otherwise attached and are not connected by a true joint.

Diastematomyelia: A developmental malformation of the spinal cord that occurs in two halves separated by cartilage or bone. This can be accompanied by spina bifida occulta or aperta, and the cleft can be partial or complete.

Diathermy: High-frequency electrical current that produces a deep heating effect.

Dick Internal Spinal Fixator: Instrumentation used for posterior spinal fusion with pedicle screws and a highly adjustable three-dimensional linkage which is internally implanted. The points at which the pedicle screws attach are adjustable and linked with a rod.

Diclofenac Potassium: A nonsteroidal anti-inflammatory drug. See Cataflam, Voltaren.

Dictionary of Occupational Titles: A publication distributed by the U.S. Department of Labor. This is a compendium of job titles and job descriptions which also includes job demands, environmental conditions, and hazards. See DOT.

Diffuse Idiopathic Skeletal Hyperostosis: A syndrome which involves diffuse ligamentous calcification and ossification seen in 5–10% of the population over 65 years of age. This is characterized by a thick "flowing" osteophyte and calcification of the anterior lateral aspect of the vertebral bodies. This has been confused on radiographs with the bamboo spine appearance of ankylosing spondylitis. See Hyperostosis, Ankylosing Hyperostosis, Forrestier's Disease, DISH.

Diffuse Myofascial Pain Syndrome: This is pain at many sites and has been defined by the American College of Rheumatology as pain at 11 of 18 tender point sites, presence of subcutaneous nodules, and a history of widespread pain for greater than 3 months. See Fibromyalgia.

Diflunisal: A nonsteroidal anti-inflammatory drug which is a derivative of salicylic acid. See Dolobid.

Digastric Line: A radiographic sign for basilar impression. An AP open-mouth view is performed. A line is drawn between the two digastric grooves just medial to the base of the mastoid processes. The distance vertically to the apex of the odontoid and the OA joints is measured. The measurement to the apex of the odontoid has a normal range of 1 to 21 mm. The odontoid should not project above this line. The measurement to the OA joint has a normal range between 4 and 20 mm. See Biventor Line.

Digastric Triangle: An anatomic triangle in the anterior portion of the neck just underneath the mandible that is used for surgical approaches. The borders are the mandible, the anterior belly of the digastric muscle, and the posterior belly of the stylohyoid muscles (submandibular triangle).

Digital Inclinometer: An electronic device used for the noninvasive quantification of range of motion. There are many different brands of electronic inclinometers which can be used for single or double inclinometry measurements of the spine or other joints. See Electronic Inclinometer, Electronic Digital Inclinometer.

Digital Palpation: "Hands-on" diagnosis of spinal disorders by feeling for spasm and bony landmarks and by eliciting pain in specific areas.

Dihydroergotamine: A potent medication used to abort migraine headache. It is supplied in many different forms and may be useful in the resolution of analgesia rebound headache. See DHE.

Dilaudid: A hydrogenated ketone of morphine. This is a powerful narcotic analgesic used at times for postsurgical pain relief. Respiratory depression, intracranial pressure increases, and significant CNS depression are possible. There is significant abuse potential. The usual adult dose is 2 mg po every 4–6 hours as necessary. See Hydromorphone.

dim: An abbreviation for *diminish*.

Direct Arteriovenous Malformation: A fistulous communication between intradural spinal arteries and a spinal vein. See Direct AVM.

Direct AVM: A fistulous communication between intradural spinal arteries and a spinal vein. The most common is the anterior spinal artery connected to the spinal medullary vein or coronal venous plexus. This AVM may lie in the cord tissue or on the cord surface. Symptoms are usually of insidious onset, and there is slow progression towards myelopathy. See Direct Arteriovenous Malformation, AVM—Direct.

Direct Current Electrical Stimulation: A type of electrical stimulation that is used to promote bony fusion. Electrodes are placed on the skin over the area to be fused or implanted into the bony area to be fused.

Direct Joint Mobilization: This is a mobilization which is carried out with direct pressure over a vertebral segment or peripheral joint. See Mobilization.

Direct Technique: An osteopathic or manual physical therapy term which describes moving a segment in the direction it does not want to go. This also sometimes refers to a manipulation. See Muscle Energy Technique.

Disability: As defined by the AMA Guides to the Evaluation of Permanent Impairment, disability is an alteration in an individual's capacity to meet personal, social, or occupational demands or statutory or regulatory requirements. Disability is defined as the gap between what an individual can do and what that individual is required or would like to do.

Disalcid: A nonsteroidal anti-inflammatory drug of the salicylic acid group. This drug does contain salicylic acid, so it is not recommended for use in patients with chickenpox, influenza or flu symptoms due to the risk of Reye's syndrome. This is contraindicated in patients with chronic renal insufficiency or peptic ulcer disease due to its renal clearance and GI side effects. It is contraindicated for use in combination with anticoagulant drugs, oral hypoglycemic drugs, and competes with a number of drugs for protein binding sites including penicillin, thiopental, thyroxine, triiodothyronine, phenytoin, sulfinpyrazone, naproxen, warfarin, methotrexate, and possibly corticosteroids. The usual dosage is 3,000 mg given daily in two or three divided doses. This drug is available in 500-mg and 750-mg tablets. See Salsalate.

Disc: The "cushion" between two vertebrae that contains a gel-filled center called the nucleus pulposus and a tough outer covering called the anulus fibrosus.

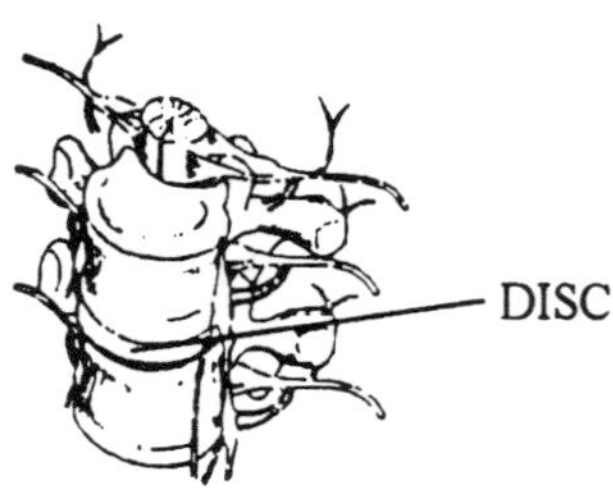

Discal: A descriptive term that refers to the intervertebral disc. See Intervertebral Disc.

Discal Ballooning: A radiographic sign in osteoporosis. The end plates become concave due to the mechanical effect of the nucleus pulposus on the osteoporotic vertebral bodies.

Disc Bulge: A diffuse expansion of the anulus fibrosus beyond the contours of the vertebral body secondary to a loss in disc height. This differs from a protruded disc in that it is not a more localized, focal expansion. In both cases, there is no herniation of the inner disc material through the anulus. See Protruded Disc.

Disc Bulge—Minor: When the nucleus of the disc ruptures through the inner annular fibers, but does not rupture through a majority of those fibers. See Disc Protrusion.

Disc Bulge—Moderate: When the nucleus of the disc ruptures through the inner annular fibers, but does not rupture through a majority of those fibers. See Disc Protrusion.

Disc Changes: Degeneration of the intervertebral disc which may represent normal aging or may be due to long-standing trauma. See Degenerative Disc Disease.

Disc Degeneration: Degeneration of the intervertebral disc which may represent normal aging or may be due to long-standing trauma. See Degenerative Disc Disease.

Disc Desiccation: When a degenerated disc loses its ability to hold water. This can be noted on MRI. See Degenerative Disc Disease.

Disc Disorders: An ICD-9 code diagnosis which is extremely nonspecific. This could mean anything from a bulging disc to a herniated disc.

Discectomy: A surgical procedure usually carried out in conjunction with a laminectomy or laminotomy in which the degenerated disc is partially or completely removed. It may be performed in combination with a foraminotomy and fusion. See Excision.

Disc Excision: A surgical procedure usually carried out in conjunction with a laminectomy or laminotomy in which the degenerated disc is partially or completely removed. It may be performed in combination with a foraminotomy and fusion. See Discectomy.

Disc Extrusion: A disc herniation through all of the annular fibers and the posterior longitudinal ligament. This is synonymous with a "herniated disc" or HNP. See Extruded Disc, Herniated Disc, Noncontained Herniation, Supraligamentous Herniation.

Disc Hernia: An extrusion of the nucleus pulposus through the anterior annular fibers. See HNP.

Disc Herniation: When the nucleus of the disc ruptures through the inner annular fibers, but does not rupture through a majority of those fibers. See Disc Protrusion.

Disc Herniation—Central: A herniation of the nucleus pulposus that occurs in the midline instead of the usual posterior lateral direction. See Central HNP.

Disc Herniation—Midline: A herniated disc that occurs in the midline. See Midline Disc Herniation.

Discitis: An inflammatory condition of the disc. Common causes are discography and surgery.

Discogenic Pain: Pain emanating from the intervertebral disc. The outer annulus is innervated, and damage to the disc through trauma or excessive disc degeneration can produce pain. This phenomenon can be demonstrated during discograms when a dye is injected into the intervertebral disc causing distension and local pain as well as different types of referred pain phenomena.

Discogram: An imaging study which shows the architecture within the disc. See Discography, Nucleogram.

Discography: An imaging study which shows the architecture within the disc. This is in contrast to MRI or CT scan which do not show internal disc architecture. This technique can also be helpful in determining whether the disc is a pain generator. Contrast dye is injected into the disc and a CT scan follows to define pathology. Pain response is recorded during the procedure and anesthetic response is frequently recorded. This technique is often used to plan for a lumbar fusion. There is some controversy as to use of routine discography. See Concordant Pain Response, P2 Response, Discordant Pain Response, P1 Response, Discogram.

Discometry: An estimate of the hydrodynamic competence of the disc. During a discogram, the resistance when the syringe plunger stops (when the disc is "full") and the volume of the fluid injected is measured. If the disc is completely incompetent, then there will be no resistance and the disc will continue to accept a large volume of fluid (much greater than the 3-ml capacity of a "normal" disc). See Intradiscal Pressure.

Discopathogenic: Abnormal function of a disc.

Discopathy: Disease of the intervertebral disc. This is also synonymous with an HNP. See Discogenic Pain.

Discordant Pain Response: A patient's pain response during discography or a provocative procedure which does not represent his or her usual symptoms. See Concordant Pain Response, P1 Response.

Disc Prolapse: When the nucleus pulposus ruptures through most of the fibers of the annulus and is contained only by a few of the outermost fibers. See Prolapsed Disc.

Disc Protrusion: When the nucleus of the disc ruptures through the inner annular fibers, but does not rupture through a majority of those fibers. See Protruded Disc.

Disc Sequestration: Material from the nucleus pulposus which is outside of the disc and separated from the disc. See Sequestered Disc, Noncontained Herniation.

Disc Space: The area between two vertebrae occupied by the intervertebral disc.

Disc Space Narrowing: A radiographic term which usually refers to narrowing of the intervertebral disc space. With disc degeneration, the disc begins to lose its ability to hold onto water and thus the size of the disc space decreases. This can be seen on x-rays. This also can imply a herniated disc. See Narrowing.

Disc Stance: A characteristic stance suggestive of the presence of a herniated disc or nerve root irritation in the lumbar spine. The patient stands with the hip or knee slightly flexed.

Disfigurement: An alteration in appearance or an abnormal appearance.

DISH: A syndrome which involves diffuse ligamentous calcification and ossification seen in 5–10% of patients over 65 years of age. See Diffuse Idiopathic Skeletal Hyperostosis.

Displaced Disc: It should be noted that discs do not "displace." Instead, the gel-like nucleus extrudes through the annulus. See HNP.

Displacement of Cervical Intervertebral Disc without Myelopathy: An ICD-9 diagnosis equivalent to a cervical HNP with or without radiculopathy. There is no compression on the cervical spinal cord.

Displacement of Intervertebral Disc without Myelopathy, Site Unspecified: An ICD-9 diagnosis which is extremely nonspecific. This roughly equates to an HNP with or without radiculopathy without pressure on the spinal cord or cauda equina. It should be noted that intervertebral discs do not "displace." Rather, the gel-like nucleus extrudes through the annulus.

Displacement of Lumbar Intervertebral Disc without Myelopathy: An ICD-9 diagnosis roughly equivalent to a lumbar HNP with or without radiculopathy and without pressure on the cauda equina.

Displacement of Thoracic Intervertebral Disc without Myelopathy: An ICD-9 code diagnosis which equates with a thoracic HNP. There is no pressure on the spinal cord.

Displacement of Thoracic or Lumbar Intervertebral Disc without Myelopathy: A nonspecific ICD-9 code which refers to a lower thoracic or high lumbar HNP with or without radiculopathy which does not cause pressure on the spinal cord.

Disruption of the Vertebral End Plate: A fracture of the vertebral end plate which can be associated with a vertebral compression fracture. See End Plate Disruption.

Dissociated Motor Loss: A radiculopathy involving the motor fibers only. There are usually no sensory symptoms, but there is motor weakness and atrophy. The most common nerve root involved is C5, causing a palsy of the deltoid muscle without sensory symptoms. This can occur secondary to HNP or as a complication of cervical spine surgery.

Distraction: Separation of the joint surfaces of the spine by traction.

Distraction Test: A physical exam maneuver similar to a manual traction test where the examiner lifts the patient's head while seated or applies traction on the patient's head while supine with a positive test being relief of radicular pain. An alternative method can be used with the patient seated. The hands are interlocked with the forearms under the patient's mandible standing behind the patient. The back of the head is fixed against the examiner's chest and a traction force is applied.

ditrx: An abbreviation for *distraction.*

Diversified Rotary Break: A chiropractic manipulation technique which is a thrust of mild acceleration and high amplitude.

Diversified Technique: A chiropractic technique that is taught at most major chiropractic colleges. The primary manipulative force is the practitioner's hands. This is a moderate to high velocity (moderately high acceleration), low-amplitude technique. Many times an audible snap or pop will be heard as a spinal correction is made. Approximately 90% of chiropractors use this technique. See Palmer Diversified.

DMD: Doctor of Medical Dentistry.

DO: Doctor of Osteopathy.

Doctor of Osteopathy: A physican who has completed a graduate course of medical education at an AOA-approved college of osteopathic medicine. Like MDs, most DOs undergo rigorous speciality training. Many DOs integrate manipulation and other hands-on treatments into their treatment regimens.

DOI: An abbreviation for *date of injury*.

Dolobid: A proprietary name for diflunisal, a nonsteroidal anti-inflammatory drug which is a derivative of salicylic acid. This drug should not be administered with indomethacin due to gastrointestinal hemorrhage. There are interactions with hydrochlorothiazide. Taken with aluminum hydroxide (common antacid) the extent of absorption is decreased. Diflunisal also increases the plasma concentration of Tylenol. It also interacts with anticoagulants resulting in prolonged prothrombin time. The most common dosage is 250–500 mg twice a day. Steady plasma levels are obtained within 3–9 days with twice daily administration. See Diflunisal.

Dolorimeter: A pressure guage used for quantifying the amount of pressure it takes to cause pain. This type of guage has been used in an attempt to objectify progress in the treatment of trigger points and tender points.

Dominant Hand: The hand with which the patient does most of his or her fine dexterity work. In most people this is the right hand. See Nondominant Hand.

Doorway Stretch: A stretching maneuver for the anterior chest and shoulder structures which includes the clavipectoral fascia, pectoralis minor, pectoralis major, subscapularis, subclavius, and other structures. See Corner Stretch.

Dorsal: Of or pertaining to the back or posterior aspect of the body. This is the opposite of ventral. See Posterior.

Dorsal Columns: Tracts of sensory nerve fibers that carry proprioceptive and vibratory information to the brain and are located in the posterior portion of the spinal cord.

Dorsal Column Stimulator: An electronic device inserted near the spinal cord which provides competitive sensory stimulation to the dorsal columns of the spinal cord in order to interfere with pain transmission. Usually, the leads are placed percutaneously initially, and preliminary testing is done with the stimulator external to the body. Often times, these patients are given a TENS trial prior to implantation of the electrodes. Patients who have a positive response to TENS may be better candidates for this type of procedure. The leads are normally placed in the epidural space. Complications of implantation can include sepsis, spinal cord compression, increased pain or discomfort, or device failure. This type of pain relief system is usually only recommended in patients with severe pain who have not responded to more conservative measures. See DCS.

Dorsal Column Theory: Referring to the posterior column in the three-column theory of spinal stability. It is thought that for gross spinal instability to occur, all three of the ligamentous columns need to be damaged. The dorsal column refers to the posterior elements such as the facet joint capsules, ligamentum flavum, and the supraspinous and interspinous ligaments.

Dorsal Glide: A stretching maneuver of the suboccipitals and anterior neck structures. The patient is asked to tuck the chin and stretch the suboccipital area upward. The stretch is first taught in the supine position. It is thought that the stretch opens the cervical intervertebral foramina.

Dorsal Horns: Posteriorly placed projections of gray matter in the spinal cord. These receive sensory input from the body. The substantia gelatinosa (see TENS) is located here.

Dorsal Osteophyte: A bone spur on the posterior vertebral body. See Osteophyte.

Dorsal Rami: The sensory nerve fibers that combine with the exiting motor fibers of the ventral ramus to form the spinal nerve. These fibers carry sensory information from the peripheral nerves back to the spinal cord. See Dorsal Ramus, Dorsal Root.

Dorsal Ramus: The sensory nerve fibers that combine with the exiting motor fibers of the ventral ramus to form the spinal nerve. These fibers carry sensory information from the peripheral nerves back to the spinal cord. See Dorsal Rami, Dorsal Root.

Dorsal Rhizotomy: A surgical or percutaneous procedure performed under fluoroscopy in which a radio frequency electrode or cryoprobe is introduced into the dorsal quadrant of the appropriate foramen to destroy the sensory portion of the nerve root. The most significant complication is destroying motor fibers. See Cryoanalgesia, Medial Branch Block.

Dorsal Root: The posterior roots that enter the spinal cord carrying sensory impulses to the dorsal horns of the spinal cord.

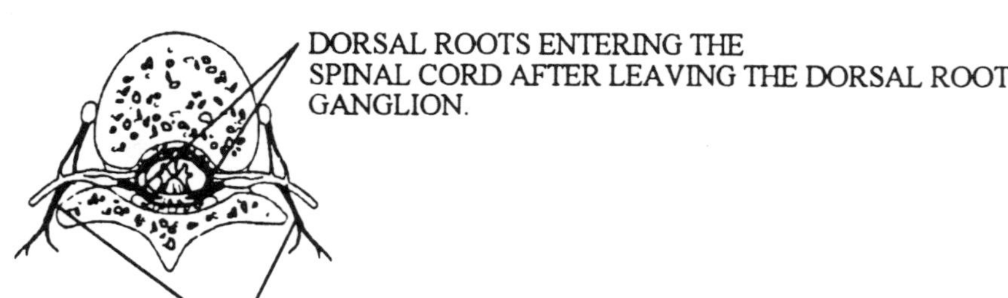

Dorsal Root Entry Lesioning: A surgical technique that destroys cell bodies in the dorsal root entry zone of the spinal cord and is performed on patients suffering from central deafferentation hypersensitivity.

Dorsal Root Ganglion: The portion of a spinal nerve root located in the intervertebral foramen where sensory nerve cells reside. The cells send projections both to the spinal cord and to the periphery.

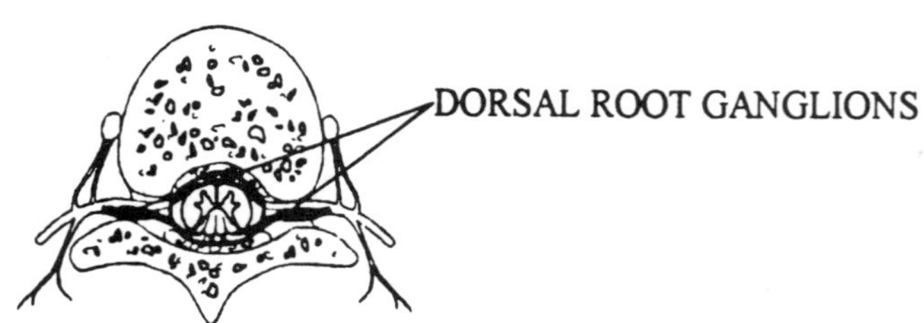

Dorsal Sacroiliac Ligament: A strong ligament on the posterior surface of the SI joint that blends deeply with the stronger interosseous SI ligament. See Dorsal SI Ligament, SI Ligaments.

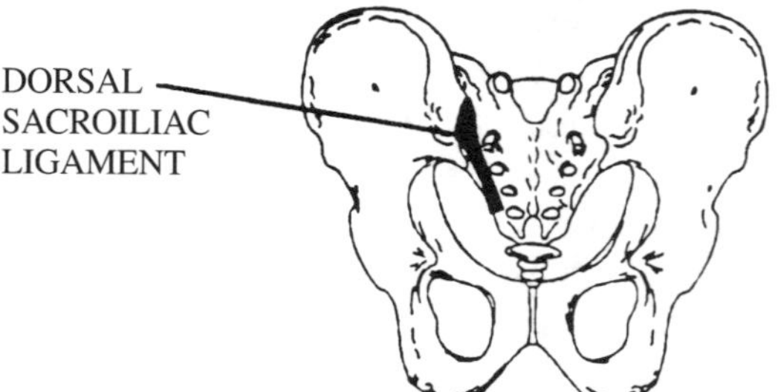

Dorsal SI Ligament: A strong ligament on the posterior surface of the SI joint that blends deeply with the stronger interosseous SI ligament. See Dorsal Sacroiliac Ligament, SI Ligament.

Dorsal Spine: Another term for thoracic spine.

Dorsomedian Septum: A plica or septum in the spinal canal between the ligamentum flavum and the posterior dura mater. This is an anatomically complex and strong ligament that seems to be involved in the biomechanics of the dura, particularly with respect to anterior/posterior movements. This ligament could be the reason why some epidural injections do not have the desired effect. If the patient has a continuous dorso-median septum, only half of the dura may be bathed in the injection material.

DOT: Department of Transportation or Dictionary of Occupational Titles.

Double Crush Syndrome: A nerve entrapment at two sites along a nerve. A common scenario is carpal tunnel syndrome that is due in part to a cervical radiculopathy. Compression of the exiting nerve root causes dysfunction in that nerve root making it more prone to entrapment distally. The implication is that an operative decompression of the carpal tunnel is unlikely to abate all of the patient's symptoms because there is still a more proximal cervical injury that needs to be addressed.

Double Curve: A scoliosis where two major curves develop of approximately equal severity. See Double Major Curve, Scoliosis.

Double Leg Lowering: A test for the strength of the external obliques and abdominals. The patient is in the supine position and is asked to lower the bilateral lower extremities or one lower extremity while keeping the lumbar spine pressed against the table. This is graded 1 through 5 and was first described by Kendall. See Lower Abdominal Progression.

Double Leg Raise Test: A physical examination maneuver in which the patient lies supine with both legs fully extended. A straight leg raising maneuver is then performed on each leg. The angle at which pain is reproduced is then noted. The examiner then raises both lower extremities together. A positive test is pain reproduced at a smaller angle when the lower extremities are raised bilaterally than when they were raised individually. It is thought that this test is positive in patients with SI joint pain. See Bilateral Straight Leg Raising Test.

Double "L" Fixation: Posterior segmental fixation with a wire that encircles the lamina in combination with a metal rod. The wire enters the spinal canal—and has inherent risks by doing so—but forms a sturdy attachment.

Double Major Curve: A scoliosis where two major curves develop of approximately equal severity. This is usually a structural scoliosis and is seen in patients with neuromuscular diseases. See Double Curve, Scoliosis, Double Major Curve.

Double Major Scoliosis: A scoliosis where two major curves develop of approximately equal severity. See Double Major Curve.

Double Spinous Sign: A radiographic sign seen on an AP x-ray associated with a clay shoveler's fracture. There is a double contour to a lower cervical spinous process. See Clay Shoveler's Fracture.

Double Thoracic Curve: A structural scoliosis with a large dominant lower thoracic curve balanced by a smaller upper thoracic curve and a compensatory nonstructural lumbar curve.

Dowager's Hump: An upper thoracic kyphosis that is commonly found in elderly women.

Downgoing Toe: A physical exam maneuver performed to detect an upper motor neuron dysfunction (brain injury or spinal cord injury above the lower lumbar area). See Babinski Sign.

Down–slip: An osteopathic movement dysfunction of the ilium which is relatively rare. The ilium is found to "ride low" on the sacrum on one side. The ASIS and PSIS are low on one side. See Inferior Innominate Shear.

Down Syndrome: The most common cause of mental retardation in children. This is an autosomal defect which results in trisomy 21. There are classic spine findings. Up to 20% of these individuals are born without a transverse ligament. Therefore, cervical flexion–extension views should be performed looking at the atlanto-dental interspace (ADI). Obviously, any type of manipulative therapy, mobilization, or muscle energy technique correction could be potentially dangerous if upper cervical instability is not ruled out prior to these procedures. See Mongolism.

Doxepin: A tricyclic antidepressant often used in chronic pain. This is a sedating antidepressant and is usually given at night to aid sleep. This medication is contraindicated in patients with glaucoma or urinary retention. There are drug interactions with MAO inhibitors, cimetidine, alcohol, and some oral hypoglycemic agents. Antidepressant doses are between 75 mg and 300 mg a day. The medication is supplied in 10-mg, 25-mg, 50-mg, 75-mg, 100-mg, and 150-mg tablets. When used in chronic pain and to aid in sleep, doses in the 10–25 mg range are more common. See Sinequan.

DPA: A technique for quantifying osteoporosis which involves using two different types of radiation. The use of two different types of energy eliminates the need for a soft tissue control. See Dual Photon Absorptiometry.

DPAT: An abbreviation for *decreased pain after treatment.*

DPM: Doctor of Podiatric Medicine.

Dripping Candle Wax: A radiographic term which describes the calcification of the ALL seen in diffuse idiopathic skeletal hyperostosis.

Drop Foot: A high-stepping gait due to weakness in the tibialis anterior musculature and commonly associated with a L4–L5 radiculopathy. This is associated with a foot slap due to weakness allowing the forefoot to suddenly hit the ground during heel strike. See Equine Gait, Steppage Gait.

Drop-Table: A type of chiropractic manipulation in which a Thompson table or similar device is used. This table contains sections which can be "dropped" suddenly to either provide or aid in a manipulative thrust.

DSCP: A somatosensory evoked potential in which a dermatome is stimulated versus a peripheral nerve. See Dermatomal Somatosensory Evoked Potential.

DSEP: A technique involving stimulation over the skin in a specific dermatome and recording over the cortex. This can be used to diagnose sensory radiculopathies. The technique is highly reader dependent and requires an experienced technician. One problem may be that dermatomal patterns have significant person to person variation. See Dermatomal Somatosensory Evoked Potential, SEP.

D-spine: An abbreviation for *dorsal spine*. Another term for thoracic spine.

DTR: A physical exam maneuver that checks the integrity of the "wiring" of the muscle being tested. See Deep Tendon Reflex.

Dual Energy X-ray Absorptiometry: One of the newer techniques for measuring osteoporosis in the spine. This technique is faster than DPA and has less radiation exposure than QCT with greater accuracy. See DEXA.

Dual Photon Absorptiometry: A technique for quantifying osteoporosis which involves using two different types of radiation. The use of two different types of energy eliminates the need for a soft tissue control. See DPA.

Duke Collar: A cervical orthosis which also extends down to the upper thoracic spine. See Long Two-Poster Orthosis.

Dura: The outer-most covering of the spinal cord. See Dura Mater.

Dural AV Fistula: An AV fistula where the nidus is the nerve root sleeve dura. These fistulas are supplied by one or more feeding vessels derived from the segmental arteries which commonly originate in the lower thoracic or lumbar region. The nidus is usually seen within the intervertebral foramen. They are commonly in the dorsal aspect of the cord and patients usually present with a subacute or acute progression of myelopathy which may become irreversible paraplegia or quadriplegia. See Type 1 AVM.

Dural Cuff: Tufts of arachnoid matter which protrude through the dura into the epidural space where they invaginate the walls of the epidural veins and drain the spinal cord and nerve root area of CSF. See Arachnoid Granulations.

Dural Leak: The leakage of CSF from the dural sac. Dural leaks can be caused by spinal injections or occasionly by spinal surgeries. A headache is common due to the decreased CSF volume. See Dural Puncture, Dural Rent, Dural Tear.

Dural Ligaments: A network of dural ligaments that attach the anterior thecal sac to the anterior and anterior lateral aspect of the spinal canal. See Hoffman Ligaments.

Dural Membrane System: The three coverings of the spinal cord: pia mater, subarachnoid, and dura mater.

Dural Mobilization: Dural mobilization involves freeing the dura from scarred restrictions. See Adverse Neural Tension, Neural Mobilization.

Dural Pain: Pain originating from the dura. The dura is innervated by the sinuvertebral nerve (recurrent meningeal nerve) and forms a mesh-like network. One of the original proponents of dural pain was Cyriax. He believed that a bulging disc which placed mechanical pressure on the dura could cause radiating lower extremity pain. See Dural Sac Impingement, Extrasegmental Referred Pain.

Dural Plexus: The mesh-work of nerves which innervate the dura through the sinuvertebral nerve.

Dural Puncture: The leakage of CSF from the dural sac. See Dural Leak.

Dural Release: Freeing the dura from scarred restrictions. See Dural Mobilization, Dural Tube Release.

Dural Rent: The leakage of CSF from the dural sac. See Dural Leak.

Dural Sac Impingement: Pressure on the dura caused by a bulging disc, HNP, or osteophyte. See Dural Pain.

Dural Signs: A concept described by Cyriax where loss of dural mobility causes pain due to a central disc protrusion or other limitation. The dura can be put on stretch through passive neck flexion, an SLR, or Slump Test. See Adverse Neural Tension.

Dural Tear: The leakage of CSF from the dural sac. See Dural Leak.

Dural Tube: Another name for the thecal sac or the dura mater. The dura is actually a tube or sac-like covering, and pain is often associated with the dura in many treatment paradigms. This terminology is used by therapists who use dural releases or dural mobilization techniques. See Dura Mater.

Dural Tube Release: Dural mobilization involves freeing the dura from scarred restrictions. See Dural Mobilization, Dura Release.

Dural Tube Restriction: Decreased mobility of the dura with movement. Cyriax postulated that the dura was a pain-sensitive structure and any decrease in movement would cause radiating pain. Maitland and Butler also thought that restriction of movement of the dura was painful. It is known that the dura is innervated along its anterior aspect with a mesh-like nerve plexus. See Dura Mater, Adverse Neural Tension.

Dura Mater: The outer-most covering of the spinal cord. This is a thick connective tissue covering. The epidural space is above the dura mater, and the subdural space is below the dura mater. This tissue provides protection and support to the spinal cord. This is a pain-sensitive structure which envelops the spinal roots and ganglia as they pass through the intervertebral foramina. See Dural Tube.

Dutchman Roll: A roll for positioning often used in Cox flexion/distraction. This can be used under the hips during a flexion/distraction maneuver.

Duverney's Fracture: A fracture of the iliac bone caused by a lateral blow. See Iliac Wing Fracture.

Dvorak Method: A radiographic technique for diagnosing segmental instability in the cervical spine. Routine flexion/extension radiographs are done, but the patient is pushed to passive end range at flexion and extension rather than just active end range. It is thought that this is a more sensitive technique for detecting segmental instability.

Dwyer Cable System: Instrumentation used for anterior interbody spinal fusion. See Dwyer Instrumentation.

Dwyer Instrumentation: Instrumentation used for anterior interbody spinal fusion in which a braided titanium cable is passed through a special screw-staple assembly which has been drilled into the vertebral body on the convex side of the curvature (for a structural scoliosis). The cable is then tightened and adjusted to reduce the scoliotic curve. See Dwyer Cable System.

Dwyer's Procedure: A surgical technique for the correction of scoliosis. See Dwyer's Technique.

Dwyer's Technique: A surgical technique for the correction of scoliosis. The technique involves removing the disc and inserting screws into the vertebral bodies on the convex side. A wire is passed through holes in the screws and tension is applied to correct the curve. See Dwyer's Procedure.

Dx: An abbreviation for *diagnosis.*

DXA: One of the newer techniques for measuring osteoporosis in the spine. See Dual Energy X-ray Absorptiometry, DEXA.

Dyck Fixator: A type of pedicle screw fixation used for a posterior spinal fusion. See Pedicle Screw Fixation.

Dynamic Listing: A chiropractic term describing abnormal movement that is characteristic of one vertebrae in relation to its adjacent segments. See Listing—Dynamic.

Dynamic Lumbar Stabilization: A rehabilitation program used to stabilize the lumbar spine through the pelvis. Neuromuscular retraining, flexibility, and strengthening are key components of the program. This is used for a variety of lumbar diagnoses including HNP, facet syndrome, SI syndrome, and others. See Pelvic Stabilization, Lumbar Stabilization, Core Stabilization, Stabilization Activities.

Dynamic Stenosis: Dynamic compression of a nerve root by an unstable spinal segment due to severe degenerative disc disease. It is thought that in the final stages of disc degeneration, there is enough excess mobility to cause recurrent compression of a nerve root.

Dynamic Thrust: This is the therapeutic force delivered during a manipulation. See Manipulation.

Dynamometer: A device which measures force. For instance, an isokenitic dynamometer measures force while the speed of a joint is controlled. A Jamar dynamometer is a device which measures grip strength.

Dysarthrosis: A deformity or malformation of a joint.

Dysesthesia: An unpleasant abnormal sensation which can be either spontaneous or evoked. See Hyperalgesia, Allodynia.

Dysesthetic Pain: Pain which is burning, tingling, crawling, or electric. This type of pain is worsened with activity and includes causalgia. An example would be the pain caused by postherpetic neuralgia.

Dysfunction Syndrome: A McKenzie physical therapy term which is used to describe low back pain with loss of range of motion in certain directions due to shortening of specific tissues. When the patient moves into the direction of lost range of motion, this will cause intermittent pain. Rehabilitation for this syndrome usually increases pain while the structures are being lengthened, with the eventual result of decreasing pain. There can be loss of flexion, loss of extension, or loss of side gliding (a combination of rotation and side bending). See McKenzie Exercises.

Dysplastic Spondylolisthesis: A congenital malformation of the upper sacrum and/or neural arch of the L5 vertebra. See Type I Spondylolisthesis.

Dysraphism: A failure of the posterior elements to fuse around the spinal cord. Spina bifida is an example of dysraphism.

Dysthymia: A chronic depressed mood that has lasted for more than two years and is associated with poor appetite or increased appetite, low self-esteem, low energy or fatigue, insomnia or hypersomnia, poor concentration and/or cognitive difficulties, and feeling of hopelessness. The patient has not had a major depressive episode during this two-year period. This differs from a major depression in that it is a more chronic condition and usually considered to be less severe.

E

E: An abbreviation for *examination.*

Eburnation: Increase in the density of bone. Also a radiologic term which implies bony sclerosis. See Sclerosis, Subchondral Sclerosis.

EBV: Epstein-Barr Virus.

Eccentric Exercise: Resistance applied to a muscle as it lengthens. Muscles can tolerate more eccentric loading than concentric. There can be greater delayed muscle soreness with eccentric exercise. See Eccentric Muscle Contraction.

Eccentric Muscle Contraction: A lengthening muscle contraction. Muscles can tolerate more eccentric loading than concentric. There can be greater delayed muscle soreness with eccentric exercise. See Eccentric Exercise.

ECRB: An abbreviation for *extensor carpi radialis brevis.*

ECRL: An abbreviation for *extensor carpi radialis longus.*

EDB: An abbreviation for *extensor digitorum brevis.*

Edwards Rods: Distraction and compression rods with hooks which are placed posteriorly. This system provides rigid fusion to the lumbar spine. It can be used to correct scoliotic deformities.

Efferent: Referring to a motor nerve. A nerve that takes impulses from the central nervous system and transmits them towards the periphery. See Efferent Nerve.

Efferent Nerve: A motor nerve. A nerve that takes impulses from the central nervous system and transmits them toward the periphery. See Efferent.

Effleurage: A stroking movement often performed in combination with massage for the purpose of removing lymphatic fluids.

Eggshell Procedure: The surgical fracture of a vertebra so that it can be collapsed and removed.

EHL: Extensor hallucis longus. This abbreviation is used to relay that the EHL has been tested for motor strength. Since the EHL is innervated by the L5 nerve root, EHL weakness can imply an L5 motor radiculopathy.

EIL: An abbreviation for *extension in lying*. A McKenzie physical therapy test maneuver in which the patient lies in a prone position performing extension on the elbows. It is then determined whether this reproduces the patient's characteristic pain pattern, or causes centralization or peripheralization of the patient's pain. See Extension in Lying.

EIS: An abbreviation for *extension in standing*. A McKenzie physical therapy test maneuver in which the patient places hands on hips and bends backward to determine if this reproduces their characteristic pain pattern. See Extension in Standing.

Eisenstein's Method: Method for determining the sagittal (anterior-posterior) diameter of the spinal canal. On a lateral lumbar spine view, a line is drawn connecting the superior and inferior articular processes of the level in question. The distance from this line to the posterior vertebral body margin at the midpoint is determined. This is the sagittal canal diameter. This method is used for L1–L4. For L5, the measurement is between the spinolaminar junction and the posterior body. The sagittal canal diameter should not be less than 14–15 mm. Any measurement below these values may represent spinal stenosis. See Canal–Body Index.

Elastic Barrier: The point in the range of motion where a vertebral segment begins to go elastic. If a vertebral segment is pushed to the end of its passive range of motion, and then pushed slightly further, it will be pushed into the elastic range. If pressure is released, the vertebral segment will "bounce back" to the end of passive range of motion.

Elavil: A tricyclic antidepressant with sedative side effects. This is used for the relief of the symptoms of depression, as well as in chronic pain patients. This medication is also used to induce sleep in patients with chronic or neuropathic pain. When used as an antidepressant, 50–100 mg of amitriptyline is given at bedtime. This can be increased by 25–50 mg to a total of 150 mg qHS. Doses up to 200–300 mg have been given in hospitalized patients. The maintenance dosage is lower, at 50–100 mg per day. For sleep, amitriptyline dosages are in the 10–25 mg range. This is the same amount used in chronic pain, but it is thought that there may be some titration of dosage upward from those levels in patients with chronic pain or neuropathic pain. Elavil is available in tablets of 10 mg, 25 mg, 50 mg, 75 mg, 100 mg, and 150 mg. See Amitriptyline Hydrochloride, Amitriptyline HCl.

Elbow Extension: A chiropractic manipulative technique. See Elbow Extension Manipulation, Elbow Extension Adjustment.

Elbow Extension Adjustment: A chiropractic manipulative technique See Elbow Extension Manipulation, Elbow Extension.

Elbow Extension Manipulation: A chiropractic manipulative technique in which the force delivered is from a sudden contraction of the triceps muscles which extends the forearm. This causes a sudden manipulative thrust. See Elbow Extension Adjustment, Elbow Extension.

Electrical Stimulation Devices: Devices which perform electrical stimulation. See TENS, MENS, Interferential E-Stim.

Electro-acupuncture: The application of electrical stimulation to acupuncture points using TENS or another electrical stimulus.

Electromyogram: A test used to determine the function of the peripheral nerves and nerve roots. See EMG, EMG/Nerve Conduction Study.

Electromyography: A test used to determine the function of the peripheral nerves and nerve roots. See EMG, EMG/Nerve Conduction Study.

Electronic Digital Inclinometer: An electronic device used for the noninvasive quantification of range of motion. See Digital Inclinometer, Electronic Inclinometer.

Electronic Inclinometer: An electronic device used for the noninvasive quantification of range of motion. See Digital Inclinometer, Electronic Digital Inclinometer.

Electrospinal Orthosis: An attempt to correct scoliosis by the application of electrical currents to the paraspinal musculature on the convex side of the curve. This current is applied transcutaneously. The clinical efficacy of this orthosis has been questioned. See TENS.

Elephant Man's Disease: An inherited disorder that affects nerve roots, cranial nerves, and peripheral nerves. Scoliosis is associated with this disease approximately 50% of the time. See Neurofibromatosis.

Ely's Heel-to-Buttock Sign: The patient lies prone and the knee is flexed with the hip externally rotated bringing the heel to the opposite buttock. This test is positive if there is irritation of the psoas musculature.

EMG: An acronym for *electromyogram.* A test used to determine the function of the peripheral nerves and nerve roots. See EMG/Nerve Conduction Study, Electromyography.

EMG/NCS: A test used to determine the function of the peripheral nerves and nerve roots. See EMG/Nerve Conduction Study, Sharp Wave.

EMG/NCV: A test used to determine the function of the peripheral nerves and nerve roots. See EMG/Nerve Conduction Study, NCV.

EMG/Nerve Conduction Study: A test used to determine the function of the peripheral nerves and nerve roots. This is often used to diagnose lumbar radiculopathy, peripheral nerve entrapments, lumbar stenosis, or peripheral neuropathy. The EMG involves placing tiny needles in different muscle groups and monitoring for electrical signs of denervation. The nerve conduction study portion involves small electrical impulses which are recorded along nerve pathways. This test can be reader dependent. This is usually performed by a physiatrist or neurologist. See EMG, Electromyogram, Electromyography, EMG/NCS, EMG/NCV, Sharp Wave.

Employability: The capacity of a worker to meet the demands of a job.

Employability Determination: An assessment by management and a physician of an individual's capacity to meet the demands of a job and the terms of employment.

Empty Feel: A type of end feel described by Cyriax in which pain limits the range of motion so that the full range cannot be obtained. The sensation is apparently one of emptiness and lacks any resistance except for the patient's pain. An example would be a shoulder with a subdeltoid bursitis being limited in abduction.

Empty Vertebra Sign: A split in the pedicle seen on an AP x-ray view of the lumbar spine due to a Chance fracture. See Chance Fracture.

End Feel: The sensation at the end point of available range of motion. This varies according to pathology. An example would be a capsular end feel secondary to a tight joint capsule. Another example would be bony end feel secondary to bony hypertrophy. In the lumbar spine, end feel can be appreciated in flexion, extension, side bending, rotation, or side glide. See Bone to Bone, Springy Block.

End Plate: A layer of cartilage approximately 1 mm thick which is located on the top and bottom of the vertebral bodies and encircled by the ring apophysis. See Vertebral End Plate.

End Plate Changes—Type 1: Changes in the bone marrow of the vertebral bodies near the intervertebral disc. These changes are seen with degenerated discs and characterized by breaks and fissures of the end plates. Also, the bone marrow becomes replaced with fibrous tissue that is well vascularized. These changes are bright on T2 weighted MRI images. See Type 1 End Plate Changes.

End Plate Changes—Type 2: The marrow becomes replaced with fat. This is associated with degenerative disc disease more severe than type 1 changes. The fatty replacement of the bone is bright on T1 weighted MRI images. See End Plate Changes—Type 1, Type 2 End Plate Changes, Type 2 Marrow Changes.

End Plate Changes—Type 3: Instead of replacement by fibrous vascular tissue or fat, there is replacement with sclerotic bone. This represents more severe degenerative disc disease than Type 1 or Type 2 changes. These are seen as low signal intensity changes on both T1 and T2 weighted MRI images. See End Plate Changes—Type 2, Type 3 End Plate Changes, Type 3 Marrow Changes.

End Plate Disruption: A fracture of the vertebral end plate which can be associated with a vertebral compression fracture. The edges are usually jagged and irregular, and this may be difficult to detect on x-ray and tomography. See Disruption of the Vertebral End Plate.

End Plate Fracture: There are three types of vertebral end plate fractures: central portion fractures, the peripheral portion fractures, or fractures that are transverse across the entire end plate. See Schmorl's Nodes, Vertebral End Plate Fracture.

End Vertebrae: A radiographic term used in the measurement of scoliosis. This is the vertebra at the superior or inferior end point of the scoliotic curve. This is determined by the vertebra whose surface point is maximally toward the concavity of the curve.

Enostosis: A sclerotic density seen on radiographs which is asymptomatic and usually not clinically significant. See Bone Island.

Enteropathic Arthritis: A group of diseases which have both GI symptoms and arthritic symptoms. The two most common are ulcerative colitis and Crohn's disease. Whipple's disease, shigella, yersinia, and salmonella are also in this group. Crohn's disease and ulcerative colitis are seen in younger adults. Involvement of the spine is almost identical to that of ankylosing spondylitis, with bilateral SI joint involvement and spondylitis. This occurs in approximately 10% of patients with ulcerative colitis and slightly less often with Crohn's disease. Bilateral SI joint involvement is much more common with Crohn's and ulcerative colitis than it is with ankylosing spondylitis. This is a seronegative arthropathy (rheumatoid factor is not present). There is a 10–12% incidence of HLA-B27 antigen. For the radiographic features of these disorders see Ankylosing Spondylitis. Involvement is more common in the thoracic, lumbar, and pelvic regions. See Enteropathic Arthropathy, Enteropathic Spondylitis, and Colitic Arthritis.

Enteropathic Arthropathy: A group of diseases which have both GI symptoms and arthritic symptoms. See Enteropathic Arthritis.

Enteropathic Spondylitis: A group of diseases which have both GI symptoms and arthritic symptoms. See Enteropathis Arthritis.

Enthesitis: An inflammatory reaction at a muscular insertion. There is a tendency toward fibrosis and calcification at this site. Movements with the effected muscle are painful. There is commonly radiographic evidence of calcification at the insertion. An example in the lumbar spine would be an enthesitis of the erector spinae as it inserts on the thoracodorsal fasciae. This process can be seen in some of the seronegative spondyloarthropathies.

Enthesopathy: Pain and inflammation at the insertion of a muscle. This is painful only when the muscle

Ext: An abbreviation for *external.*

Ext. c. rad. B: An abbreviation for *extensor carpi radialis brevis.*

Ext. c. rad. L: An abbreviation for *extensor carpi radialis longus.*

Ext. dig. brev.: An abbreviation for *extensor digitorum brevis.*

Ext. dig. comm.: An abbreviation for *extensor digitorum communis.*

Ext. dig. long.: An abbreviation for *extensor digitorum longus.*

Extension: A movement that brings two parts of a joint toward a straight position. In the spine, this is starting in a forward bent position and returning to a straight position.

Extension Bias: A term often used by therapists who practice some form of spinal stabilization. This refers to the spine being held in an extension posture to avoid symptoms during the stabilization exercises.

Extension—Craniosacral: Motion that occurs during craniosacral rhythm when the sacrum nutates (flexes forward) and the sphenobasilar symphysis descends. See Craniosacral Extension.

Extension Dysfunction of the Sacrum: An osteopathic or manual physical therapy term used to denote a sacral position such that the sacral base is extended or posterior and the apex is anterior. See Bilaterally Flexed Sacrum.

Extension in Lying: A McKenzie physical therapy test maneuver. See EIL.

Extension in Standing: A McKenzie physical therapy test maneuver. See EIS.

Extension Malposition: A chiropractic term which refers to a vertebra which is "extended" relative to the adjacent vertebrae. The anterior portion of the vertebral body is superior and the spinous process is inferior. The spinous will be noted to be closer to the spinous below. See Posteroinferior Subluxation.

Extension Restriction Side Bending: An osteopathic or manual physical therapy term used to describe a restriction in movement of the spine in flexion and side bending to one side. See ERS.

Extension—Sacral: When the base of the sacrum (top of the sacrum) moves posteriorly in relation to the ilia. See Sacral Extension, Sacral Counternutation, Sacral Backwards Bending.

External Skeletal Fixator: An external frame that holds percutaneous pins in place and provides external fixation of bone fragments or portions of the spinal column.

Externally Rotated Innominate: An osteopathic or manual physical therapy term which usually refers to the ilium being externally rotated or turned out relative to the sacrum. See Outflare.

Ext. hall. long.: An abbreviation for *extensor hallucis longus.*

Ext. poll. brev.: An abbreviation for *extensor pollicis brevis.*

Ext. poll. long.: An abbreviation for *extensor pollicis longus.*

Extr.: An abbreviation for *extremity.*

Extra-articular Limitation: When the amount of limitation at one joint is controlled by the position of another joint. One example is a straight-leg raising maneuver. There is limitation of hip flexion when the knee is extended, but not when the knee is flexed.

Extradural Defect: A radiographic term used to describe a disc bulge or bony protrusion that indents the thecal sac. Since the thecal sac (dura) is innervated along with the nerve root sheaths, this may represent a site of pain generation.

Extradural Meningioma: An extradural primary tumor of the spine which represents approximately 7% of all meningiomas. These lesions tend to be vascular and may erode bony structure giving the appearance of an extradural metastases. They are rare and when excised have a tendency to recur. Whenever an extradural meningioma is encountered, an intradural lesion must be ruled out. They are almost always associated with intradural components, and the communication between the extradural space and intradural space is sometimes, but not always, demonstrated.

Extradural Steroids: The delivery of local anesthetic and steroids extrathecally through a lumbar route.

Extrapyramidal System: Tracts in the central nervous system which fine-tune motor function. For instance, Parkinson's disease, with its tremor, rigidity, and abnormal posturing, is a dysfunction of the extrapyramidal system.

Extrasegmental Referred Pain: A concept that apparently originated with Cyriax. He believed that low lumbar dural pain could spread to the legs, the abdomen, and into the mid-thoracic spine. He also believed that the cervical dura could refer pain to the head and mid-thoracic spine. See Dural Pain.

Extraspinal: Outside the spine.

Extra Strength Tylenol: Double-strength acetaminophen tablets containing 650 mg (instead of 325 mg) of Tylenol.

Extravasated Dye: Dye during a discogram which has traveled outside of the confines of the disc. It is "extravasated" through complete tears in the annulus.

Extruded Disc: A disc herniation through all of the annular fibers and the posterior longitudinal ligament. This is synonymous with a "herniated disc" or HNP. See Disc Extrusion, HNP, Herniated Disc.

F

FABER Test: A test for SI joint syndrome which puts the hip into flexion, abduction, and external rotation, usually by placing the ankle on the opposite knee. A downward pressure can be placed on the flexed knee, with the other hand stabilizing the opposite pelvis. The patient should report pain in the SI joint area. See Flexion Abduction External Rotation, Patrick's Test.

Facetal Asymmetry: Facet joints that are asymmetrical with respect to the plane of articulation. See Facet Tropism.

Facet Arthrosis: Degeneration of the facet joints. This occurs as decreased disc height places more load on the posterior elements (facets) causing degeneration. See Facet Hypertrophy.

Facet Asymmetry: Facet joints that are asymmetrical with respect to the plane of articulation. See Facet Tropism.

Facet Block: Injection of local anesthetic and steroid into the facet joints (usually lumbar) under fluoroscopic guidance. This is performed diagnostically and therapeutically for facet pain. The needle is advanced toward the target until bony or cartilaginous resistance is appreciated. The needle is then readjusted until it is felt to slip into the joint space. Contrast medium is injected (0.3–0.5 cc) producing an arthrogram of the facet joint. It is possible to burst the facet capsules during this procedure so care must be taken while injecting. The typical volume injected in the typical lumbar facet joint is usually about 1 ml. See Zygapophyseal Blocks, Facet Blocks, Facet Injection.

Facet Capsular Adhesions: A term that refers to scarring of the facet joint capsules which can restrict movement. See Capsular Adhesions.

Facet Dislocation—Bilateral: A cervical spine injury involving extensive ligamentous destruction including tearing of the interspinous, intertransverse, capsular ligaments, ligamentum flavum, and some portion of the annulus. See Bilateral Facet Dislocation.

Facet Dislocation—Unilateral: A cervical spine injury involving dislocation of one facet which occurs as a result of a flexion and rotation injury. See Unilateral Facet Dislocation.

Facetectomy: Excision of all or a portion of a facet joint.

Facet Hypertrophy: Enlargement of the facet joints due to degeneration. As we age, or as the intervertebral disc is traumatized, the disc itself loses height, thus placing more pressure on the facet joints. This increased load causes degeneration of the cartilage within the facet joints and leads to bony enlargement. This can narrow the space within the intervertebral foramen and cause foraminal stenosis or lateral recess stenosis. See Degenerative Proliferative Disease, Facet Arthrosis.

Facet Imbrication: Abnormal joint movement. See Subluxation.

Facet Injection: Injection of local anesthetic and steroid into the facet joints (usually lumbar) under fluoroscopic guidance. See Facet Block.

Facet Joint: A synovial joint about the same size as the PIP joints (small joints at the end of the fingers). There are two joints at the back of each vertebra that articulate with the vertebra above and vertebra below. The facet joints help control movement of the spine and as such are oriented differently in every spinal region. The facet has long been thought to be a cause of spinal pain. See Apophyseal Articulation, Apophyseal Joints, Facet Joint, Superior Articular Process, Z-joint.

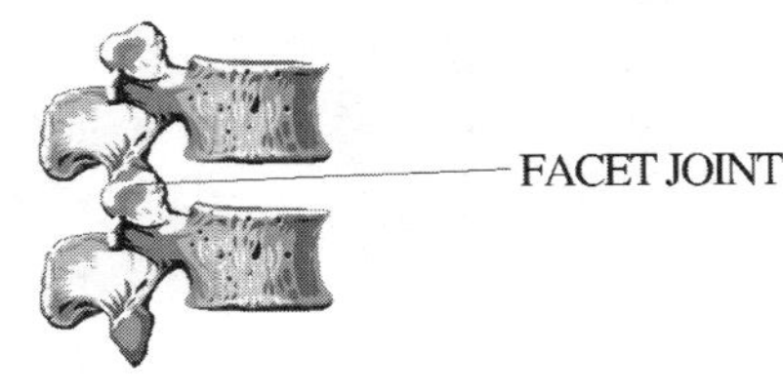

Facet Joint Dysfunction: A chiropractic term used to denote a vertebral segment that does not move freely in all directions. See Subluxed Vertebra.

Facet Joint Nerve Ablation: A technique of destroying the medial branch nerves to the facets for the purpose of controlling severe chronic facet pain. See Facet Rhizotomy.

Facet Rhizolysis: A technique of destroying the medial branch nerves to the facets for the purpose of controlling severe chronic facet pain. See Facet Rhizotomy.

Facet Rhizotomy: A technique of destroying the medial branch nerve supply to the facets for the purpose of controlling severe chronic facet pain. This can be performed surgically, with radio frequency current, and with cryoanalgesia. The major risk is anterior ramus damage. It should be noted that the facets should be absolutely identified as the pain generator before pursuing this type of destructive procedure. See Facet Joint Nerve Ablation, Facet Rhizolysis.

Facet Syndrome: Pain emanating from the lumbar facet joints. The facet joints occur in pairs in the posterior portion of the lumbar spine where one vertebral segment stacks upon the other. With disc degeneration and a decrease in the height of the disc, the facet joints often bear more weight and become degenerated and hypertrophied. These enlarged facet joints can press on the exiting nerve roots and cause radiculopathy or lumbar stenosis. Facet joint pain can also refer to the gluteal region or lower extremities. Acute facet syndromes may be more responsive to manual medicine than chronic facet syndromes. See Acute Facet Syndrome.

Facet Tropism: Facet joints that are asymmetrical with respect to the plane of articulation. This is usually seen on CT scan or axial MR images. There is some controversy as to whether this is associated with increased incidence of low back pain. This can also be seen on an AP view of the spine. See Tropism, Facet Asymmetry.

Facilitated Positional Release: The type of manipulation performed by most osteopaths and manual physical therapists. See OMT.

Facilitated Segment: Hyperactivity within a spinal segment and within the muscles and structures innervated by that segment. Abnormal afferent or sensory input to a particular area of the spinal cord is kept in a constant state of increased excitation. This then causes the musculature innervated by that segment to be maintained in a state of increased tone. "Osteopathic lesions" and "somatic dysfunctions" are associated with this phenomena. It has also been postulated that myofascial trigger points occur in facilitated segments. Correction of the lesion or somatic dysfunction either through manipulation, mobilization, muscle energy techniques, or strain/counterstrain may cause the facilitated segment to resolve.

Facilitation: Hyperactivity within a spinal segment and within the muscles and structures innervated by that segment. See Facilitated Segment.

Facilitative Lesion: Hyperactivity within a spinal segment and within the muscles and structures innervated by that segment. See Facilitated Segment.

FACO: Fellow of the Academy of Chiropractic Orthopedists.

FACS: Fellow of the American College of Surgeons.

Factitious Disorder: A medicolegal term which represents the conscious and willful misrepresentation of illness or symptoms in order to escape work duties and/or receive financial compensation. True malingering is thought to be rare. See Malingering.

FADIRE Test: An acronym for *f*lexion, *ad*duction, *i*nternal *r*otation, and *e*xtension which is used in evaluating a hip disorder. This is different from the FABER test used to evaluate SI disorders. See FABER Test.

Failed Back: Chronic and disabling pain thought to be secondary to a laminectomy or laminectomy and discectomy done for HNP or a disc bulge. See Failed Back Syndrome.

Failed Back Syndrome: Chronic and disabling pain thought to be secondary to a laminectomy or laminectomy and discectomy done for HNP or a disc bulge. The etiology of this syndrome is unclear. Some think this is secondary to instability caused by a facetectomy performed with a laminectomy. Others believe this syndrome is caused by chronic arachnoiditis. See Failed Back, Postlaminectomy Syndrome.

Fajersztajn Sign: A physical exam maneuver in which one leg is raised with the patient in the supine position. See Crossed Straight-Leg Raising Test, Well Leg Raising.

Far Lateral Disc: An HNP in which the root entrapment is lateral to the central canal in the foramen. This occurs ten times less often than the classic posterolateral HNP. Unlike classic posterolateral disc herniations, the most common level is L4–L5 with L3–L4 being the next most common, and L5–S1 occurring less than 25% of the time. This type of disc herniation tends to occur in an older population. See Far Lateral Herniated Disc, Far Lateral HNP.

Far Lateral Disc Herniation: A disc sequestration (free fragment) or disc extrusion which extends into the intervertebral foramen. See Far Lateral Disc, Foraminal Disc Herniation.

Far Lateral Herniated Disc: An HNP in which the root entrapment is lateral to the central canal in the foramen. See Far Lateral Disc, Far Lateral HNP.

Far Lateral HNP: An HNP in which the root entrapment is lateral to the central canal in the foramen. See Far Lateral Disc, Far Lateral Herniated Disc.

Fascial: Of or referring to the fascia. The fascia covers muscles and makes up the tissue planes of the body.

Fascic: Involuntary twitching of muscle fibers. See Fasciculation Potentials.

Fasciculation Potentials: Involuntary twitching of muscle fibers which can be seen electromyographically and can be associated with denervation. This is also associated with anterior horn cell diseases such as ALS. See Fascic.

Fast Spin-Echo Sequence: A modification of the standard spin-echo sequence in MRI. Rather than a single 180° pulse, a series of 180° pulses are applied, thus generating many echoes.

Fast Twitch Fiber: A skeletal muscle fiber with a fast reaction time that is anerobic. Muscles rich in fast twitch fibers are called phasic. These are muscles responsible for moving joints rather than holding posture. See Fast Twitch Muscle Fiber.

Fast Twitch Muscle Fiber: A skeletal muscle fiber with a fast reaction time that is anerobic. See Fast Twitch Fiber.

FB: An abbreviation for *foreign body*.

FCE: A test of physical strength and stamina used to determine working restrictions and work tolerance. See Functional Capacity Evaluation.

FCER: Foundation for Chiropractic Education and Research.

FCR: An abbreviation for *flexor carpi radialis*.

FCU: An abbreviation for *flexor carpi ulnaris*.

Feldene: A nonsteroidal anti-inflammatory drug. Piroxicam is in a nonsteroidal class by itself. The most common dosage is 20 mg once a day. Both 10- and 20-mg capsules are available. Aspirin and this drug should not be taken together. Patients receiving oral anticoagulants should be monitored carefully. There is an interaction with lithium in that there are increased lithium plasma concentrations. See Piroxicam.

Feldenkrais: A movement approach used to retrain the body into more efficient movement patterns. Moshi Feldenkrais was an Israeli engineer and physicist. The approach is based on the idea that abnormalities of movement occur in response to past trauma. The approach focuses on programming the brain to develop more efficient movement patterns. There are two approaches: "awareness through movement" and "functional integration." In the Feldenkrais approach, gentle sequences of movement allow for slow, deliberate alterations of inefficient movement patterns into more efficient movement patterns. See Movement Patterning.

Femoral Avascular Necrosis: A loss of blood supply to the femoral head which leads to destruction and necrosis of the bone. See Avascular Necrosis of the Femoral Head.

Femoral Nerve: A nerve that arises from the second, third, and fourth lumbar nerve roots. It provides innervation to the iliacus, psoas, sartorius, pectineus, and quadriceps. It provides sensation to the anterior surface of the thigh and through an internal saphenous branch to the entire inner surface of the leg and the anterior medial surface of the knee. It has been postulated that irritation in this nerve can produce pain in the anterior thigh.

Femoral Nerve Stretch Test: An adverse neural tension test performed with the patient in the prone position while the knee is flexed passively. See PKB, Nachlas' Knee Flexion Sign.

Femoral Nerve Traction Test: A traction test in which the patient lies on one side. The lower limb is extended at the hip and flexed at the knee. This test can be sensitized by adding flexion of the cervical spine to increase traction on the upper lumbar nerve roots and cauda equina. This is very similar to a slump maneuver with a prone knee bend maneuver. The test is positive in mid-lumbar radiculopathies if pain or numbness radiates down to the anterior thigh. See PKB, Slump Test.

Femoral Neuropathy: Dysfunction of the femoral nerve which can be associated either with an acute traction injury or diabetes. The femoral nerve arises from the second, third, and fourth lumbar nerve roots and provides innervation to the iliacus, psoas, sartorius, pectineus, and quadriceps. It provides sensation to the anterior surface of the thigh and through an internal saphenous branch to the entire inner surface of the leg and anterior medial surface of the knee. Therefore, common symptoms include numbness in the anterior thigh and weakness in the quadriceps (knee extensors). This has been confused with a high lumbar HNP or high lumbar radiculopathy.

Femoral Triangle: An anatomic triangle bounded by the inguinal ligament, the adductor longus, and the sartorius which contains the femoral nerve, artery, and vein. See Scarpa's Triangle.

Femur Head Line: An x-ray marking technique which involves placing a dot at the upper most portion of the femoral head bilaterally. A line is then used to connect these two dots. This is used to look for leg length discrepancies or inequalities that might be causing a pelvic tilt. See FHL.

Fenoprofen: A nonsteroidal anti-inflammatory drug in the benzeneacetic acid class. It possesses anti-inflammatory, analgesic, and antipyretic properties. See Nalfon.

Ferguson Method: One technique for measuring a scoliotic curve on AP radiography. A method for quantifying scoliosis. See Risser-Ferguson Method.

Ferguson's Angle: A radiographic measurement of the angle between the superior endplate of L2 and the base of the sacrum. See Lumbosacral Angle, Lumbosacral Lordotic Angle.

Ferguson's Gravitational Line: A radiographic term which refers to a plumb line which represents the center of gravity of the spine. See Ferguson's Weight Bearing Line.

Ferguson's Weight Bearing Line: A radiographic term which refers to a plumb line which represents the center of gravity of the spine. A shift of the spine in the anterior-posterior direction or in a lateral direction is thought to occur due to spinal subluxations or muscular spasm. See Lumbar Gravity Line.

FHL: An x-ray marking technique which involves placing a dot at the upper most portion of the femoral head bilaterally. A line is then used to connect these two dots. This is used to look for leg length discrepancies or inequalities that might be causing a pelvic tilt. See Femur Head Line.

Fhx: An abbreviation for *family history*.

Fibrillation Potentials: An EMG finding which usually corresponds to loss of partial or complete nerve supply in a given muscle. These findings must be seen across several muscles to find the common nerve root that is involved in a radiculopathy.

Fibromyalgia: A term which is roughly equivalent with diffuse systemic myofacial pain. This is pain at many sites and has been defined by the American College of Rheumatology as pain at 11 of 18 tender point sites, presence of subcutaneous nodules, and a history of widespread pain for more than 3 months. This diffuse muscular pain has no known etiology. There have been some studies connecting this to decreased REM sleep and fatigue. There may or may not be associated trigger points. This is somewhat of a catchall term which may represent many different musculoskeletal disease states. See Diffuse Myofascial Pain Syndrome, Nonarticular Rheumatism.

Fibromyositis: Pain emanating from the muscles. See Myofascial Pain.

Fibrositis: A somewhat ambiguous term with multiple meanings. This can have essentially the same meaning as myofascial pain. This term is also synonymous with tendonitis, bursitis, capsulitis, and tenosynovitis. Used in some contexts, it can have the same meaning as fibromyalgia. This includes widespread pain with local tenderness at 11 of 18 sites, skin roll tenderness over the upper scapular region, and sleep disturbances. This was first introduced by Gowers in 1904 as a term for muscular rheumatism.

Fibular Allograft: A cadaveric bone graft which is made up of a section of the fibula.

Fibular Graft: A graft for fusion that is taken from the fibula which is usually much stronger in resisting compression than iliac crest grafts. The graft is resorbed slowly and provides structural support longer than other grafts.

Fick Method: A method for measuring flexion deformity. On a standing lateral radiograph a line is drawn through the base of the sacrum and through the femur. The angle at the intersection of these two lines is the sacrofemoral angle. See Sacrofemoral Angle, Sacral Femoral Angle.

Figure of Four Hip Test: A test for SI joint syndrome which puts the hip into flexion, abduction, and external rotation usually placing the ankle on the opposite knee. See FABER Test.

FIL: A McKenzie test maneuver which involves bringing the patient's legs to the chest to determine if this reproduces the patient's characteristic pain. An observation is also made as to whether centralization or peripheralization of pain occurs with this maneuver. See Flexion in Lying.

Filling Defect: During a myelogram, dye is injected into the subarachnoid space and outlines the nerve roots. If there is pressure on a nerve root, often that nerve root will not fill with dye. See Nerve Root Filling, Filling—Nerve Root.

Filling—Nerve Root: During a myelogram, dye is injected into the subarachnoid space and outlines the nerve roots. If there is pressure on a nerve root, often that nerve root will not fill with dye. See Nerve Root Filling, Filling Defect.

Filum Terminale: The "terminal thread" of the pia mater, which extends from the tip of the spinal cord to blend with the periosteum on the posterior coccyx. The function is likely to anchor the spinal cord and dura. There are two portions: the externum and the internum. The former is surrounded by dura, while the latter is merged with the dura.

Filum Terminale Syndrome: A progressive neurologic deficit seen in patients with spina bifida and myelomeningocele. See Tethered Cord Syndrome.

Fioricet with Codeine: A Fioricet tablet with 30 mg of codeine phosphate. The common dosage includes one to two capsules every 4 hours, and total daily dosage should not exceed six capsules. See Codeine.

Fiorinal: A medication used for the relief of the symptom complex of headache and is classified as an abortive. This contains butalbital (a barbiturate), acetaminophen, and caffeine. This is contraindicated in patients with porphyria and can be addictive due to the barbiturate component. The common dosage is one or two capsules every 4 hours as needed. Total daily dosage should not exceed six tablets. Using this medication more than two days a week may cause rebound headache. See Muscle Contraction Headache, Tension Headache.

Fiorinal with Codeine: A Fiorinal capsule which also contains 30 mg of codeine phosphate. Common dosage is one to two capsules every four hours with a total daily dosage not to exceed six capsules. See Fiorinal, Codeine.

First Rib Mobilization: A gentle mobilization of the first rib used to treat thoracic outlet syndrome. In this case, it is thought that decreased first rib mobility irritates the brachial plexus. By increasing first rib available range of motion, brachial plexus irritation decreases. This technique can be performed as a direct technique using the scalenes with direct pressure over the first rib or as an indirect technique.

First Thoracic Nerve Root Test: A physical exam maneuver performed with the patient in the seated position. The patient then abducts the shoulder to 90° with the forearm pronated. The elbow is then flexed to 90°. The forearm is then pronated fully and the elbow fully flexed with the pronated hand placed behind the neck or head. Pain elicited in the scapular regions suggests a T1 nerve root involvement.

FIS: A McKenzie test maneuver in which the patient flexes forward at the spine while standing to see if this reproduces the usual symptom complex. See Flexion in Standing.

Fish Mouth Sign: A radiology term used to denote an extruded disc on MRI. On sagittal proton density images, the outermost annulus appears as a dark band. When the nucleus pulposus breaks through the outer most annulus, it resembles a fish mouth.

Fish Vertebra: An increase in concavity of the end plates seen at multiple continuous levels and commonly associated with osteoporosis. This makes the individual vertebral segments look like the vertebra of a normal fish. This occurs due to structural weakness in the end plates and mechanical stress from the nucleus pulposus. This is also associated with Paget's disease and hyperparathyroidism. See Cod Fish Vertebra, Hourglass Vertebra.

Fixateur Interne: Spinal instrumentation used for limited pedicle fixation of a thoracolumbar spine fracture.

Fixation: A chiropractic term used to denote a vertebral segment that does not move freely in all directions. Fixations are usually addressed by manipulating into the direction of lost movement. See Subluxation, Interosseous Disc Relationship, Spinal Subluxation.

Fixation Dysfunction: A chiropractic term which refers to restricted motion in the functional spinal unit. Put more simply, this refers to restricted motion in one or more directions. See Fixation.

Fixation Subluxation: A chiropractic term which refers to a vertebral segment which is hypomobile on motion palpation. See Fixation.

fix/dys: A chiropractic term which refers to restricted motion in the functional spinal unit. See Fixation Dysfunction, Subluxation.

Fixed Stenosis: A type of lateral recess stenosis which occurs when degenerative disc disease has advanced to the level of "stabilization." Significant bony hypertrophy has occurred.

Flaccid Paralysis: A paraplegia or quadriplegia that affects the lower motor neurons and results in complete loss of muscle tone and deep tendon reflexes. This is secondary to a lower motor neuron lesion.

Flat Low Back Posture: A standing posture that demonstrates a decreased lumbosacral angle, a decreased lumbar lordosis, hip extension, and backward tilting of the pelvis. This is usually caused by lack of a normal lumbar curve and places much stress on the posterior longitudinal ligament. The abdominals are usually tight along with the hip extensors. The lumbar extensors are usually stretched and weak.

Flat Upper Back Posture: A standing posture characterized by a decrease in the thoracic curve, low riding scapulae, depressed clavicles, and a flat neck. It looks similar to a military posture. There can be fatigue in the muscles required to maintain the posture, and thoracic outlet syndrome may develop. The thoracic erector spinae and scapular retractors are tight. The scapular protractors and muscles of the anterior thorax are weak.

Flex. c. rad.: An abbreviation for *flexor carpi radialis*.

Flex. c. uln.: An abbreviation for *flexor carpi ulnaris*.

Flex. dig. prof.: An abbreviation for *flexor digitorum profundus*.

Flex. dig. subl.: An abbreviation for *flexor digitorus sublimis*.

Flex. dig. supr.: An abbreviation for *flexor digitorum superficialis*.

Flexeril: A muscle relaxant which acts at the brain-stem level to decrease muscular activity without acting directly on muscle contraction. It is related to the tricyclic antidepressants. This drug is not effective in spasticity due to central nervous system disorders such as CVA. It cannot be used in conjunction with MAO inhibitors or in the acute recovery phase of MI, patients with arrhythmias, heart block, or conduction disturbances, or in patients with congestive heart failure. It is also contraindicated in hyperthyroidism. It may enhance the effects of alcohol, barbiturates, and other CNS depressants. The usual adult dosage is 10 mg three times a day and should not exceed 60 mg a day. The use of this drug for periods greater than 2–3 weeks is not recommended according to the PDR. See Cyclobenzaprine.

Flexibility: The ability of a muscle or connective tissue to yield to stretching.

Flexion: A movement that brings two parts of a joint or body into a bent position. In the spine, this is starting straight and moving into forward bending.

Flexion Abduction External Rotation: A test for SI joint syndrome which puts the hip into flexion, abduction, and external rotation. See FABER Test.

Flexion Bias: A term often used by therapists who use spinal stabilization as treatment. This refers to a stabilization program where the spine is held in a flexion posture to avoid symptoms and during the stabilization exercises.

Flexion—Craniosacral: Motion that occurs during craniosacral rythym when the sacrum counternutates and the sphenobasilar symphysis ascends. See Craniosacral Flexion.

Flexion-Distraction: A chiropractic technique which involves traction force to reduce disc bulging into the intervertebral foramen and/or spinal canal. See Cox Flexion-Distraction.

Flexion Dysfunction of the Sacrum: An osteopathic or manual physical therapy term used to denote a sacral position such that the sacral base is anterior and inferior and the apex is posterior and superior. See Bilaterally Extended Sacrum.

Flexion–Extension Injury: A sprain/strain syndrome of the cervical spine caused by a hyperextension–hyperflexion injury. See Acceleration–Deceleration Injury, Whiplash Injury.

Flexion–Extension Views: X-rays taken in the extremes of flexion and extension to detect abnormal segmental movement of the vertebral bodies. This technique can be used with spondylolisthesis to determine if there is "slipping" of one vertebral segment on another. This is also used to look for segmental instability (small abnormal movements in the vertebral segments). After serious trauma these views can help to rule out large abnormal movements of the vertebral column (instability) that might lead to possible spinal cord damage or radiculopathy. See Stress Evaluation.

Flexion in Lying: A McKenzie test maneuver which involves bringing the patient's legs to the chest to determine if this reproduces the patient's characteristic pain. See FIL.

Flexion in Standing: A McKenzie test maneuver in which the patient flexes forward at the spine while standing to see if this reproduces the usual symptom complex. See FIS.

Flexion Left: Bending to the left. See Side Bending.

Flexion Malposition: A chiropractic term which refers to a segment which is noted to be statically "flexed" relative to the adjacent vertebrae. This means that the anterior portion of the vertebra is inferior and the spinous process is superior. The spinous will be noted to be closer to the spinous above. The spinous and both transverse processes appear more prominent. See Posterosuperior Subluxation.

Flexion-Relaxation Phenomenon: A change in EMG activity of the paraspinal muscles that occurs as a person bends forward from standing. See FRP.

Flexion Restriction Side Bending: An osteopathic or manual physical therapy term which describes a restriction of movement of a vertebral segment into extension and side bending to one side. See FRS.

Flexion Right: Bending to the right. See Side Bending.

Flexion—Sacral: When the base of the sacrum (top of the sacrum) moves anteriorly in relation to the ilia. See Sacral Flexion, Sacral Nutation, Sacral Forward Bending.

Flip Angle: In gradient echo recalled MRI images, the signal intensity (image contrast) not only varies as a function of TR and TE but also depends on the flip angle selected. Altering the flip angle may be helpful in looking at tissue interfaces such as fat–muscle, muscle–fluid, and fat–fluid. See GRE.

Flip Test: A physical exam maneuver used to test for radiculopathy. The patient sits on an examination table with the back straight and the legs extended. If there is a radiculopathy, the patient will not be able to maintain this position without flexing the knee or raising the hip from the table in order to relieve nerve root tension.

Floor Lift: A lift from the ground which is commonly tested by computerized isometric equipment. The patient is in a full flexed posture with the knees bent, crouching to lift from the floor.

Floor to Knuckle: A type of lift tested during a functional capacity evaluation. The patient is asked to lift from floor height to just below waist level.

Flowing Hyperostosis: A radiographic term which describes the calcification of the ALL in diffuse idiopathic skeletal hyperostosis.

Fluori-Methane Spray: An organic solvent spray which evaporates quickly and is used in spray and stretch technique. This produces a sensation of cold on the skin and is used to provide a neurophysiologic distraction while a stretch is applied. See Spray and Stretch.

Fluoroscopically Guided: The use of a fluoroscope (real time x-ray) to determine correct needle placement in spinal injections. For instance, an SI joint injection is often done under fluoroscopic guidance.

Fluoroscopy: A type of real time x-ray imaging which allows bony anatomy to be viewed during injection procedures. A C-arm is used to allow the fluoroscope beam to be convienently placed over the area to be viewed. See C-arm.

Fluoxetine: An antidepressant. See Prozac.

FmHx: An abbreviation for *family history.*

Focal Arachnoiditis: An inflammatory reaction of the arachnoid membrane (one of the coverings of the spinal cord and brain) which is localized and usually seen adjacent to disc herniations. This focal inflammatory response may lead to scarring in that area. See Focal Spinal Arachnoiditis, Intradural Arachnoid Irritation.

Focal Arachnoid Scarring: An inflammatory reaction of the arachnoid membrane (one of the coverings of the spinal cord and brain) which is localized and usually seen adjacent to disc herniations. See Focal Arachnoiditis, Focal Spinal Arachnoiditis.

Focal Cervical Dystonia: An abnormal twisting posture of the head and cervical spine. See Torticollis, BOTOX.

Focal Spinal Arachnoiditis: An inflammatory reaction of the arachnoid membrane (one of the coverings of the spinal cord and brain) which is localized and usually seen adjacent to disc herniations. See Focal Arachnoiditis, Intradural Arachnoid Irritation.

Foix-Alajouanine Syndrome: The subacute or acute progression of myelopathy caused by the spontaneous thrombosis of a spinal cord AVM. See AV Fistula.

Fold and Hold: A technique of treatment which is advocated for the treatment of acute and subacute muscular strain. See Strain-Counterstrain.

Foot—Pronated: A foot that is turned outward (sole of the foot points to the outside). See Pronated Foot.

Footrest: A supporting device for the feet which is used while sitting or standing. While sitting, supporting the lower extremities is thought to decrease the lordosis in the low back. Also, this provides a derotation to the pelvis. While standing, the non–weight bearing foot is placed on the footrest.

Foramen: The space through which the nerve root and nerve root sheath must pass to exit the spinal canal. There are two foramens per level which are composed of arches in the vertebrae above and below. They are the "window" through which the nerve roots pass. The size of the foramen can be decreased with degenerative disc disease or an acute disc herniation. The size can also be decreased by pseudohypertrophy of the ligamentum flavum, spondylosis, or facet joint hypertrophy. See Intervertebral Foramen, Neural Foramina, Vertebral Foramen.

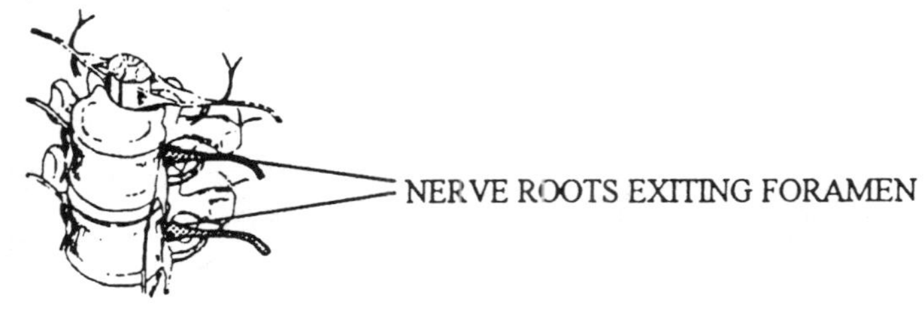

Foramen Arcuale: A relatively uncommon syndrome characterized by dizziness, light-headedness, vertigo, vasomotor face disturbances, retro-orbital pain, disturbances of vision, and other symptoms. See Syndrome of Barre-Lieou.

Foramen Magnum: The hole in the base of the skull through which the brain stem passes.

Foramen Magnum Line: A line drawn between the anterior and posterior margins of the foramen magnum on a lateral skull. See McRae's Line.

Foraminal Compression Test: A physical examination maneuver used to close off the foramen and compress the exiting nerve root. The test is performed as a screen for nerve root irritation, HNP, or foraminal stenosis. The patient is seated with the head and neck in a neutral position. The examiner exerts progressively increasing compression on the head and neck. A positive test is reproduction of a radicular pain pattern (radiation of numbness or tingling into a dermatome of the upper extremity). Another testing technique has also been described. For this maneuver, the head is rotated toward the side of the complaint and then compression is applied. See Jackson's Lateral Compression Test.

Foraminal Disc Herniation: A herniated disc that extends into the foramen (the window through which the nerve roots pass). Since the nerve root passes through this area, nerve root compression is common. See Far Lateral Disc Herniation.

Foraminal Stenosis: A decrease in the overall size of the intervertebral foramen (the bony window through which the nerve roots pass) caused by enlargement of the superior facet or a degenerative disc. The nerve root passing through the foramen can become irritated or compressed. Severe foraminal stenosis can cause radiculopathy. Conservative management tends to be less effective. Surgical management can include enlarging the foramen by removing bone, a decompressive laminectomy, and/or fusion to reduce continued facet joint degeneration. See Bony Compression, IVF Encroachment, Neuroforaminal Compromise.

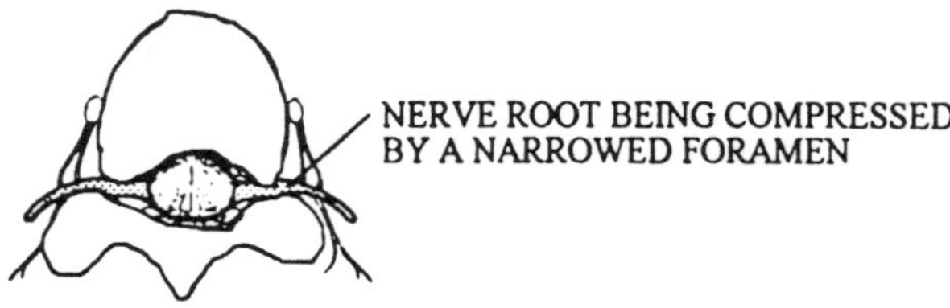

Foraminotomy: A "cleaning out" of the intervertebral foramen to provide more space for the nerve root. A foraminotomy can be combined with other procedures, such as laminectomy, discectomy, or fusion, in an attempt to cause further nerve root or cord decompression or add stability. See Laminectomy, Laminoforaminotomy.

Force Couple: Muscles which act together to rotate a part about its axis. For instance, force couple between the upper and lower trapezius muscles rotates the scapula in abduction.

Forrestier's Bowstring Sign: A physical exam maneuver in which the patient stands and the examiner observes any asymmetry in the spinal musculature and posture. The patient is then asked to laterally bend to one side. If there is tightening or contracture of the ipsilateral musculature, this suggests ankylosing spondylitis. Lateral flexion is compared bilaterally, and asymmetrical motion is identified in the thoracic spine. This is nonspecific test in that any thoracic spine involvement could give a positive test.

Forrestier's Disease: A syndrome which involves diffuse ligamentous calcification and ossification seen in 5–10% of patients over 65 years of age. See DISH, Ankylosing Hyperostosis.

Forward Bending: Flexion of the spine. See Bending—Forward.

Forward Bent Sacrum: An osteopathic or manual physical therapy term used to denote a sacral position such that the base is anterior and inferior and the apex is posterior and superior. See Bilaterally Flexed Sacrum.

Forward Flexion View: The flexion portion of a flexion/extension x-ray series. See Flexion–Extension Views.

Forward Head: A head and neck position often seen after whiplash injuries.

Forward Head Position: A head and neck position often seen after whiplash injuries. The head is displaced forward with extension at the atlanto-occipital joint and flexion in the lower cervical spine. The sternocleidomastoid and suboccipital muscles can be shortened and thus prevent the head from being brought back into normal alignment. See Forward Head Posture, Forward Head, Gooseneck Deformity, Forward Head.

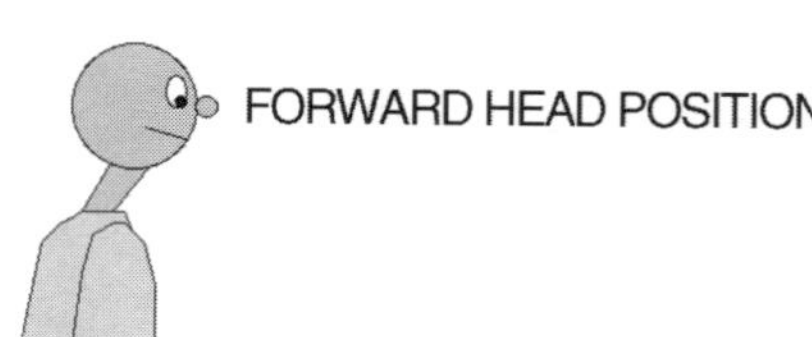

Forward Head Posture: A head and neck position often seen after whiplash injuries. See Forward Head Position.

Forward Ilium: A movement dysfunction of the pelvis in which the ilium is noted to be anterior-inferior relative to the sacrum. See Anterior Ilium, Forward Innominate, Forward Innominate Rotation, Anterior Iliac Rotation, Anteriorly Rotated Ilium, Anterior Innominate, Anteriorly Rotated Innominate.

Forward Innominate: A movement dysfunction of the pelvis in which the ilium is noted to be anterior-inferior relative to the sacrum. See Forward Innominate Rotation, Forward Ilium, Anterior Ilium, Anterior Iliac Rotation, Anteriorly Rotated Ilium, Anterior Innominate, Anteriorly Rotated Innominate.

Forward Innominate Rotation: A movement dysfunction of the pelvis in which the ilium is noted to be anterior-inferior relative to the sacrum. See Forward Innominate, Forward Ilium, Anterior Ilium, Anterior Iliac Rotation, Anteriorly Rotated Ilium, Anterior Innominate, Anteriorly Rotated Innominate.

Forward Sacral Torsion: An osteopathic or manual physical therapy term which describes a sacral torsion along an oblique sacral axis (from one sacral base to the opposite ILA). The dysfunction is named "left on left" or "right on right." The sacral base becomes more asymmetrical in flexion with the side opposite the torsion moving forward (left on left with the right sacral base moving forward). The lumbar spine is concave to the side of the torsion (for example, left on left with the left lumbar concave to the left) and because of this the same side leg is short (in this example, left). This is caused by tightness or spasm in the piriformis and can be named as right on right or left on left. Treatment is through muscle energy technique correction, strain–counterstrain, or myofascial release to the piriformis. See Anterior Torsion, Left-Facing Sacrum, Right-on-Right Sacral Torsion.

Four-poster Orthosis: A cervical orthosis which extends down to the upper thoracic spine and is intermediate in its effectiveness in controlling overall cervical range of motion. Four metal rods add to its stability. It does control all three axes of cervical range of motion and provides better overall stability than a Philadelphia collar or a Thomas collar.

Fractured Dens: A fracture of the tooth-like process of C2. See Odontoid Fracture.

Fracture Dislocation of the Thoracic Spine: A fracture of the thoracic spine with separation of the fractured segment. This most commonly occurs in the T4–T7 region. Fractures of the lamina, facets, and vertebral bodies are seen. Paraplegia is a frequent complication, and the most common etiology is a significant impact motor vehicle accident.

Fractured Odontoid: A fracture of the tooth-like process of C2. See Odontoid Fracture.

Fracture of the Posterior Arch of the Atlas: A fracture of the posterior portion of the arch of the atlas. See Fracture of the Posterior Arch of C1.

Fracture of the Posterior Arch of C1: A fracture of the posterior portion of the arch of the atlas. This is usually caused by an axial load or compressive force and can be associated with a hangman's fracture. A lateral cervical x-ray can be used for diagnosis. The vertebral artery may be involved, and this fracture can be associated with symptoms of vertebrobasilar insufficiency. See Posterior Arch of C1 Fracture, Fracture of the Posterior Arch of the Atlas, Hangman's Fracture.

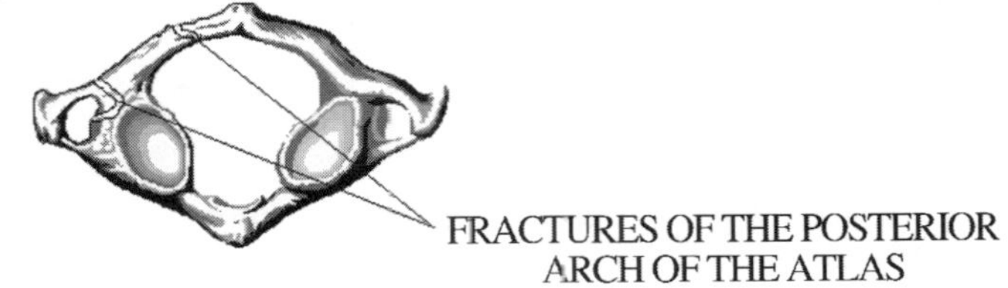

Fracture Sacral—Vertical: A fracture of the sacrum which usually occurs due to indirect trauma to the pelvis. See Vertical Fracture of the Sacrum, Sacral Fracture—Vertical, Vertical Sacral Fracture.

Free Fragment: A fragment of an extruded disc that becomes disconnected from the parent disc and can migrate into the subligamentous space, retroligamentous space, or rarely intradurally. See Sequestered Disc.

Free Weights: Weights used for strength training which are not part of any machinery. A standard dumbbell is an example of this type of weight-lifting equipment.

Freeze-dried Bone: Bone which is preserved through rapid freezing and then dehydrating in a vacuum. This bone is commonly used for allograft fusions. See Allograft, Fusion, Bank Bone.

Frontal Headaches: A type of headache which occurs in the forehead.

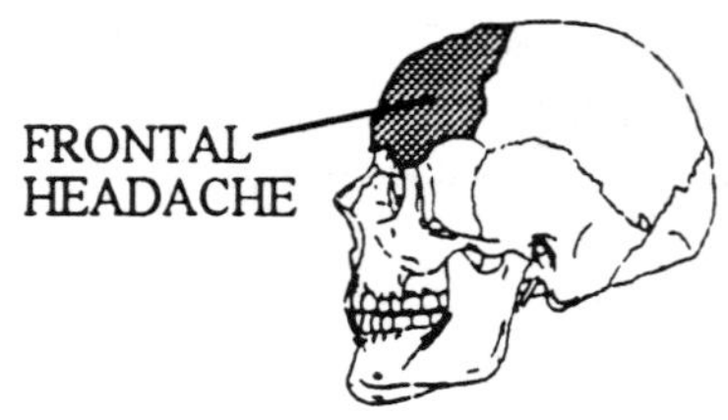

Frontal-Occipital Headaches: Pain which is usually described as starting at the base of the skull or in the back of the head and radiating to the forehead. This type of headache is commonly seen after whiplash injuries. It has been associated with trigger points in the semispinalis capitus, rectus capitus posterior minor, and upper trapezius. It also seems to be associated with biomechanical abnormaities at the OA or AA joints.

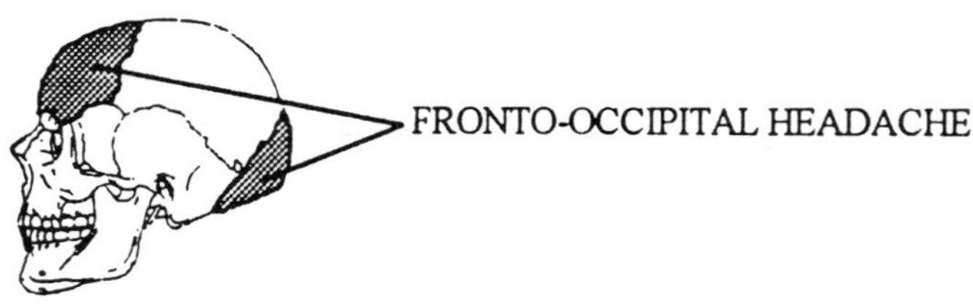

Frozen Shoulder: A marked decrease in range of motion, usually in one shoulder and of unknown etiology. See Adhesive Capsulitis, Scaphohumeral Periarthritis.

FRP: A change in EMG activity of the paraspinal muscles that occurs as a person bends forward from standing. At first, EMG activity increases as the load increment increases and the muscles support the spine. Later, as the ligaments take over, the muscles relax to a level below that obtained when the subject was standing. See Flexion-Relaxation Phenomenon.

FRS: An osteopathic or manual physical therapy term which describes a restriction of movement of a vertebral segment into extension and side bending to one side. Common treatments: muscle energy techniques, joint mobilization, manipulation, Jones strain-Counterstrain. This may be associated with a facet syndrome. See Flexion Restriction Side Bending.

FRSL: An osteopathic or manual physical therapy term which describes a vertebral segment that is flexed, rotated to the left, and side bent to the left. This means that the motion of the segment is restricted in extension, rotation to the right, and side bending to the right.

FRSR: An osteopathic or manual physical therapy term which describes a vertebral segment that is flexed, rotated to the right, and side bent to the right. This means that the motion of the segment is restricted in extension, rotation to the left, and side bending to the left.

Fryette's Laws: Three laws governing lumbar or thoracic spinal motion. The first law (type 1 behavior) states that when the lumbar or thoracic spine is in a neutral position, side bending and rotation occur in opposite directions. The second law (type 2 behavior) states that when the lumbar or thoracic spine is flexed (discal control) or extended (facet control), side bending and rotation will occur in the same direction. It should be noted that the second law also pertains to the cervical spine with the exception of C0–C1 and C1–C2. The third law (closed system mechanics) states that when motion is introduced in one direction, movement in all other directions will be reduced.

FS: An abbreviation for *full spine.*

FSCO: Federation of Straight Chiropractic Organizations.

Fulcrum Fracture: A horizontal fracture through both the vertebral body and the posterior elements produced by a hyperflexion injury. See Chance Fracture.

Full Curve: A scoliotic curve which encompasses the entire spine such that the only horizontal vertebra is at the apex.

Full Spine: A chiropractic technique which considers all spinal levels. This is in contrast to techniques which consider only specific areas of the spine.

Full Spine Radiography: A technique for evaluation of the entire spinal column on one 14″ × 36″ AP x-ray film.

Functional Activities: Those self-care functions that an individual must perform every day for normal hygiene. See Activities of Daily Living, ADL.

Functional Capacity Assessment: A test of physical strength and stamina used to determine working restrictions and work tolerance. See FCE, Functional Capacity Evaluation.

Functional Capacity Evaluation: A test of physical strength and stamina used to determine working restrictions and work tolerance. This is usually combined with some form of computerized dynamometry (computerized strength testing). Statements are made about lift/carry abilities, push/pull abilities, and postures to be avoided at work. A coefficient of variance is often given in an attempt to determine the validity of the patient's effort. A high coefficient of variance (> 15%) can mean that the patient has not given a true maximal effort. This can be due to either self-limiting pain behaviors or, rarely, malingering. A job strength index is often quoted, which is the patient's maximum lift relative to the maximum lift that the patient must perform at work. See FCE, Physical Capacity Evaluation, Work Capacity Evaluation, WCE, Work Tolerance Screening.

Functional Curve: A compensatory scoliotic curve above or below a structural curve. This curve does not have a bony rotational component. See Nonstructural Scoliosis.

Functional Leg Length: The functional length of a lower extremity measured from the umbilicus to the medial malleolus. See Apparent Leg Length.

Functional Leg Length Discrepancy: A short leg due to an SI joint dysfunction or adaptive curve of the lumbar spine and not a difference in length of the leg bones. There is usually a small, subtle change in length. See Apparent Leg Length, Structural Leg Length Discrepancy, Functional Leg Length Inequality, Functional Short Leg, Shoe Lift.

Functional Leg Length Inequality: A short leg due to an SI joint dysfunction or adaptive curve of the lumbar spine and not a difference in length of the leg bones. See Functional Leg Length Discrepancy.

Functional Radiology: Use of x-ray motion studies to look for instability.

Functional Scoliosis: A reversible scoliosis of the spine which is not caused by bony changes. A functional scoliosis is usually due to one-sided muscle weakness or functional tightness which can be a compensatory mechanism for biomechanical problems elsewhere. See Scoliosis—Functional, Scoliosis, Nonstructural Scoliosis.

Functional Short Leg: A short leg due to an SI joint dysfunction or adaptive curve of the lumbar spine and not a difference in length of the leg bones. See Functional Leg Length Discrepancy.

Functional Technique: An osteopathic treatment approach during which the provider guides the dysfunctional part through movement with continous feedback. The dysfunctional joint is moved away from the barrier to movement to "unwind" the joint until the tissue tension is equal in all planes.

Fusion: A surgical procedure performed to eliminate movement over painful or unstable spinal segments. Spinal fusion is often used to treat degenerative disc disease but is also used to treat scoliosis, kyphosis, fractures, and tumors. A bone graft is placed across a spinal segment (anterior, posterior, or posterolateral). The graft then, ideally, grows together with the patients bone and the area is immobilized. The graft can be an autograft (bone taken from the patient) or an allograft (cadaver bone). The bony graft placed for fusion sometimes does not fuse. Many devices have been designed to aid fusion rates including magnetic stimulators and rigid instumentation (to hold a section of spine in place to allow it to fuse). Also, posterior fusion rates seem to be lower in smokers. See Spinal Fusion, Spinal Arthrodesis.

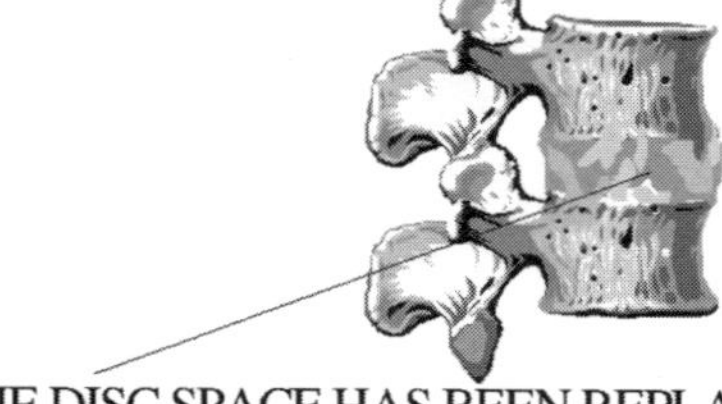

THE DISC SPACE HAS BEEN REPLACED WITH BONE GRAFT. THIS BONE GRAFT HAS FUSED WITH THE SURROUNDING BONE, PREVENTING THE TWO VERTEBRAE FROM MOVING.

Fusion—Intertransverse: The fusion of two spinal segments using bone graft placed between decorticated transverse processes. See Intertransverse Fusion.

Fusion Nonunion: A spinal fusion surgery with bone graft which has failed to heal together and fuse.

Fusion—SI Joint: A surgical procedure. See SI Joint Fusion, SI Arthrodesis, Sacroiliac Arthrodesis, Sacroiliac Fusion.

F-wave: A portion of a nerve conduction study which involves stimulating distally (i.e., near the wrist) and recording the response of a distal muscle (i.e., in the hand). The electrical impulse travels to the spinal cord and back down again stimulating the distal muscle. This differs from an H-reflex in that there is no reflex arc involved. This technique can be used to determine gross slowing in the nerve being tested but can not localize the slowing.

Fx: An abbreviation for *fracture*.

G

GAD: Gadopentetate dimeglumine. This is an intravenous contrast agent used in MRI which enhances scar tissue and other structures that are well vascularized. See Gadolinium.

Gadolinium: Gadopentetate dimeglumine. This is an intravenous contrast agent used in MRI which enhances scar tissue and other structures that are well vascularized. The most common use for gadolinium with MRI scanning of the spine is to evaluate postoperative scarring versus recurrent disc herniations. See GAD, Gadopentetate Dimeglumine.

Gadopentetate Dimeglumine: This is an intravenous contrast agent used in MRI which enhances scar tissue and other structures that are well vascularized. See Gadolinium, GAD.

Gaenslen's Sign: A physical exam maneuver for SI joint dysfunction. The test is performed by bringing one knee to the chest while the other hip is placed in extension off the edge of the table. A positive test would be pain in the SI joint region on the side of hip flexion. See Gaenslen's Test.

Gaenslen's Test: A physical exam maneuver for SI joint dysfunction. See Gaenslen's Sign.

Gait: The manner in which a patient walks. There are many different types of gaits depending on pathology.

Gait Evaluation: An examination technique in which the examiner observes the patient while walking. The type of gait is noted. For instance, if the patient's right hip drops, the left gluteus medius is suspected.

Gait Training: A technique used in spine rehabilitation to teach proper biomechanical techniques while walking. Usually, neutral spine posture is emphasized.

Gallie Fusion: A technique for posterior atlantoaxial fusion which involves wiring the posterior arch of the atlas and spinous process of the axis together. A bone graft is placed between the atlas and axis. One potential complication involves neurologic damage secondary to sublaminar wire placement. See Gallie Method.

Gallie Method: A technique for posterior atlantoaxial fusion which involves wiring the posterior arch of the atlas and spinous process of the axis together. See Gallie Fusion.

Gantry: The circular entrance or "doughnut" of a CT scanner or MRI scanner. The patient passes through the gantry when being scanned.

Gardner-Wells Tongs: A device used for skeletal traction of the cervical spine which is U-shaped with pins which are designed to follow the coronal contour of the skull. This is used to treat fractures of the cervical spine.

Garland-Thomas Line: A radiographic line for determining if there is anterolisthesis of L5 on S1 (spondylolisthesis). See Ullmann's Line.

Gas in Nucleus Pulposus: Gas noted to be within the disc space on radiographs. See Vacuum Sign.

Gastroc: Abbreviation for the *gastrocnemius muscle*, a muscle that makes up the bulk of the calf which is responsible for dorsiflexion of the foot. See Gastrocnemius, Calf Muscle.

Gastrocnemius: A muscle that makes up the bulk of the calf which is responsible for dorsiflexion of the foot. It crosses both the knee and ankle joints and is thus also capable of flexing the knee when the foot is not fixed, or maintaining extension of the knee in standing. Its two heads originate from the posterior medial and lateral femoral condyles and come together to join with the achilles tendon which inserts at the posterior calcaneus. It is innervated by the S1 and S2 roots and the tibial nerve. See Calf Muscle, Gastroc.

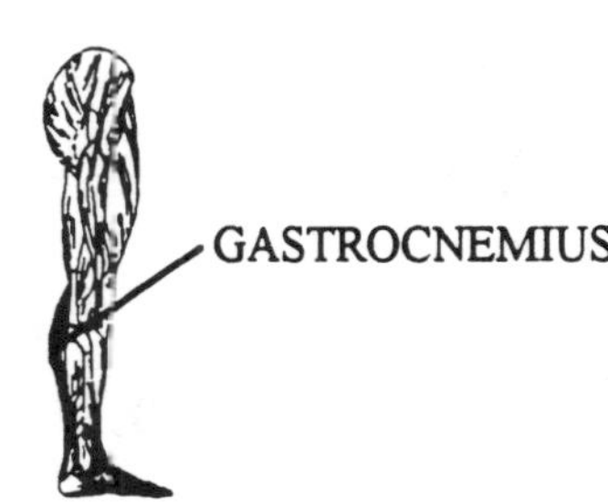

Gastroc Stretch: A physical therapy stretch performed against a wall. The patient places the leg to be stretched back and the other leg forward. The back leg is kept straight with the heel on the floor and turned slightly outward. The patient then leans into the wall until a stretch is felt in the gastrocnemius.

Generalized Back Pain: A nonspecific term for diffuse pain and tenderness within the low back.

Genitofemoral Nerve: A lower extremity peripheral nerve that originates from the second lumbar root and is primarily sensory. It carries sensation from the inner thigh and scrotum. Irritation of this nerve in the abdominal wall can cause painful hyperesthesia at the upper inner thigh and scrotum.

Genu Recurvatum: Hyperextension of the knee. This is commonly referred to as "back-kneed."

Genu Valgum: A valgus deformity at the knee. The feet are apart and the knees touch in this type of stance. This is commonly referred to as "knock-kneed."

Genu Varum: A varus deformity at the knees in which the knees are apart and the feet are closer together. This is commonly referred to as "bowlegged."

Geode: A focal region of bone loss. See Subchondral Cyst.

George's Line: A radiographic sign used to detect abnormal vertebral alignment. A lateral cervical view is taken. The posterior surfaces of the vertebral body are connected with a continuous line. Normally, a straight line cannot be drawn owing to the cervical lordosis. However, the key landmarks are the alignment of the superior and inferior posterior body corners. In normals, there is a smooth alignment of each posterior body corner. Flexion–extension films are often added. See Posterior Vertebral Alignment Line, Posterior Body Line.

GHJ: An abbreviation for *glenohumeral joint.*

Ghost Joint: An x-ray sign in late stage ankylosing spondylitis. This is an obliterated SI joint space due to SI joint fusion.

Giant Cell Tumor: A benign bony tumor of the spine which is slow growing but locally aggressive. The tumor is detected in the third or fourth decades of life and radiographs demonstrate an area of focal "rarification" (in contrast to a lytic appearance or marginal sclerosis). The most common site of involvement is the vertebral body, and the surrounding cortical bone is expanded as the tumor enlarges. A CT scan is helpful in diagnosis, and complete excision is recommended for treatment. A CT scan is also used to detect recurrences, and the patient should have routine CT follow-up. Radiation therapy is sometimes used following excision. Even though these tumors are considered benign, they are locally aggressive and do predict a bad prognosis including death. Management of this tumor can be tricky. A disease free margin should always be attempted; however, the extensive excision required may require instrumentation.

Gibbus: A sharp angular kyphotic deformation in the spine. This appears as a hump.

Gibbus Angle: An angle measured on lateral radiographs which determines the degree of kyphosis. The upper end plate of the normally positioned vertebra above and the lower end plate of the normally positioned vertebra below are determined. Lines are then drawn from these points, and an angle is measured between the two intersecting lines.

Gibbus Deformity: A severe form of thoracic kyphosis in which there is a significant hump in the thoracic spine.

Gillet SI Move: A chiropractic manipulation technique for the SI joint which is a long lever arm adjusting maneuver.

Gillet's Test: A common physical exam test used to detect SI joint dysfunction (abnormal SI joint movement). The patient stands while both PSISs are palpated with the thumbs. The patient then lifts one leg and the PSIS on that side should move inferiorly if that SI joint is normal. However, if the joint is hypomobile, the PSIS will be stationary or more superior. The joint is also assessed for a "feel" to see if one side is less mobile than the other. See March Test, Stork Test.

Gill Procedure: A technique of spinal decompression for spondylolisthesis. The "free floating" neural arch is excised to decompress L5 and S1. No fusion is performed.

Give Away Weakness: A nonphysiologic physical exam finding characterized by the patient's muscle "giving way" suddenly when resistance is applied. This is thought to be associated with symptom magnification or malingering.

Glasgow Coma Scale: A system for determining neurologic function after a traumatic injury to the head. Eye opening, verbal response, and motor response are graded. The lowest score is 3 and a normal score is 15.

Glide: A joint movement on a plane parallel to the joint surface. The spine can be "glided" from side to side to simulate a combination of lateral bending and rotation.

Glomus AVM: A glomus-type intradural, arteriovenous malformation. See Type 2 AVM.

Gluteal Gait: Weakness in the gluteal musculature that causes a tilting of the pelvis and trunk towards that side during the stance phase of walking. See Trendelenburg Gait.

Gluteal Muscles: The major extensors and external rotators of the hip. These muscles also play a major role in re-extension of the spine from a flexed postion. The group consists of the gluteus maximus, gluteus medius, and gluteus minimus. There can be decreased recruitment of these muscles with SI joint dysfunction, tight anterior hip capsule, and deconditioning.

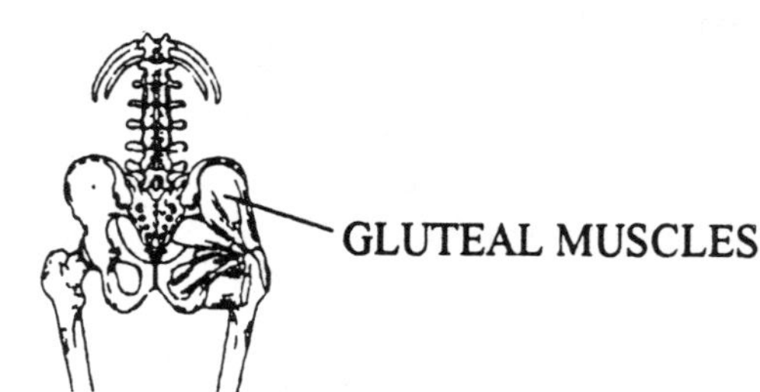

Gluteal Skyline Test: A physical exam test used to screen for lower lumbar radiculopathy. The test is based on the idea that the L5, S1, and S2 nerve roots innervate the gluteal musculature. The patient is viewed from the lower end of the table while lying prone. The patient is asked to contract the gluteals. Asymmetry of the gluteal musculature is considered a positive test.

Gluteus Maximus Muscle: One of the two major extensors of the spine, the other being the erector spinae. The gluteus maximus is involed in re-extension of the spine from 90 to 45°. It originates from the sacrum, the dorsal SI ligaments, the ilium near the PSIS, the thoracodorsal fascia, and the sacrotuberous ligament and inserts for the most part into the iliotibial tract with some fibers attaching to the linea aspera. Where the tendon passes over the greater trochanter, there is a bursa. It is a major extensor and external rotator of the hip with the foot free. With the hip in extension, it also acts as an adductor. The gluteus maximus is innervated by the inferior gluteal nerve from the sacral plexus (L5–S2).

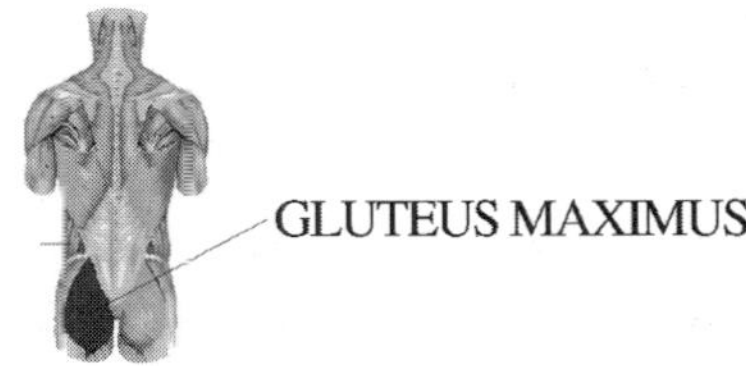

Gluteus Medius Gait: Weakness in the gluteal musculature that causes a tilting of the pelvis and trunk toward that side during the stance phase of walking. See Trendelenburg Gait.

Gluteus Medius Lurch: Weakness in the gluteal musculature that causes a tilting of the pelvis and trunk during the stance phase of walking. See Trendelenburg Gait.

Glut. max.: An abbreviation for *gluteus maximus.*

Glut. med.: An abbreviation for *gluteus medius.*

Gluts: Referring to the gluteal muscles. See Gluteal Muscles.

Goading: Deep pressure placed over a muscle similar to ischemic compression or deep massage.

Golfer's Fracture: When a golfer's swing is abruptly halted, a rib fracture may ensue. These usually occur at the lateral margin of the rib.

Golgi End Organs: Receptors found in the joint capsules which adapt slowly and continue to discharge. Unlike the ruffini end organs, golgi end organs can deliver information independently of the state of muscular contraction. These end organs have a major proprioceptive function and give information to the body about the position of a joint.

Golgi Tendon Receptors: Receptors located in the tendinous attachments of a muscle that detect excessive overload. When these receptors fire they inhibit the muscle in which they are located. They are tension-sensitive and not length-sensitive. Their function is to prevent muscular damage due to overload.

GON: An abbreviation for *greater occipital nerve.* See Greater Occipital Nerve.

Goniometer: A device used for measuring joint angle and range of motion. This is usually a simple protractor instrument.

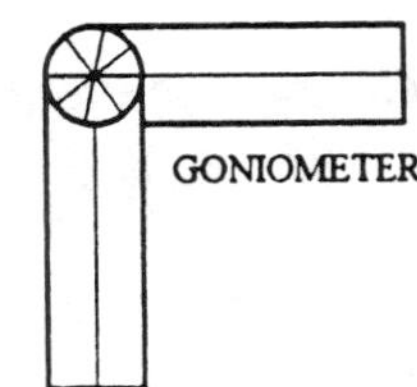

Gonstead Pelvic Marking System: A chiropractic system for full spine x-ray analysis which is a method of measuring innominate length and width, femoral head height (leg length and equality), and sacral rotation. A complicated series of dots are placed along various bony landmarks and perpendicular lines are drawn to measure distances.

Gonstead Technique: A chiropractic technique that uses the practitioner's hands to make corrections of the spine. This is a high-velocity (high-acceleration), low-amplitude adjusting technique. A side posture position is used to adjust the lumbar spine. This is the technique taught in most major chiropractic colleges and is used by more than half of the U.S. chiropractors.

Gooseneck Deformity: A head and neck position often seen after whiplash injuries. See Forward Head Position.

Gore Procedure: A surgical technique for anterior cervical fusion similar to the Simmon's procedure. See Simmon's Procedure.

Gout: An acutely painful, inflammatory arthritis characterized by the formation of crystals in the joint space due to hyperuricemia. The arthritis is caused by interarticular deposits of sodium monourate. Some patients develop aggregations of these crystals which may lead to a destructive arthropathy (tophi). Classically, the most common clinical manifestation is extreme pain in the feet, and more commonly, the big toe. However, there is spine involvement and radiographic changes in advanced long-standing disease. In approximately 15% of patients, the SI joint will be involved. Articular erosions and sclerosis are commonly seen on radiographs. Both SI joints are usually involved. Upper cervical involvement is also possible with odontoid erosions and atlantoaxial and subaxial instability. End plate erosions and facet joint degeneration of the lumbar spine is also seen.

Gower's Sign: A clinical observation traditionally made in patients with muscular dystrophy in which the patient must "climb up his or her legs" to re-extend at the hips. This can also be observed in patients with severe low back strain or low back pain.

GP: An abbreviation for *general practitioner*.

Grade 1 Manual Muscle Test: The inability of a muscle to move a joint through any part of its range of motion. See Manual Muscle Test—Grade 1.

Grade 1 Mobilization: A very small-amplitude movement applied to a joint at the beginning of the available range of motion. See Mobilization—Grade 1.

Grade 2 Manual Muscle Test: The ability of a muscle to move a joint against gravity through only part of its available range of motion. See Manual Muscle Test—Grade 2.

Grade 2 Mobilization: A large-amplitude mobilization in the middle of the available range of a spinal segment. See Mobilization—Grade 2.

Grade 3 Manual Muscle Test: The ability of a muscle to move a joint against gravity (without resistance) through its full range of motion. See Manual Muscle Test—Grade 3.

Grade 3 Mobilization: A large-amplitude mobilization at the end of the available range of motion of a spinal segment. This pushes the segment to the end of range of motion for that segment. See Mobilization—Grade 3.

Grade 4 Manual Muscle Test: The ability of a muscle to move a joint (against resistance) through its full range of motion. See Manual Muscle Test—Grade 4.

Grade 4 Mobilization: A small-amplitude mobilization at the end of the available range of motion for a spinal segment. This pushes that segment up to the end of range of motion. See Mobilization—Grade 4.

Grade 5 Manual Muscle Test: Normal muscle strength. See Manual Muscle Test—Grade 5.

Grade 5 Mobilization: Essentially the same thing as a manipulation. See Mobilization—Grade 5, Manipulation.

Gradient-Recalled Echo Image: An MR imaging sequence which is helpful because it depicts bony margins well. See GRE Imaging.

Graft Resorption: A surgical term referring to a bone graft for fusion which has been resorbed by the body. A pseudoarthrosis should be ruled out at this level (excessive motion).

Gravitational Line: The imaginary line that represents a plumb line dropped from the vertex of the head in a patient with perfect posture. This line passes through the external auditory canal, lateral head of the humerus, third lumbar vertebra, anterior third of the sacrum, greater trochanter, lateral condyle of the knee, and just anterior to the lateral malleolus. See Weight Bearing Line of L3.

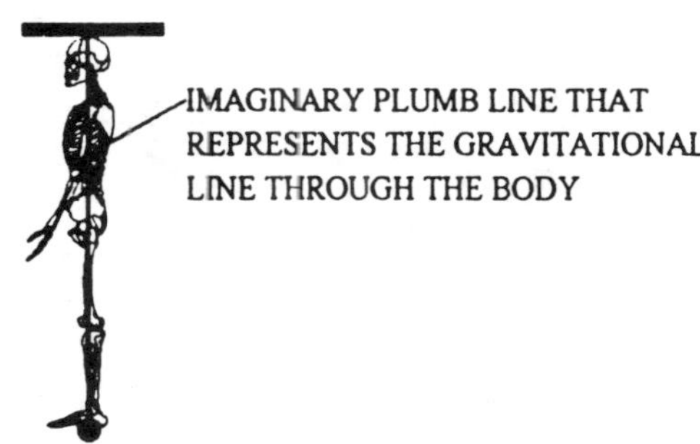

Gravity Unloading: A rehabilitation technique used in patients unable to tolerate exercises in normal gravity without pain. This can be accomplished either through pool therapy/aquatic therapy or through mechanical unloading, using traction devices. The proprietary name for this system is the Zuni unloading system or SOMA system. See Medical Exercise Therapy, SOMA, Zuni, Unloading Therapy.

Gray Matter: Central nervous system tissue which contains nerve cell bodies and neurons. These are unmyelinated structures (nerve fibers without insulation) which are gray against the myelinated white matter.

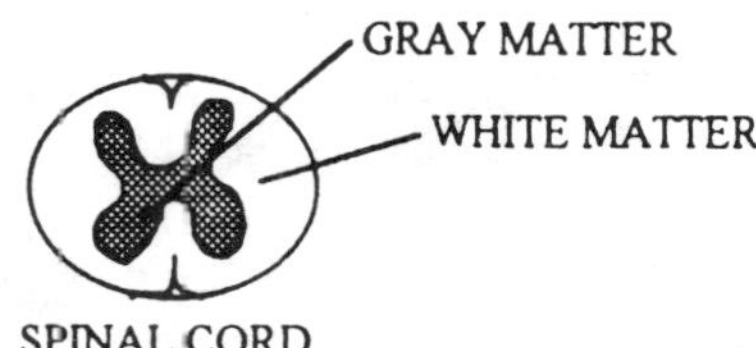

Gray Rami Communicantes: Postganglionic fibers that emerge from the sympathetic ganglia and connect to corresponding spinal nerves or to other fibers in the sympathetic chain. They serve as communicating pathways for the autonomic nervous system and merge with the sinuvertebral nerve. See Rami Communicantes.

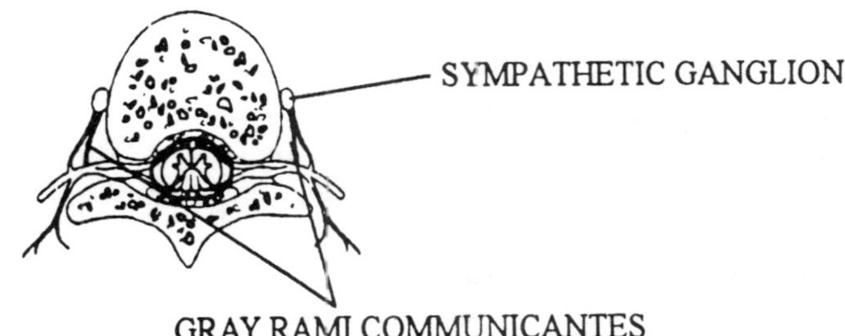

grd: An abbreviation for *grade*.

Greater Occipital Nerve: A clinical syndrome involving irritation of the greater occipital nerve as it passes through the semispinalis capitis and trapezius (according to Travell). See GON, Greater Occipital Neuralgia.

Greater Occipital Neuralgia: A clinical syndrome involving irritation of the greater occipital nerve as it passes through the semispinalis capitis and trapezius (according to Travell). This includes occipital headaches which can often radiate anteriorly. Entrapment is due to trigger point activity in the semispinalis capitis that produces taut bands that compress the nerve as it penetrates the muscle. This is commonly seen with chronic cervical myofascial pain or after whiplash injuries. Treatments include icing, spray and stretch, postural exercises, deep tissue work including myofascial release, ischemic compression or myotherapy, injection and stretch, and cervicothoracic stabilization techniques. This syndrome may be related to an upper cervical dysfunction which has similar symptoms. See Occipital Neuralgia, GON, Greater Occipital Nerve.

DISTRIBUTION OF GREATER OCCIPITAL
HEADACHES
GREATER OCCIPITAL NERVE EXIT SITE
THE PAIN CAN USUALLY BE EXACERBATED
OR MADE LESS BY APPLYING PRESSURE
IN THIS AREA.

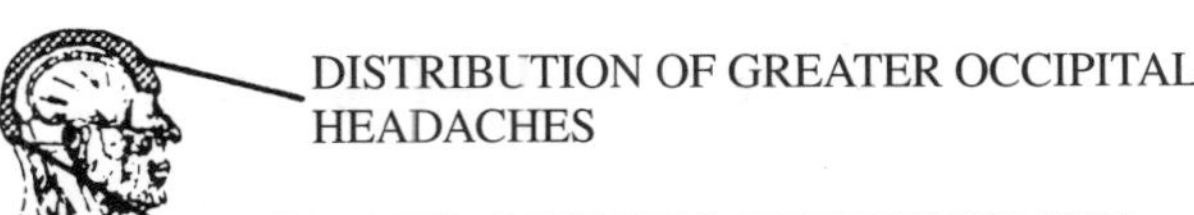

Greater Trochanter: A bony prominence on the femur which can be easily palpated in the lateral hip.

This is the insertion for the gluteus medius, gluteus minimus, obturator externus, gemelli, piriformis, and obturator internus. The trochanteric bursa overlies the greater trochanter.

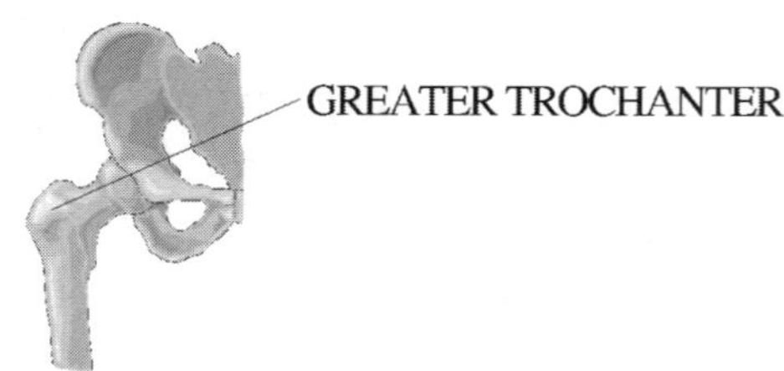

GRE Imaging: An MR imaging sequence which is helpful because it depicts bony margins well. For this reason, it is the imaging sequence of choice for viewing osteophytes or bony stenosis. This imaging sequence reduces total imaging time. See Gradient-Recalled Echo Image, Flip Angle.

Grip Dynamometer: A grip strength measuring device often used to determine if a patient is giving a maximum effort during functional capacities testing. See Jamar Dynamometer.

Grip Strength Measurements: The use of a hand dynamometer to quantify the amount of strength in the hand while gripping. See Grip Strength Testing.

Grip Strength Testing: The use of a hand dynamometer to quantify the amount of strength in the hand while gripping. This can also be used during a functional capacity evaluation to determine the coefficient of variation for a set of measurements. This in turn can be used to help identify when a patient is giving less than maximal effort. See Coefficient of Variation, Grip Strength Measurements.

Griswold Brace: A three-point brace with two pads anteriorly over the sternum and pubis and one pad posteriorly over the thoracolumbar area. This system restricts flexion of the thoracic and lumbar spine. See Jewett Brace.

Gross Instability: An orthopedic spine term which refers to excessive motion between two vertebral segments. Instability worsens with the progression of degenerative disc disease. Gross instability is defined as an angular deformity of 16° or greater or a translational deformity of greater than 10% of the end plate length (or 5 mm) on lateral flexion/extension radiographs.

Gross Motion: The overall motion of the joint.

Gross Range of Motion: A term that usually refers to the overall range of motion of a spinal region, for instance, overall cervical range of motion. This term can also be used to imply the total range of motion of any body part.

Grostic Technique: An upper cervical chiropractic technique that utilizes specific measured analysis of the cervical spine together with manual adjusting to re-establish a biomechanical balance of the spine. Sustained manual traction is used.

Guillford Collar: A cervical orthosis which also extends down to the upper thoracic spine. See Long Two-poster Orthosis.

Gymnastic Ball: A large, brightly colored rubber ball used in many lumbar stabilization programs. See Swiss Ball.

Gymnic Ball: A brand name for a Swiss ball. See Swiss Ball.

H

H/A: An abbreviation for *headache.*

HA: An abbreviation for *headache.*

Hackett Technique: A prolotherapy injection technique which was developed by Hackett in the 1930s. Dextrose is used almost exclusively as the proliferant. Injections are given every 6–12 weeks.

HADD: The deposition of hydroxyapatite crystals in multiple locations. See Hydroxyapatite Deposition Disease.

Halcion: A benzodiazepine used to induce sleep in insomnia. In clinically depressed patients, the worsening of depression, including suicidal ideation, is possible. As with all benzodiazepines, clearance in the elderly is decreased so a lower dosage should be given. There is significant abuse potential, so short-term use is recommended. Recommended adult dose is 0.25 mg every hour of sleep. The drug is supplied in 0.125 mg and 0.25 mg tablets. See Triazolam.

Halifax Fixation: A surgical technique and instrumentation designed for C1–C2 fusion. Interlaminar clamps are used. This technique provides superior stabilization to a Gallie fusion and approximately equal fixation to a Brooks fusion.

Hall-Pike Maneuver: This is a Dekleyn's test performed with the patient lying supine and the head extended off the end of the examination table. The examiner then adds extension, rotation, and lateral flexion checking for nystagmus or other neurovascular signs. See Dekleyn's Test.

Halo: A device used for immobilization of the cervical spine. A halo ring is placed just below the maximum diameter of the head and four pins are screwed into the skull. This is then connected to a vest-type orthosis through metal rods, which provide absolute stabilization of the cervical spine. This is often used in the treatment of cervical spine fractures or cervical spine instability.

Halo-Femoral Traction: A halo ring combined with pins placed in the distal femoral diaphyses to provide spinal traction. The halo ring is fixed to the skull by four pins.

Halo-Pelvic Device: A cervical, thoracic, lumbar, sacral orthosis used for immobilization of the thoracic and thoracolumbar spines. This provides the most stabilization and almost absolute control over flexion/extension, lateral bending, and axial rotation. This is used to treat clinical instability due to fractures, especially when neurologic compromise is a factor.

Halo-Pelvic Traction: A halo ring combined with a pelvic ring for use in providing spinal traction. The pelvic ring is secured through pins into the pelvis.

Halo Placement: The use of a halo orthosis following a surgical procedure or an unstable fracture. This is used after a cervical fusion without instrumentation or to provide stability to an unstable fracture.

Hamstring Stretch: A physical therapy stretch used to increase length in the hamstrings. There are many different techniques described for stretching hamstrings. Usually, the patient lies in a supine position supporting the spine on the floor. One technique has the patient bring one knee to the chest with the knee in flexion. The patient is asked to extend the knee and control the stretch by the degree of extension. Another technique uses a towel with the above technique to add tension. The patient can also perform this stretch through a doorway. The rationale behind stretching the hamstrings is that tight hamstrings will shunt biomechanical work to the erector spinae musculature and overload these muscles.

Hamstring Wall Stretch: A stretch for the hamstrings musculature that is performed through a doorway. One leg is extended and propped up against the side of the doorway. The opposite leg is through the doorway. The buttocks are moved slowly toward the wall until a stretch is felt in the back of the thigh.

Hand Dynamometer: A grip strength measuring device often used to determine if a patient is giving a maximum effort during functional capacities testing. See Jamar Dynamometer.

Handicap: A patient is handicapped if he or she has an impairment that substantially limits one or more of life's activities, has a record of such impairment, or is regarded as having such an impairment. This is obviously a very broad definition. Handicap can also be thought of as a barrier or obstacle to some activity.

Hangman's Fracture: A fracture of the second cervical vertebra. This fracture represents a traumatic spondylolisthesis. Fracture usually occurs in the most anterior portion of the lateral masses or into the pedicle. Neurologic symptoms vary. The most common cause of this fracture today is a motor vehicle accident. Stability and neurologic integrity should be assessed focusing on the integrity of the anterior elements. Facet joint dislocation and the alignment of C2 should also be assessed. Treatment depends on stability, neurologic status, facet joint status, and positioning. Common treatments include cervical collar, halo orthosis, traction, closed reduction, open reduction internal fixation, and removal of bony pieces from the spinal canal. See Type IV Spondylolisthesis.

Hard Disc: An HNP with osteophytes causing nerve root impingement. See Soft Disc.

Harrington Compression Rods: A surgical rodding system that applies a compressive force instead of distractive force in the correction of scoliosis. The rods tend to produce lumbar extension and thus are not used to treat lumbar degenerative disc disease. These rods are similar to Harrington distraction rods, but the hooks are turned in the opposite directions. See Harrington Distraction Rods.

Harrington Distraction Rods: A rodding system classically used in the surgical management of scoliosis that applies a distractive force to correct spinal curvature and provide stabilization. They are also used to treat spondylolisthesis and trauma. However, they are not classically used to treat degenerative disc disease. The complications can include problematic attachment of the lower end and loss of the lumbar lordosis. See Harrington Rods.

Harrington Rods: Rods which can be placed posteriorly in the lumbar spine and can add either compression or distraction forces in order to straighten a scoliotic spine. This system offers a broad range of stiffness, but generally requires longer fusion times. Similar systems include Cotrel-Dubousset, Edwards, and Jacobs rods and TSRH instrumentation. Disadvantages include the need for postoperative stabilization and obliteration of the normal sagittal curves.

Harrison Technique: A chiropractic technique which is considered "biophysics." This is one of the cervical techniques which uses an instrument to adjust.

Hartsill Fixation: Posterior segmental fixation with a wire that encircles the lamina in combination with a metal rod. The wire enters the spinal canal—and has inherent risks by doing so—but forms a sturdy attachment.

Hautant's Test: A test for vertebral artery insufficiency. The patient is seated and the shoulders are flexed to approximately 90° with the elbows extended and the forearms supinated. The patient is instructed to rotate his head fully to the right with eyes closed. The examiner is in front of the patient and monitors tendency for pronator drift of one extremity. If this occurs, the test is positive. The test is then repeated on the opposite side.

HE: An abbreviation for *hyperemic*.

Headache: Pain experienced in the head. The pain location can be periorbital, frontal, temporal, on the vertex, or occipital. With respect to the spine, headaches can be caused by abnormal cervical spine mechanics. One of the most common of these is an upper cervical dysfunction at the C0–C2 complex. Myofascial pain of many of the cervical muscles, including the sternocleidomastoid, suboccipitalis, semisplenius capitis, and upper trapezius, can also cause headache. TMJ syndrome can also cause headache either through a primary joint dysfunction or through the associated myofascial syndromes. Headaches can also be vascular in origin, such as migraine and cluster headaches. Treatment for an upper cervical dysfunction usually involves muscle energy technique correction of the biomechanical abnormality and/or strain-counterstrain. Manipulation or mobilization can also be helpful. Myofascial release, spray and stretch, ischemic compression, and trigger point injections are also common treatments. Often, after whiplash injury, there is excess OA extension and shortening of the suboccipitals with weakness of the deep cervical rotators, which can all lead to headache. See Tension Headache, Migraine Headache.

Heavy Work: A NIOSH work category which involves lifting up to 100 pounds frequently and/or carrying objects of up to 50 pounds.

Heel Lift: An orthotic or shoe insert which increases the height of the heel while walking. This is used commonly to correct a structural short leg. It is thought that an anterior ilium will be found on the side of the short leg. A heel lift can be used in an attempt to correct this dysfunction. See Inshoe Lift, Shoe Lift.

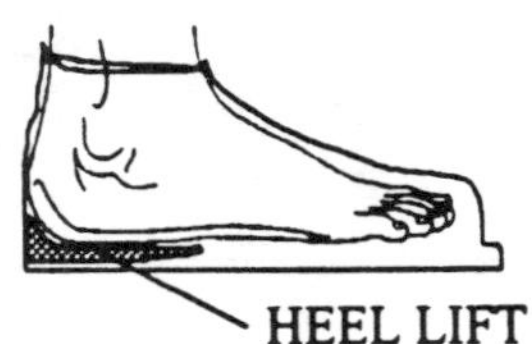

Heel–Toe Gait: A physical examination maneuver in which the patient is asked to walk on heels and then walk on toes across the room. This stresses the tibialis anterior and then gastrocsoleus in an antigravity fashion and is a screen for L4, L5, or S1 motor radiculopathies. If the patient cannot walk on the heels, an L4–L5 motor radiculopathy is suspected due to the tibialis anterior weakness. If the patient cannot walk on the toes, an S1 radiculopathy is suspected due to gastrocsoleus weakness. See Heel-to-Toe Gait.

Heel-to-Toe Gait: A physical examination maneuver in which the patient is asked to walk on heels and then walk on toes across the room. See Heel-Toe Gait.

Heel–Toe Walk Test: A physical examination maneuver positive in patients with significant motor involvement in the L4, L5, or S1 nerve roots. The patient is instructed to walk on the toes, while the examiner observes for heel drop during walking. The patient is then asked to walk on the heels and is observed for foot drop. Evidence of heel drop indicates gastrocsoleus weakness and a possible S1 motor radiculopathy. Evidence of foot drop indicates tibialis anterior and EHL weakness and possible L4 or L5 motor radiculopathy.

Heifetz Tong: A device used for cervical traction that is applied to the vertex of the skull.

Hellerwork: A system of deep tissue body work involving eleven 1-hour sessions. This technique is used to realign the body's myofascial planes in three dimensions. Dialogue is stressed during the sessions to allow the patient to become aware of emotional stress that may be related to physical tension. There is an element of movement training included in this system. Similar to rolfing, each session covers a specific area of the body. However, each session also includes a specific emotional focus.

Hemangioma: A common benign tumor of the spine. These occur in approximately 10% of all people, but are rarely symptomatic or of any clinical significance. Reports of deformity or pain related to vertebral hemangiomas are rare, but neurologic compromise has been reported. Diagnosis is usually made on plain radiographs and prominent vertical striations are usually seen. These lesions are frequently picked up on CT or MRI. Excision is performed only in rare cases and often requires identifying the vascular supply of the tumor before embolization or operative ligation can take place. See Vertebral Hemangioma.

Hemicord Syndrome: An incomplete form of spinal cord injury usually seen after a penetrating knife wound or gunshot wound. See Brown-Sequard Syndrome.

Hemilaminectomy: Removal of only half of the lamina during surgical decompression of a nerve root.

Hemisacralization: Congenital fusion of L5 to the sacrum which occurs only on one side.

Hemispherical Annular Degeneration: Degeneration of the intervertebral disc which may represent normal aging or may be due to longstanding trauma. See Degenerative Disc Disease.

Hemivertebra: The incomplete development of one side of a vertebra. There is a triangular deformity of the vertebral body that results in a scoliotic deformity. These deformities have been associated with other vertebral anomalities. See Lateral Hemivertebra.

HEP: An abbreviation for *home exercise program.*

hern: An abbreviation for *herniation.*

Herniated Disc: A "slipped disc." The term "slipped disc" is actually not correct since there is nothing to slip out of place. Instead, the disc is like a gel-filled, tough fibrous sack that gets a hole in it, causing the toothpaste-like gel to squirt out or herniate. This can cause pressure on the exiting nerve root and/or cause a significant inflammatory reaction that can lead to radiculopathy (dysfunction of the nerve root that can cause weakness, numbness, and/or tingling in one extremity). This term can mean anything along a spectrum of disc injury, including a disc bulge, a disc protrusion, an extruded disc, or a sequestered disc. See HNP, Herniated Nucleus Pulposus, Slipped Disc, Ruptured Disc, Extruded Disc, Disc Extrusion, Disc Hernia.

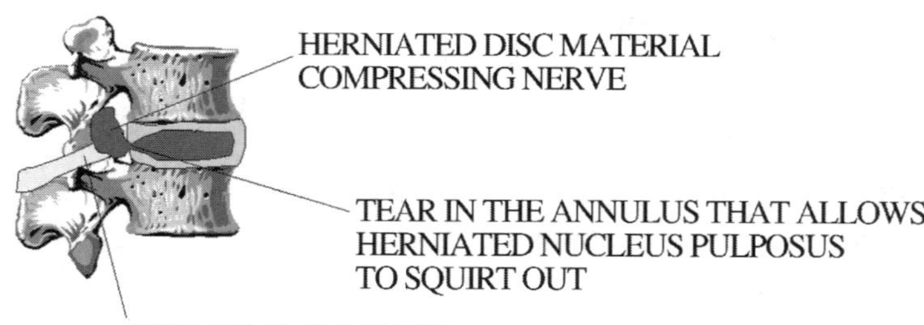

Herniated Nucleus Pulposus: A "slipped disc." See Herniated Disc, Disc Extrusion, HNP.

Heterograft: This ususally refers to a bone graft used for spinal fusion that was taken from an animal other than man. See Xenograft.

Hibb's Spinal Fusion: One of the first surgical techniques for spinal fusion, which involved placing bone grafts across the lamina and articular processes to achieve stabilization at four points.

Highet's Scale: One of the standard scales used throughout the medical community to grade muscle strength. It is graded 0–5 with a 5 being normal muscle strength. A 3/5 is defined as complete range of motion against gravity. A 4/5 is complete range of motion against gravity with some resistance. See Manual Muscle Testing.

High Far Lift: A type of lift commonly tested during an evaluation of work capacity. The patient's arms are away from the body at shoulder height as the patient pushes upwards. See High Near Lift.

High First Rib: A manual medicine term which is often associated with thoracic outlet syndrome. The first rib moves higher on inspiration than normal due to direct trauma to the supporting ligamentous structures or to hypertonicity or tightness in the anterior and/or middle scalenes. Since the first rib is the floor of the thoracic outlet, the brachial plexus (and/or subclavian artery) is irritated or compressed between the first rib and the roof of the thoracic outlet, the clavicle. Treatment is through direct or indirect muscle energy technique to the first rib, myofascial release of the scalenes, or mobilization of the clavicle or SC joint.

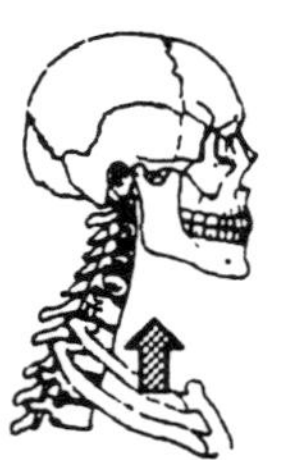

High Near Lift: A type of lift commonly tested during an evaluation of work capacity. The patient is in a standing position with elbows flexed and close to the body. The patient then pushes upward from approximately shoulder height. See High Far Lift.

High-velocity Thrust: A chiropractic or osteopathic manipulative procedure in which a low-amplitude, quick manipulation is delivered.

High-velocity Thrusting: The application of a force to a joint that takes it beyond its normal range of motion into its elastic range. See Manipulation.

Hilton's Law: Any nerve crossing a joint gives a branch to that joint.

HIO: Hole in one upper cervical adjusting technique. See HIO Technique, Palmer Upper Cervical Technique.

HIO Technique: A chiropractic technique that utilizes the x-ray analysis and adjusting techniques developed by B.J. Palmer to correct subluxations in the upper cervical spine (C1–C2). See Palmer Upper Cervical Technique.

Hip Extension—Prone: A lumbar stabilization exercise. See Prone Hip Extension.

Hip Flexion—Bilateral Isometric: A lumbar stabilization exercise. See Bilateral Isometric Hip Flexion.

Hip Flexion—Unilateral Isometric: A lumbar stabilization exercise. See Unilateral Isometric Hip Flexion.

Hip Flexor Stretch: A physical therapy exercise used to stretch the hip flexors (rectus femoris and iliopsoas). The patient takes a half-kneeling stance with one leg flexed forward at the hip and kneels with the other on the floor. Pelvic tilt is maintained as the patient is asked to stretch forward. This can also be performed with a foot on a chair (knee on the floor side) to stretch the rectus femoris more aggressively.

Hip Pointer: Contusion of the iliac crest or anterior superior iliac spine (ASIS). This may be associated with an evulsion of the muscles from the iliac crest. There is pain and swelling over the iliac crest or ASIS and there may be a hematoma. There may be limited side bending to the opposite side. Common treatments include icing, heat, injection of corticosteroids, anti-inflammatory medications, stretching after the acute stage, protection of this area, and decreasing activities.

Hip Rolls: A lumbar rotation exercise which involves starting in the hook lying position and rolling the flexed knees from side to side allowing small amounts of lumbar rotation.

Hip Scouring: An exam maneuver which is used to detect hip pathology presenting as low back pain. The examiner takes the patient's knee and thigh and pushes toward the acetabulum while sweeping the hip through all hip motions (internal rotation, external rotation, flexion, extension, abduction, and adduction). Pain or restrictions are noted.

Histaminic Cephalgia: A headache caused by excessive dilatation of the arteries in the brain. This is considered a vascular headache, and the etiology is unknown. See Migraine Headache.

HLA-B27: A laboratory blood test helpful in confirming the diagnosis of the spondyloarthropathies (ankylosing spondylitis [AS] and Reiter's syndrome). A positive test increases the likelihood of an ankylosing spondylitis significantly, and a negative test reduces the likelihood of this diagnosis. This test is usually ordered in patients with low back pain of insidious onset, with equivocal radiographic findings for anklyosing spondylitis with morning stiffness. A positive HLA-B27 antigen is found in over 87.5% of American caucasians with AS, while only 8% of American caucasians without AS have a positive HLA-B27. See Ankylosing Spondylitis.

HMO: Health maintenance organization.

HNP: An abbreviation for *herniated nucleus pulposus*, commonly called a "slipped disc." An extrusion of the nucleus pulposus through the anterior annular fibers. See Anterior HNP, Anterior Disc Herniation, Anterior Herniated Disc, Extruded Disc, Herniated Disc, Intervertebral Disc Displacement, Intervertebral Disc Rupture, Soft Disc.

HNP Central: A herniation of the nucleus pulposus that occurs medially instead of the usual posterior lateral direction. See Central HNP.

HP: An abbreviation for *hot pack*.

Hoffa Massage: A massage technique based on Hoffa's text published in 1900 and later revised by Max

Bohm in 1913. This represents classical massage techniques such as effleurage, petrissage, tapotement, and vibration. Focus is on mobilization of the myofascial system.

Hoffman Ligaments: A network of dural ligaments that attach the anterior thecal sac to the anterior and anterorolateral aspect of the spinal canal. These ligaments have a tethering effect on the neuraxis. In the lumbar spine, these ligaments are well developed and are tethered to the dura not only centrally but also in the lateral recess. These ligaments are thickest in the lumbar region and become more wispy in the thoracic spine. In the cervical spine, they are shorter and thicker. In essence, these ligaments act as an anchoring mechanism of the neuraxis to the rest of the body. A disc bulge can put compressive forces on the dura through these ligaments. See Dural Ligaments.

Hold-Relax: A proprioceptive neuromuscular facilitation (PNF)-muscle energy technique. See Contract-Relax.

Hold-Relax-Contract: A variation of the contract-relax technique. See Contract-Relax-Contract.

Hole in One: A chiropractic technique that utilizes the x-ray analysis and adjusting techniques developed by B.J. Palmer to correct subluxations in the upper cervical spine (C1–C2). See Palmer Upper Cervical Technique.

Hook Lying: Lying supine (on the back) with the knees at approximately a 90° angle. This position is used in a lumbar stabilization program as the correct position for sit-ups and abdominal strengthening. This is also used in other physical therapy programs as a starting position for many activities.

Hook-Lying Arm Raise Overhead: A lumbar stabilization exercise in which the patient starts in the hook-lying position. The patient is asked to tighten the stomach and squeeze the buttocks as one arm is lowered overhead. The arm is lowered until the patient feels the back begin to arch. This exercise is then repeated with the other arm. See Arm Raise Overhead—Hook-Lying.

Hook-Lying Bent Leg Lift: A lumbar stabilization exercise in which the patient starts in the hook-lying position. The patient is asked to tighten the stomach and squeeze the buttocks as one leg is raised approximately 3–4 inches off the floor. Neutral spine position is maintained throughout this exercise. This exercise is then repeated with the opposite leg. See Bent Leg Lift—Hook-Lying.

Hook-Lying Combination: A lumbar stabilization exercise where the patient starts in the hook-lying position. The patient is asked to tighten the stomach and squeeze the buttocks as one leg is raised 3–4 inches off the ground while the opposite arm is raised over the head and lowered. The exercise is repeated with the opposite arm and leg.

Hoover's Test: A test used to detect symptom magnification or malingering. The examiner places the patient's heels in his hands and asks the patient to lift one leg. Normally, there will be a downward pressure in the opposite leg to compensate for lifting the one leg off the table. However, the test is positive if there is no downward pressure on the opposite leg, because the patient is only feigning an attempt to lift the leg.

Horizontal Displacement: The loss of the ability of the spine under physiologic loads to maintain its pattern of normal movement. See Spinal Instability.

Horizontal Fracture of the Sacrum: The most common type of sacral fracture usually seen at the level of the third and fourth sacral segments near the lower end of the SI joint. If the fracture line is horizontal, it can be difficult to identify on an AP view. This is due to gas and fecal material in the bowels, and an enema may be helpful to aid in visualization. A lateral radiograph can be helpful in demonstrating the fracture. The lower segment can be displaced or angled forward. See Transverse Fracture of the Sacrum, Sacrum Fracture—Transverse, Horizontal Sacral Fracture, Sacrum Fracture—Horizontal, Transverse Sacral Fracture, Suicide Jumper's Fracture.

Horizontal Sacral Fracture: The most common type of sacral fracture usually seen at the level of the third and fourth sacral segments near the lower end of the SI joint. See Horizontal Fracture of the Sacrum, Suicide Jumper's Fracture, Transverse Sacral Fracture.

Hot Packs: A form of moist heat which consists of several sizes of segmented canvas bags filled with silicon dioxide. This allows this modality to use the large heat capacity of water to transfer moist heat to the body for up to 30 minutes. Indications for this type of superficial heating modality include pain, muscle spasm, bursitis, tenosynovitis, and myofascial pain. Heat is delivered very superficially and likely causes a vasodilatation with increased blood flow to the surface of the skin. However, it has also been postulated that reflex vasoconstriction and cooling occurs in deeper tissues. See Hydrocollator Packs, Hydro.

Hourglass Vertebra: An increase in concavity of the end plates seen at multiple continuous levels and commonly associated with osteoporosis. See Fish Vertebra, Cod Fish Vertebra.

H-reflex: The electronic representation of an Achilles' reflex. This is a long latency nerve conduction study. A delayed H-reflex (or decreased amplitude of the response) points to prior dysfunction or ongoing compression of the S1 nerve root or proximal sciatic nerve.

HT: An abbreviation for *hypertonic*.

Hunchback: A severe thoracic kyphosis that may be caused by severe scoliosis causing a large posterior thoracic rib hump.

Hurdler's Fracture: Avulsion of the apophysis of the ischial tuberosity as a result of a large contraction of the hamstrings. See Avulsion Fracture of the Ischial Tuberosity.

Hx: An abbreviation for *history*.

Hydro: An abbreviation for *hydrocollator packs*. See Hot Packs, Hydrocollator Packs.

Hydrocodone Bitartrate with APAP: The generic equivalent of Lortab and Vicodin. This is available in 2.5/500, 5.0/500, 5.0/750, 7.5/650, 7.5/750, and 10/650. The 7.5-mg hydrocodone tablet contains 750 mg of acetaminophen instead of the 500 that would be found in the equivalent Lortab tablet. See Lortab.

Hydrocollator Packs: A form of moist heat which consists of several sizes of segmented canvas bags filled with silicon dioxide. See Hot Packs.

Hydrocortisone Phosphate Injection: A synthetic adrenal corticosteroid which is used for intramuscular injection. For contraindications and drug interactions, see Steroid. This is available in an injectable solution of 50 mg per ml. This is a rapid-onset, but short-duration steroid. See Hydrocortone Acetate.

Hydrocortone Acetate: A synthetic adrenal corticosteroid which is used for intra-articular and soft tissue injection. This is a depot preparation which is longer-acting than hydrocortisone phosphate. For contraindications and drug interactions, see Steroid. A dose of 25–37.5 mg is used in the larger joints such as the knee; 10–25 mg is used in the small joints; 25–37.5 mg is used in the bursa; 5–12.5 mg is used in tendon sheaths; 25–50 mg is used for soft tissue infiltration; and 12.5–25 mg is used in ganglia. The drug is supplied in a 25 mg per ml form. A 50 mg per ml form is also available. See Hydrocortisone Phosphate Injection.

Hydromorphone: A hydrogenated ketone of morphine. See Dilaudid.

Hydroxyapatite Deposition Disease: The deposition of hydroxyapatite crystals in multiple locations. This disease effects both men and women equally from the middle-aged to the elderly. The most common joint involvement is at the shoulder, but involvement of the cervical and lumbar spine is not uncommon. Clinical features include pain, tenderness, lumbar swelling, and decreased range of motion. In the spine, these depositions are seen along the longus colli, nucleus pulposus, and anulus fibrosus. The patient complains of a painful stiff neck, muscle spasm, painful dysphasia, and sense of fullness in the throat. There is calcification just anterior to the C2–C3 vertebral bodies. The intervertebral disc becomes calcified, and when this occurs in the nucleus pulposus it mimics a normal discogram on x-ray. However, calcification of the annulus is more common than calcification of the nucleus. See Calcifying Tendinitis, Calcifying Bursitis, Tendinitis Calcarea, Periarthritis Calcarea, Hydroxyapatite Rheumatism, HADD.

Hydroxyapatite Rheumatism: The deposition of hydroxyapatite crystals in multiple locations. See Hydroxyapatite Deposition Disease.

Hyperabduction Maneuver: A physical exam test for thoracic outlet syndrome. Hyperabduction of the arm with the shoulder abducted and extended in an attempt to cause the neurovascular bundle to be compressed underneath the pectoralis minor and coracoid process. If the radial pulse decreases with this maneuver or numbness and tingling are found, this is considered a positive test. There are several different varieties of this test. See Wright's Hyperabduction Maneuver, Hyperabduction Test.

Hyperabduction Syndrome: Compression of the neurovascular bundle by the pectoralis minor or clavipectoral fascia. See Pectoralis Minor Syndrome.

Hyperabduction Test: A physical exam test for thoracic outlet syndrome. See Hyperabduction Maneuver.

Hyperalgesia: An increased response to a stimulus that is normally painful. See Allodynia, Hyperpathia, Dysesthesia.

Hyperesthesia: Increased sensitivity to stimulation. There is a diminished threshold to any stimulus and an increased response. This is similar to dysesthesia.

Hyperextension Brace: A three-point brace with two pads anteriorly over the sternum and pubis and one pad posteriorly over the thoracolumbar area. This system restricts flexion of the thoracic and lumbar spine. See Jewett Brace, Griswold Brace.

Hyperextension Orthosis: A TLSO that maintains the spine in slight extension and prevents flexion.

Hyperextension Subluxation: A chiropractic term which denotes a retrolisthesis. This is a minor movement of one vertebra back on another. It is believed that this can be associated with a facet syndrome.

Hyperextension Test: A physical exam maneuver used to rule out femoral nerve tension or irritation. The patient is prone and the knees are extended. The examiner then places the palm of the hand in the L5–S1/sacrum area to stabilize the spine. With the other hand, the examiner then slowly extends the hip of the affected leg. The test is deemed positive if the patient experiences radiating pain in the anterior thigh. This is very similar to a PKB (prone knee bend) maneuver or a femoral nerve stretch test. See PKB.

Hyperflexion Sprain: An injury secondary to sudden hyperflexion. There is temporary or partial luxation of the facet joints with total or partial rupture of the posterior ligaments and joint capsules, but without dislocation. This most often occurs in the cervical spine.

Hyperkyphosis: A spinal curve in which the apex points posteriorly. More than normal kyphosis. See Kyphosis.

Hyperlordosis: An exaggerated lumbar lordosis.

Hypermobile Subluxation: An abnormal intervertebral joint position in which the supporting tissues have been stretched or degenerated such that there is excess movement at that level. See +++, Subluxation.

Hyperostosis: This is thick new bone formation within the anterior longitudinal ligament. This gives the spine a bumpy contour, which is characteristic of diffuse idiopathic skeletal hyperostosis. See Diffuse Idiopathic Skeletal Hyperostosis.

Hyperostosis Triangularis Ilii: An isolated SI arthropathy usually found in women of child-bearing age. See Osteitis Condensans Ilii.

Hyperparathyroidism: Hyperactivity of the parathyroid gland causing an increase in the bone building hormone known as parathormone (PTH). Females are affected predominantly, with a ratio of 3:1. Common symptoms are weakness, lethargy, polydipsia, and polyuria. There is a serum calcium elevation in primary hyperparathyroidism but low to normal levels in secondary hyperparathyroidism. Calculi can be seen in the kidneys at times on an AP view of the abdomen. Parathormone levels will be high. With respect to the spine, bone density is decreased, trabecular patterns are accentuated, and there is a slight increase in the concavity of the end plates. Widened SI joints can also be seen.

Hyperpathia: An increased reaction to a stimulus, especially a repetitive stimulus. See Hyperalgesia, Allodynia.

Hyperreflexia: An abnormally increased deep tendon reflex (DTR) or other reflex. In the case of a deep tendon reflex, a 3+ DTR is considered hyperreflexic (when using the standard 0–4+ scale). This can be normal for the patient if symmetrical, or it could indicate upper motor neuron dysfunction if assymetrical (stroke, brain injury, or spinal cord compression above the level being tested).

Hypertonia: Increased muscle tone. This can either be due to an upper motor neuron dysfunction such as a CVA or something as simple as spasm.

Hypertonicity: A synonym for *muscle spasm.*

Hypertrophy: An increase in the cross-sectional size of a structure. This is most commonly experiened in muscles after strength training. Muscle hypertrophy in rehabilitation programs usually does not occur for 4–5 weeks after a strength training program has begun. It is hypothesized that strength gains during the first 4–5 weeks are due to increased neurologic recruitment of muscle fibers. See Muscle Hypertrophy.

Hypesthesia: Decreased sensitivity to touch or other stimuli. See Hypoesthesia.

Hypnotic: A medication used to promote sleep.

Hypoalgesia: A raised threshold of pain with a lowered pain response.

Hypochondriasis: Excessive preoccupation with illness that interferes with daily functioning. No organic cause can be found to explain the patient's symptoms.

Hypoesthesia: Decreased sensitivity to touch or other stimuli. See Hypesthesia.

Hypokyphosis: Less than normal kyphosis. See Kyphosis.

Hyporeflexia: A decrease in deep tendon reflexes. This is a 1+ deep tendon reflex that may be normal for the patient or may indicate an incomplete flaccid paralysis (spinal cord, nerve root, or peripheral nerve entrapment).

Hypotonia: A decrease in overall muscle tone or tension. See Hypotonicity.

Hypotonicity: A decrease in overall muscle tone or tension. See Hypotonia.

Hysterical Neurosis: A pain disorder which involves pain or loss of bodily function without a physical cause. See Conversion Disorder, Conversion Hysteria, Conversion Reaction.

Hysterical Scoliosis: A lateral curvature of the spine that develops due to a conversion reaction.

I

Iatrogenic: A disorder (problem or complication) caused by the medical profession. For instance, if a patient developed a gastric ulcer due to long-term NSAID use, this would be considered an iatrogenic disease.

Iatrogenic Spondylolisthesis: A stress fracture of the pars interarticularis one level above or below a spinal fusion. This likely occurs due to shunting of biomechanical forces to the pars above and/or below the fused segment. See Postsurgical Spondylolisthesis.

IBD: An abbreviation for *inflammatory bowel disease*. In the context of spinal problems, IBD is associated with a spondyloarthropathy in about 15–20% of the cases. See Inflammatory Bowel Disease.

Ibuprofen: A nonsteroidal anti-inflammatory drug which is in the propionic acid class. The usual dosage is between 200 and 800 mg taken three times a day. The common prescription dosage is between 400 and 800 mg three or four times a day. Over-the-counter Advil tablets contain 200 mg. See Motrin, Advil.

IC: An abbreviation for *intercostal.*

ICA: International Chiropractors Association.

Ice Packs: The use of ice applied to the surface of the body after injury. See Cryotherapy.

ICS: An abbreviation for *intercostal space.*

ICSM: International Conference on Spinal Manipulation.

Idiopathic: A condition or disease which has an unknown cause.

Idiopathic Adolescent Scoliosis: A lateral curvature of the spine which is structural in nature (altered shape of the individual vertebral bodies) for which the etiology is unclear. This is the most common type of scoliosis. See Idiopathic Scoliosis.

Idiopathic Scoliosis: A lateral curvature of the spine which is structural in nature (altered shape of the individual vertebral bodies). The etiology for this is unclear. See Idiopathic Adolescent Scoliosis.

ILA: An osteopathic or manual physical therapy term that refers to the inferior lateral angle of the sacrum. This is used as a reference point in the diagnosis of SI joint dysfunctions. The sacrotuberous and sacrospinous ligaments insert in this area. The ILA is the area where the narrow sacral apex begins to widen (just superior to the apex). See Inferior Lateral Angle.

Iliac Apophysis: The epiphysis (growth plate) along the wing of the ilium which has been used in scoliosis to estimate growth remaining. The complete closure of the apophysis signals the end of skeletal growth and a dramatic decrease in the risk of progression of the scoliosis.

Iliac Crest: The uppermost part of the iliac "wings." This is the superior border of the ilium which is easily palpable above the lateral hip. This point is commonly used as a landmark during many different physical exam maneuvers and is also used as a site for autogenous bone graft.

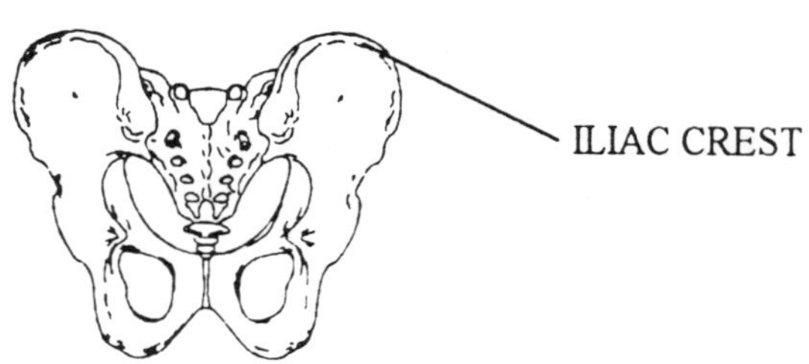

Iliac Crest Bone Graft: An autograft taken from the iliac crest which is usually tricortical in configuration (cortex on three sides). This procedure is performed in order to obtain a graft to promote bony fusion elsewhere. This type of graft is considered by many to be the best quality graft for achieving fusion.

Iliac Crest Height: A physical exam maneuver which involves comparing the heights of the iliac crests by palpating bilaterally with the thumb or index finger. This is a test for pelvic obliquity that may be positive in patients with a leg length discrepancy or SI joint dysfunction.

Iliac Fossa: The origin of the iliacus muscle. A concave depression in the iliac wing.

Iliac Inflare: An osteopathic or manual physical therapy term that is used to describe an SI joint dysfunction where the ilium is internally rotated or turned in toward the midline with respect to the sacrum. See Inflare.

Iliac Outflare: An osteopathic or manual physical therapy term which usually refers to the ilium being externally rotated or turned out relative to the sacrum. See Outflare.

Iliac Spine: A bony projection along the surface of the iliac crest which has four protuberances which are palpable on exam. These are the posterior superior iliac spine (PSIS), the posterior inferior iliac spine (PIIS), the anterior superior iliac spine (ASIS), and the anterior inferior iliac spine (AIIS).

Iliac Tuberosity: The attachment site for the posterior sacroiliac ligaments. This is a large roughened protuberance on the posterior aspect of the ilium.

Iliacus Muscle: One of the two muscles that make up the iliopsoas muscle. This is a major flexor which also internally rotates the hip. It takes its origin from the iliac fossa and the lateral aspect of the sacrum and inserts on the lesser trochanter. The innervation is the femoral nerve.

Iliac Wing Fracture: A fracture of the iliac bone caused by a lateral blow. There is splitting of the iliac wing, and the fracture line is best imaged on oblique x-ray films. There is usually very little separation of the fractured halves due to the strong muscular attachments. This is considered a stable fracture, but if the halves are displaced, ORIF may be necessary. See Duverney's Fracture.

Ilial Rotation: A manual medicine term that denotes an ilium which is noted to be in an abnormal position on exam. It is thought that damage to the SI ligaments causes abnormal movement between the ilium and sacrum. See Innominate Rotation.

Iliofemoral Ligament: One of the strongest ligaments of the body. It resembles an inverted Y and is sometimes referred to as the Y Ligament of Bigelow. This ligament is found in the anterior hip and attaches proximally to the anterior inferior iliac spine and to an area on the ilium just proximal to the superior and posterior superior rim of the acetabulum. The ligament checks internal rotation and extension of the hip. It is one of the major supporting ligaments in standing.

Iliohypogastric Nerve: A mixed motorsensory nerve that originates from the upper most part of the lumbar plexus. It is derived from the twelfth thoracic and first lumbar roots. It carries sensation from the outer and upper part of the buttocks and lower part of the abdomen. It innervates the internal oblique and transversalis muscles. Lesions of this nerve are rare.

Ilioinguinal Nerve: A branch of the lumbar plexus that arises from the twelfth thoracic and first lumbar roots. It carries sensation from the upper inner portion of the thigh, the pubic region, and the external genitalia. It innervates the transversalis, internal oblique, and external oblique muscles. Injuries to this nerve are usually associated with injuries to the iliohypogastric nerve. Some believe that this nerve can be irritated with SI joint syndromes and other lumbar disease processes causing pain and paresthesias in the inner thigh, pubic region, and external genitalia.

Iliolumbar Ligament: The ligament connecting the transverse processes of the fifth lumbar vertebra to the ilium bilaterally. There is also an iliolumbar ligament extending from the transverse processes of L4 in most individuals. These ligaments act as a stabilizing force for the lower lumbar spine, especially in rotation. The anterior iliolumbar ligament is attached to the lower end of the quadratus lumborum muscle. The superior iliolumbar ligament is formed by thickenings in the fascia that surround the base of the quadratus lumborum. The posterior portion of the ligament is also intimate with the quadratus lumborum. Pain in the iliolumbar ligament is referred to the L1 sclerotome as well as to the L3 and L4 sclerotomes. The referral pattern is to the anterior medial upper thigh. From a manual medicine perspective, the iliolumbar ligament provides stability to the ilium on the sacrum and can be strained in ilial rotations.

Iliolumbar Ligament Strain: Tearing of the iliolumbar ligament fibers usually caused by a rotational injury to the lumbar spine. The iliolumbar ligament is thought to stabilize the L5 segment. There is tenderness in the regions of the origin and insertion of the ligament, and there may also be associated annular tears. Sclerotherapy and injection of corticosteroids have been used. Also, muscle energy technique, lumbar stabilization, manual medicine, and other techniques may be helpful. Radiation of pain to the anterior thigh is thought to be the referral pattern of this ligament.

Iliolumbar Ligament Test: A test used to identify the iliolumbar ligament as a pain generator. The patient lies prone, and the examiner blocks the spinous process on the side nearest the examiner. The opposite ASIS is then lifted from the table. For instance, to test the left iliolumbar ligament, the spinous process is blocked on the right, and the left ASIS is lifted. Pain should be felt in the iliolumbar ligament being tested and/or possibly in a pain referral pattern. Because stress is placed on the L5–S1 facet joint on the side tested, pain may be originating from this structure as well. To rule out facet involvement, springing of the spinous process of L5 with a PA force is necessary. If pain is reproduced, the facet joint is thought to be involved. If there is no pain, the ligament is thought to be involved.

Iliopectineal Line: A bony ridge on the anterior inlet of the pelvis. This divides the pelvis into the greater and lesser pelvis.

Iliopsoas Muscle: One of the major flexors of the hip that also assists in external rotation and abduction of the hip. This muscle is actually made up of both the iliacus and psoas muscles. The origin of the iliacus portion is the iliacus fossa and anterior sacrum. The origin of the psoas portion is the anterior portion of the second through fourth vertebral bodies and transverse processes.

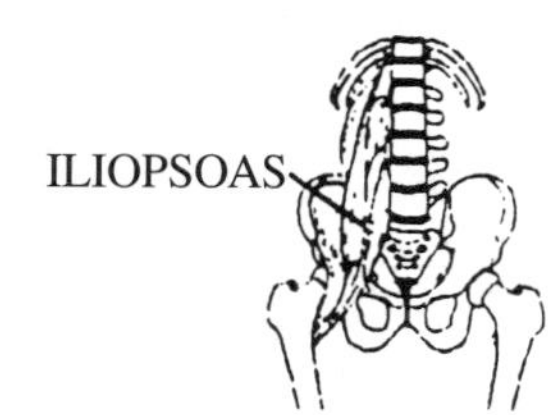

Iliopubic Eminence: A raised ridge on the pelvis which is caused by fusion of the ilium and pubis.

Iliosacral Dysfunction: An osteopathic or manual physical therapy term which refers to a dysfunction of the ilium on the sacrum. This would include an upslip, a downslip, an anterior ilial rotation, a posterior ilial rotation, an outflare, or an inflare. See IS, ISD.

Iliosacral Motion: Motion of the ilia on the inferior transverse axis of the sacrum that occurs with walking. See Transverse Axes of the Sacrum.

Iliotibial Band: A fascial tract that runs laterally from the iliac crest to the lateral tibial tubercle. The gluteus maximus and tensor fasciae lata insert posteriorly and anteriorly into the iliotibial tract. This arrangement has been called the "deltoid" of the hip. Tightness in the iliotibial tract can cause relative abduction of the hip. Tightness can also be found with an SI joint syndrome or trochanteric bursitis. Tightness in the iliotibial band has also been proposed as a cause of knee pain. See Ober's Test, Iliotibial Tract, ITB.

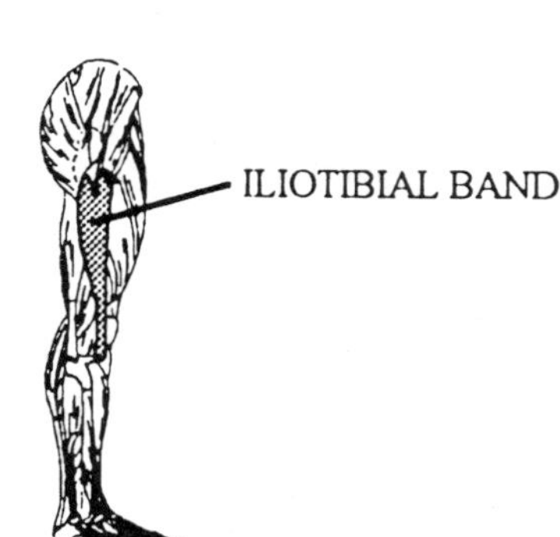

Iliotibial Band Syndrome: An inflammatory condition of the iliotibial band. This develops secondary to tightness which causes friction as the iliotibial band passes over the lateral femoral condyle. There is localized pain at this site. Friction can also develop between the iliotibial band and the greater trochanter. See Trochanteric Bursitis, Ober's Test, Iliotibial Band Friction Syndrome.

Iliotibial Tract: A fascial tract that runs laterally from the iliac crest to the lateral tibial tubercle. See Iliotibial Band.

Ilium: The superior aspect of the innominate bone. This is a large, flat, curved bone which makes up the lateral pelvis.

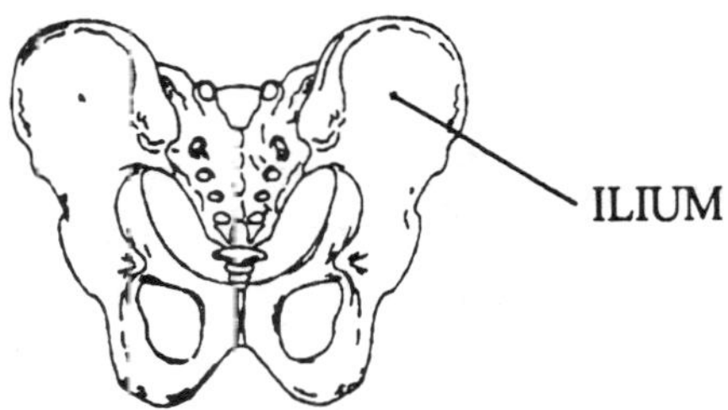

IM: An abbreviation for *intramuscular*.

Imipramine: A tricyclic antidepressant which is used in chronic pain. It probably acts by blocking uptake of norepinephrine at nerve endings. It is contraindicated for use in conjunction with MAO inhibitors, and it does have anticholinergic side effects. Patients with any evidence of cardiovascular disease require cardiac surveillance. The antidepressant dose is 75–150 mg a day starting at 75 mg. Dosages for chronic pain are 10–25 mg orally every hour of sleep. It is available in 10-mg, 25-mg, and 50-mg tablets. See Tofranil.

Imitrex: An injectable selective 5-HT receptor agonist used for vascular and migraine headaches. It is thought that 5-HT receptors are present in cranial arteries and in the dura mater. Imitrex activates this receptor and causes vasoconstriction. Imitrex should not be given intravenously. It also should not be given to patients with ischemic heart disease or Prinzmetal's angina. Imitrex may also cause small increases in blood pressure so should not be given to patients with uncontrolled hypertension. It should not be used concomitantly with ergotamine-containing preparations. It is contraindicated and should not be given to patients who are on MAO inhibitors. It is also contraindicated in patients with basilar or hemiplegic migraine. Chest, jaw, or neck tightness is relatively common following Imitrex injection and the first dose should be given in a physician's office. Six milligrams are injected subcutaneously, and the maximum recommended dose is two 6-mg injections in a 24-hour time span. Lower doses than 6 mg can also be used. Imitrex is supplied in a 6-mg injection form and is sold in cartons of two syringes. There is an Imitrex SELFdose system kit containing two unit-of-use syringes, one Imitrex SELFdose Unit, and instructions for usage. See Sumatriptan.

Impairment: As used in the AMA Guides to the Evaluation of Permanent Impairment, this is defined as an alteration of an individual's health status that is assessed by medical means. Impairment can be either temporary or permanent. It can also be either partial or total. Impairment is what is physically wrong with a body part or organ system and its functioning. Impairment leads to disability only when the medical condition limits the patient's capacity to meet the demands of life and activities. Refer to the AMA Guides to the Evaluation of Permanent Impairment. See Impairment Rating.

Impairment Rating: The degree of impairment assigned to a patient with residual pain loss of function once MMI has been reached. This usually corresponds to a percentage number in upper extremity units or whole person units as described by the AMA Guides to the Evaluation of Permanent Impairment. This number is derived by using range of motion loss, neurologic loss, strength loss, diagnosis, amputation, and other factors. It is applied after MMI has been reached (worker's compensation) and if there is residual disability. There are currently four editions of the AMA Guides with additional revisions, and each state determines which edition or revision it currently uses. See Impairment, MMI, Permanent Impairment.

Impingement: The compression of a structure by another structure. For instance, a nerve can be impinged as it travels through a tight bony space. See Impingement Syndrome.

Impingement of the Rotator Cuff: The compression of a structure by another structure. See Impingement Syndrome.

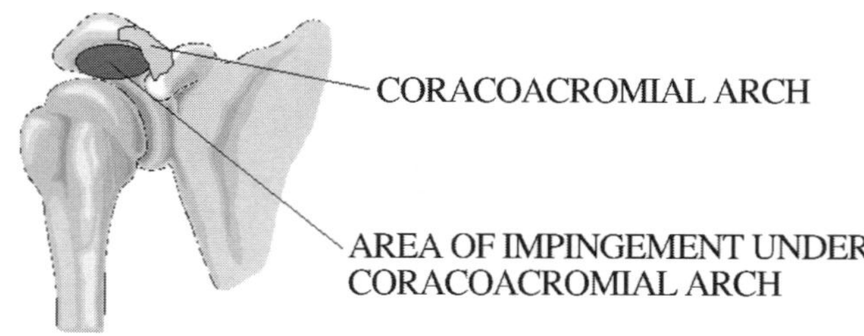

Impingement Syndrome: Compression of the supraspinatus and subacromial bursa underneath the coracoacromial arch. There is compression of the supraspinatus muscle at point of decreased vascularity, and this can lead to degeneration within the tendon and a partial or complete rotator cuff tear. Physical exam findings commonly noted are positive empty can test, pain in the supraspinatus muscle on palpation, positive impingement signs, and positive/negative drop test. There is almost always associated weakness in the rotator cuff musculature. Treatments include injection of the subacromial bursa, strengthening of the rotator cuff, strengthening of the muscles that stabilize the scapula, increased recruitment of the musculature that stabilizes scapula to avoid dyskinesis between the glenohumeral and scapulothoracic articulations, mobilization of the clavicle, stretching and mobilization for increased range of motion of the glenohumeral joint, axillary rib corrections, and thoracic spine segmental corrections. See Rotator Cuff Impingement, Impingement of the Rotator Cuff, Impingement, Rotator Cuff Tendinitis, Supraspinatus Tendinitis, Subacromial Bursitis, Shoulder Bursitis.

In: A chiropractic term used to denote an ilium which has rotated internally. See In Ilium.

In-Ex Ilium: A chiropractic notation for an SI joint dysfunction in which one ilium is internally rotated and the opposite ilium is externally rotated. This would be equivalent to the osteopathic terminology of an inflare combined with an outflare. This is rotation along the y-axis with one ASIS more medial and the other ASIS more lateral.

In Ilium: A chiropractic term used to denote an ilium which has rotated internally. This would be equivalent to the osteopathic inflare. The axis of rotation is the y-axis with the ASIS found medially.

Incisal Distance: The amount of opening of the mouth. This is the tip-to-tip distance between incisors when the mouth is opened. It is thought that in TMJ dysfunction or in TMJ syndrome, this distance will be less.

Incisal Path: The path of the mandible in relation to the center of the upper incisors during jaw opening. This is usually followed along a sagittal plane and is said to be abnormal if there is significant deviation from midline with opening or closing of the jaw.

Inclination: Another word for flexion at the atlanto-occipital joint.

Inclinometer: This term most commonly refers to a bubble inclinometer. This is a measurement device which measures the angle of a body part. For instance, bubble inclinometers are used in the ROM measurements described in the AMA Guides. To measure lumbar flexion, one end of the device is placed at T12 and the other over the sacrum. The patient is asked to flex forward and the angles are read. The T12 measurement is subtracted from the sacral measurement to give a true lumbar flexion measurement. The device consists of a round dial which contains a circular tube filled with colored water. The dial has measurements in degrees which are zeroed to the top of the meniscus of the circular tube. This is then read against the dial once the patient has moved from the initial position in order to read the degrees of movement. See Bubble Inclinometer.

Increased Interosseous Spacing: A chiropractic term which refers to increased space between vertebral segments when compared with the spacing of the segment above and the spacing of the segment below. This occurs after initial disc injury as the disc takes on water and swells. See Superior Subluxation.

Inderal: A beta blocker drug normally used for hypertension which is also used for the prevention of migraine headache. It is not indicated as an abortive (a drug which would decrease headache pain once the attack has started). It is not indicated for use in patients with cardiac failure, angina pectoris, bronchospastic diseases, diabetes and hypoglycemia, thyrotoxicosis, or Wolff-Parkinson-White syndrome. There are drug interactions with verapamil, aluminum hydroxide, ethanol, phenytoin, phenolbarbital, rifampin, chlorpromazine, antipyrine, lidocaine, thyroxine, cimetidine, and theophylline. Inderal is available both in a short-acting form and a long-acting (LA) form. The initial dosage for migraine is 80 mg in divided doses, usually twice a day. The usual effective dose is 160–240 mg per day in divided doses. If satisfactory response is not obtained within 4–6 weeks, Inderal should be discontinued. It is advisable to withdraw the drug gradually over a period of several weeks. The LA form can also be given for migraine prophylaxis. Initial dose is again 80 mg, but once a day. The usual effective dose range is 160–250 mg once a day. See Inderal-LA, Propranolol.

Inderal-LA: A beta blocker drug normally used for hypertension which is also used for the prevention of migraine headache. See Inderal, Propranolol.

Indirect Technique: An osteopathic or manual physical therapy term which describes a treatment in which a joint is moved in the direction of least muscular or capsular resistance. A good example would be strain-counterstrain. In this technique, the musculature is shortened to "break" the neurophysiologic cycle of increased tone. See Strain-Counterstrain.

Indocin: A nonsteroidal anti-inflammatory drug in the indole class. This is one of the drugs of choice in the treatment of ankylosing spondylitis. Indocin does interact with anticoagulants in that it may prolong prothrombin time. Probenecid may increase plasma levels of Indomethacin (Indocin). There may be an interaction with Lasix and triamterene. There also may be an interaction with beta blockers. Common dosages include 25 mg two to three times a day. A 50-mg capsule is also available. See Indomethacin.

Indomethacin: A nonsteroidal anti-inflammatory drug in the indole class. See Indocin.

Indurated: The hardening of tissue which can occur through fibrosis, infection, or edema. See Induration.

Induration: The hardening of tissue which can occur through fibrosis, infection, or edema. See Indurated.

Industrial Back Brace: A soft low back support with or without metal stays with an anterior Velcro closure. There are usually suspenders or supports to prevent the brace from riding too low.

inf: (1) An abbreviation for *inferior*. (2) A chiropractic notation for hyperextension of the vertebral body. The vertebral body is noted to be posterior and the spinous process is found inferior.

Infantile Scoliosis: A lateral curvature of the spine that develops before age 3.

Inferior Arcuate Ligament: One of the supporting ligaments of the pubic symphysis.

Inferior Articular Process: The specialized mass of bone which extends downward from the lower lateral corner of the lamina. There is a smooth surface covered with cartilage on the lateral portion of each inferior articular process that makes up a portion of the facet joint. If the vertebra is viewed from the side or obliquely it looks like a dog. The inferior articular process would represent the paw, the spinous process the nose, and the superior articular process the ear. See Facet Joint.

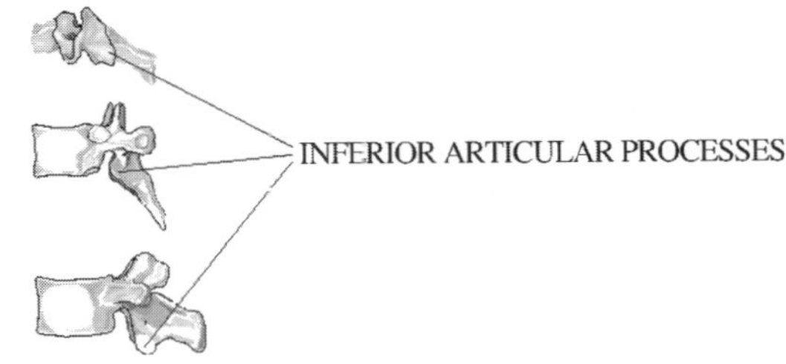

Inferior Innominate Shear: An osteopathic movement dysfunction of the ilium which is relatively rare. See Down-slip.

Inferiority: A chiropractic term which means that a part is inferior or downward in relation to another.

Inferior Lateral Angle: An osteopathic or manual physical therapy term that refers to the inferior lateral angle of the sacrum. See ILA.

Inferior Nutation: A Latin term meaning "nodding." In the lumbar spine, nutation usually refers to the ilium or the sacrum. See Nutation.

Inferior Pube: A pelvic dysfunction in which one side of the pubic symphysis is noted to be inferior relative to the other due to a shearing force in the sagittal plane. See Inferior Pubic Bone.

Inferior Pubic Bone: A pelvic dysfunction in which one side of the pubic symphysis is noted to be inferior relative to the other due to a shearing force in the sagittal plane. There is increased mobility in an inferior direction and increased mobility in a superior direction. See Inferior Pube, Inferior Pubic Shear, Inferior Shear.

Inferior Pubic Ramus: The inferior and medial portion of the pubic ring that joins the ischial ramus laterally. This encloses the lower portion of the obturator foramen.

Inferior Pubic Shear: A pelvic dysfunction in which one side of the pubic symphysis is noted to be inferior relative to the other due to a shearing force in the sagittal plane. See Inferior Pubic Bone.

Inferior Shear: A pelvic dysfunction in which one side of the pubic symphysis is noted to be inferior relative to the other due to a shearing force in the sagittal plane. See Inferior Pubic Bone.

Inferior Subluxation: A chiropractic term which refers to a vertebral segment that has undergone degenerative changes. There is decreased disc height so this spinous process is noted to be closer to the spinous process below and farther from the spinous process above. The spinous process is noted to be more inferior.

Inf. glut.: An abbreviation for *inferior gluteal.*

Inflammatory Bowel Disease: In the context of spinal problems, IBD is associated with a spondyloarthropathy in about 15–20% of the cases. There is a higher incidence of spondyloarthropathies with Crohn's disease than with ulcerative colitis. See IBD.

Inflare: An osteopathic or manual physical therapy term that is used to describe an SI joint dysfunction where the ilium is internally rotated or turned in toward the midline with respect to the sacrum. This can occur if the articular surface of the sacrum is convex instead of the usual concave. This is a rare condition. See Iliac Inflare.

Infrared Lamp: A passive modality which utilizes a standard heat lamp over the exposed area. This is a superficial heating modality used for superficial pain relief and general relaxation of the superficial musculature.

Inguinal Ligament: The ligament that extends from the ASIS to the pubic tubercle bilaterally. The neurovascular structures of the thigh pass under the inguinal ligament.

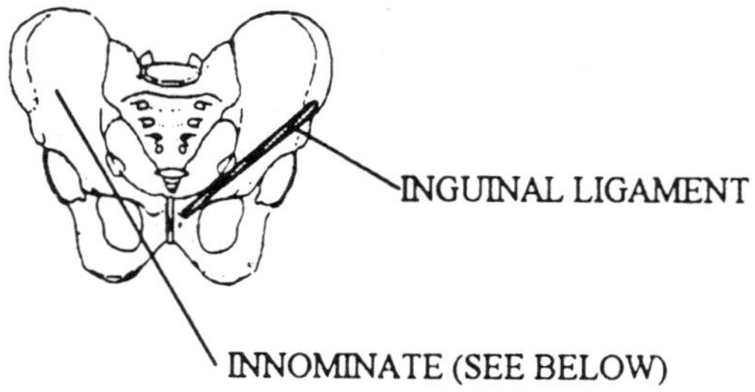

INGUINAL LIGAMENT

INNOMINATE (SEE BELOW)

Inhalation Restriction: Abnormal movement of the rib cage. A rib or series of ribs that move more freely toward exhalation (collapse of the rib cage) than toward inhalation (expansion of the rib cage). See Pump Handle Restriction, Bucket Handle Restriction, Exhalation Rib.

Inhalation Rib: Abnormal rib motion. See Exhalation Restriction, Inhalation Rib, Pump Handle Restriction, Bucket Handle Restriction.

Inlet of the Pelvis: The large opening in the pelvic ring. See Pelvic Inlet.

Inlet View: An x-ray view of the pelvis used for evaluating the positioning of pelvic fractures. The x-ray beam is directed at an angle of 25° toward the feet.

Innominate: The ilium, ischium, and pubis named as one unit. This is a term often used by manual physical therapists, chiropractors, and osteopaths to name an iliosacral dysfunction. See Pelvic Bone.

Innominate Rotation: A manual medicine term that denotes an ilium which is noted to be in an abnormal position on exam. See Ilial Rotation.

ins: An abbreviation for *inspection*.

Insertional Activity: The amount of irritation of the muscle membrane noted during a needle EMG exam. Excessive irritation is associated with injury of the nerve supplying that muscle.

In-shoe Lift: An orthotic or shoe insert which increases the height of the heel while walking. See Shoe Lift, Heel Lift.

Instability: (1) Ligamentous instability seen at L5–S1 usually demonstrated on flexion–extension views of the lumbar spine. See Lumbosacral Instability. (2) Excessive vertebral motion that is beyond normal physiologic motion. This can be due to a traumatic disruption of the ligamentous supporting structures, degenerative disc disease, or fracture. See Vertebral Body Instability.

Instability—Postlaminectomy: Segmental instability which occurs after a laminectomy due to removal of the medial portion of the facet joints. See Failed Back Syndrome, Postlaminectomy Instability.

int: An abbreviation for *intermittent*.

Intensive Outpatient Pain Program: Usually a five-day-a-week, eight-hour-a-day program designed to reintegrate patients with chronic pain syndrome back into a more functional lifestyle. Group psychotherapy is often used to help focus these patients away from their somatic complaints. Biofeedback can be included to help with relaxation. Also, physical activity is emphasized to help restore patients back to baseline physical functioning. Self-reliance and methods for pain relief that can be performed without assistance are taught. See IOP.

Interbody Fusion: The placement of a bone graft into the intervertebral space for the purpose of fusing two vertebral segments.

Intercalary Bone: A radiographic sign which represents calcification within the fibers of the anulus fibrosus.

Intercostal: The space between individual ribs.

Intercostal Muscles: The muscles that occupy the intercostal space between individual ribs.

Interferential E-stim: A form of electrical stimulation in which two or three different currents are passed through a specific area. Portions of each current are cancelled by the other, resulting in a characteristic net current applied to the target area. See Interferential Stim.

Interferential Stim: A form of electrical stimulation. See Interferential E-Stim.

Intermedullary Vein: One of the segmental veins draining the spinal cord into the longitudinal veins in the epidural space.

Intermittent Traction: Traction that is alternatively applied and then released at short intervals. Intermittent traction is usually more comfortable for the same amount of traction force applied and is the most common type of traction used. It is usually applied with a mechanical device and set for a specific traction force and interval. This technique is used for the relief of nerve root pressure due to foraminal stenosis, HNP, and other nerve root compression syndromes. See Traction—Intermittent.

Internal Disc Disruption: A fissure that extends perpendicular to the fibers of the annulus. See Radial Tear of the Annulus, Annular Tear.

Internally Rotated Innominate: An osteopathic or manual physical therapy term that is used to describe an SI joint dysfunction where the ilium is internally rotated or turned in toward the midline with respect to the sacrum. See Inflare.

International System: A technique for naming chiropractic vertebral subluxations which is rarely used in clinical practice. This is a right-handed orthogonal coordinate system which has been proposed for defining movements and positions of the functional spinal unit. The x, y, and z axes are used. For instance, +Z indicates forward movement along the z-axis which would be otherwise be termed anterior. −Y would mean downward movement along the y-axis which would otherwise be inferior.

Interosseous Disc Relationship: A chiropractic term used to denote a vertebral segment that does not move freely in all directions. See Subluxation, Fixation.

Interosseous Sacroiliac Ligament: Extremely strong ligaments contained within the SI joint that blend with the dorsal SI ligaments to form the posterior border of the joint. These ligaments bind the sacrum and ilium together and are the strongest of all the SI ligaments. For instance, when the joint is forced apart the ligament rarely fails in midsubstance and usually fractures a portion of bone from either side.

Interpedicular Distance: The distance between the pedicles measured on an AP x-ray view.

Interpediculate Distance: The distance between the pedicles on an AP view of the spine. This can be helpful in diagnosing spinal stenosis. This distance varies greatly, and there are normal values published.

Intersegmental Range of Motion Palpation: A chiropractic technique of palpating vertebral position which can be performed either statically or with motion added. See Motion Palpation, IRMP.

Interspace: An orthopedic term referring to the disc space. For instance, the L4–L5 interspace would mean the L4–L5 disc space.

Interspinous Ligament: The ligamentous attachment between adjoining spinous processes. This is one of the checks to spinal flexion (these ligaments limit forward bending). See ISL.

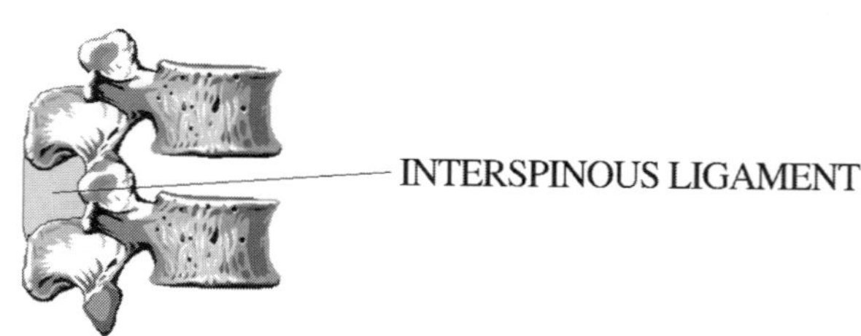

Interspinous Ligament Sprain: Tearing in the fibers of the interspinous ligament (ligaments between adjoining spinous processes). Patients with degenerative disc disease may be more prone to this type of injury as they have more intrinsic biomechanical creep that would place the interspinous ligaments at their end range in long-standing flexion. There is localized tenderness in the interspinous space, and range of motion is decreased in flexion. Extension is usually not painful. See Interspinous Ligament Syndrome.

Interspinous Ligament Syndrome: Tearing in the fibers of the interspinous ligament (ligaments between adjoining spinous processes). Patients with degenerative disc disease may be more prone to this type of injury as they have more intrinsic biomechanical creep that would place the interspinous ligaments at their end range in long-standing flexion. See Interspinous Ligament Sprain.

Intertransverse Fusion: The fusion of two spinal segments using bone graft placed between decorticated transverse processes. This is often combined with instrumentation. See Fusion—Intertransverse.

Intertransverse Ligaments: Sheets of connective tissue extending from the upper border of one transverse process to the lower border of the transverse process above. These are not considered true ligaments. These connective-tissue sheets separate the anterior musculature of the spine from the posterior musculature.

Interval Change: The amount of change (usually on x-rays) in the condition since the last examination.

Interval Degeneration: A radiographic term which refers to two or more x-rays which show progressive degeneration of the spine.

Interval Training: A training program alternating heavy work with periods of rest or lighter training.

Intervertebral: Between two adjacent vertebrae.

Intervertebral Disc: The gel-filled sac between two vertebral segments. There is a tough outer covering (anulus fibrosus) and a soft, water-rich center (nucleus pulposus) which is the consistency of hard, gel toothpaste. With aging, the amount of water that the nucleus pulposus can retain decreases and the disc dries out. Also, small tears develop in the annulus and can lead to a degenerated disc or a herniated disc. See Discal, HNP, IVD .

Intervertebral Disc Disorder: An ICD-9 diagnosis code which is nonspecific. This can refer to degenerative disc disease, a disc bulge, or HNP.

Intervertebral Disc Disorder with Myelopathy: An ICD-9 diagnosis code. This may refer to a large herniated disc causing direct pressure on the spinal cord or spondylosis in which a large bone spur causes direct compression on the spinal cord. See Myelopathy.

Intervertebral Disc Displacement: An extrusion of the nucleus pulposus through the anterior annular fibers. See HNP.

Intervertebral Disc Rupture: An extrusion of the nucleus pulposus through the anterior annular fibers. See HNP.

Intervertebral Foramen: The bony window through which the nerve root passes. It is composed of the superior and inferior vertebral foramen. See Foramen, Vertebral Foramen.

Intervertebral Joint: The joint formed as two vertebral bodies are stacked on top of each other. This joint is made up of the intervertebral disc joining the vertebral bodies above and below. Along with the facet joints, this allows movement between the two vertebrae.

Intervertebral Space: The space occupied by the intervertebral disc between individual vertebral bodies. Bone grafts are often placed in the intervertebral space to provide intersegmental fusion.

Intoeing: A condition in which the feet point inward. This can occur with antiverted hips or can be secondary to either femoral or tibial torsion. See Pigeon-toed.

Intradiscal Pressure: The pressure inside the intervertebral disc. This increases with sitting, flexion, and standing and decreases with lying supine and traction. See Discometry.

Intradiscal Scarring: A term synonymous with degenerative disc disease. See Degenerative Disc Disease.

Intradural Arachnoid Irritation: An inflammatory reaction of the arachnoid membrane (one of the coverings of the spinal cord and brain) which is localized and usually seen adjacent to disc herniations. See Focal Spinal Arachnoiditis, Focal Arachnoiditis.

Intraneural Fibrosis: Scar tissue that forms within a nerve.

Intraspinal: Located within the spinal canal.

Intrathecal: Located within the thecal sac and the subarachnoid space.

Iohexol: A nonionic contrast medium used in myelography.

Iontophoresis: The delivery of a medication through the skin (usually an anesthetic or anti-inflammatory steroid) by an electrical current. The medication is charged with an ion, and an electrical current is used to drive the medication into the area being treated. Penetration of the substance is superficial and likely does not travel more than 1 cm, so it is not reccomended for the treatment of deep structures. This modality can be very helpful in treating bursitis or tendonitis. Some patients are not able to tolerate iontophoresis secondary to skin reaction, and improper application of the electrodes can cause burning of the skin. See Trochanteric Bursitis.

IOP: Usually a five-day-a-week, eight-hour-a-day program designed to reintegrate patients with chronic pain syndrome back into a more functional lifestyle. See Intensive Outpatient Pain Program, Pain Clinic.

Iopamidol: A nonionic contrast medium used in myelography.

IOPP: Usually a five-day-a-week, eight-hour-a-day program designed to reintegrate patients with chronic pain syndrome back into a more functional lifestyle. See Intensive Outpatient Pain Program.

Ipsilateral: Pertaining to the same side.

IRMP: A chiropractic technique of palpating vertebral position which can be performed either statically or with motion added. See Motion Palpation, Intersegmental Range of Motion Palpation.

IS: An osteopathic or manual physical therapy term which refers to a dysfunction of the ilium on the sacrum. See Iliosacral Dysfunction.

Ischemic Compression: The application of progressively stronger pressure on a trigger point. This pressure causes ischemia within that portion of the muscle followed by a hyperemic response on the release of pressure. This is thought to "release" the trigger point. See Shiatsu, Myotherapy, Acupressure, Massage.

Ischemic Myelopathy: Myelopathy associated with spinal cord ischemia (lack of blood flow to the spinal cord). Causes include anterior spinal artery occlusion or a glomus or juvenile AVM.

Ischial Bursitis: An inflammation of the ischial bursa. Pain usually occurs with sitting and is relieved by standing. There is palpable tenderness over the ischial bursa. Treatment usually includes icing, ultrasound, anti-inflammatory medications, and an ischial relief pad. See Weaver's Bottom.

Ischial Ramus: A portion of the pubic ring which extends from the ischial tuberosity anteriorly to meet the inferior ramus of the pubis.

Ischial Spine: A raised area on the posterior border of the body of the ischium that forms the lower border of the sciatic notch. See Spine of the Ischium.

Ischial Tuberosity: The inferior portion of the ischium used for sitting. This is also used for a landmark in many manual medicine techniques.

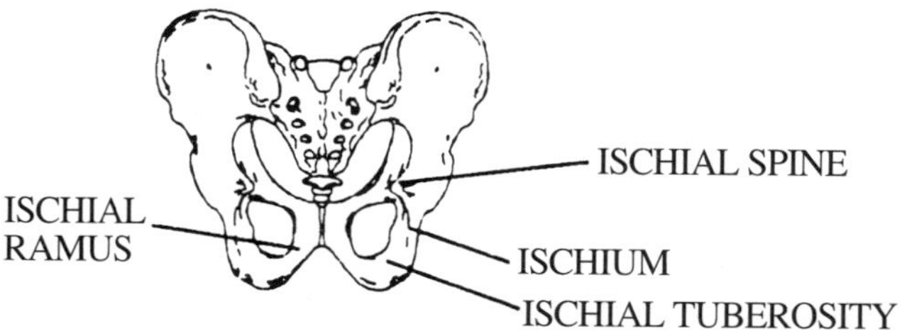

Ischial Tuberosity Avulsion Fracture: Avulsion of the apophysis of the ischial tuberosity as a result of a massive contraction of the hamstrings. See Avulsion Fracture of the Ischial Tuberosity.

Ischiosacral Dysfunction: A movement dysfunction of the pelvis in which the ischium is noted to be displaced. This is thought to cause a change in tension in the sacrotuberous and sacrospinous ligaments.

Ischium: The inferior bone of the pelvis that supports the body while sitting. It makes up the inferior wall of the obturator foramen. There are two main prominences, the ischial spine and the ischial tuberosity, both important attachment sites for SI ligaments (sacrospinous and sacrotuberous).

ISD: An osteopathic or manual physical therapy term which refers to a dysfunction of the ilium on the sacrum. See Iliosacral Dysfunction.

ISL: The ligamentous attachment between adjoining spinous processes. See Interspinous Ligament.

Isokinetic: A muscle contraction where the speed of contraction is held constant. See Isokinetic Testing.

Isokinetic Dynamometry: Strength testing in which the velocity of the movements is controlled. See Isokinetic Testing.

Isokinetic Exercise: Exercise in which the speed of muscular contraction is held constant.

Isokinetic Testing: Strength testing in which the velocity of the movements is controlled. The patient is asked to move against resistance in which the speed at which the patient can move is limited in degrees per second. This is commonly performed at 30° per second, 60° per second, or 90° per second. Force is then measured during this movement. A Cybex lumbar testing station is an example of an isokinetic dynamometer. See Isokinetic Dynamometry, Isokinetic, ISTU.

Isometric Exercise: Exercise in which the length of the muscle is held constant and no motion is produced within the joint. This is used where active movement of the joint would increase pain. Isometric exercise is performed to increase recruitment of muscle fibers (the amount of the muscle that can be activated by the nerves) in the muscle being strengthened.

Isometric Resistance Exercise: A static form of exercise where the patient contracts a muscle without an appreciable change in the length of the muscle or without joint motion. For example, in the lumbar spine, this is commonly performed in extension with the patient contracting the lumbar extensors without movement. See Isometrics.

Isometrics: A static form of exercise where the patient contracts a muscle without an appreciable change in the length of the muscle or without joint motion. See Isometric Resistance Exercise.

Isometric Strength Testing Unit: A type of force-measuring device. See ISTU.

Isostation B-200: A proprietary name for a computerized low back testing machine. See B-200.

Isotonic Exercise: Exercise that is carried out against a constant force as the muscle lengthens or shortens. See Isotonic Resistance.

Isotonic Muscle Contraction: Exercise that is carried out against a force weight as the muscle lengthens or shortens. See Isotonic Resistance.

Isotonic Resistance: Exercise that is carried out against a constant force as the muscle lengthens or shortens. One example is free weight exercise where the load does not vary through the range of motion. Another example is a standard pulley weight machine used for strengthening. See Isotonic Exercise, Isotonic Muscle Contraction.

Isotrak: An electromagnetic device for measurement of low back movements. This measures movements kinematically in three dimensions.

Isotrunk Machine: A computerized strength testing device that focuses on the measurement of trunk movement.

Isthmic Spondylolisthesis: Spondylolisthesis due to fracture or elongation of the pars interarticularis. See Type II Spondylolisthesis, Spondylolisthesis—Isthmic.

ISTU: A type of measuring device which calculates the amount of force a patient can apply in a given position against a nonmoveable object. See Isometric Strength Testing Unit, Isokinetic Testing.

ITB: A fascial tract that runs laterally from the iliac crest to the lateral tibial tubercle. See Iliotibial Band.

ITBS: An inflammatory condition of the iliotibial band. See Iliotibial Band Syndrome.

ITB Stretch: A stretch for the iliotibial band. The patient lies on one side and flexes the bottom knee. The patient then grabs the ankle of the top leg and brings this knee back and down. This position is held for about five seconds with a stretch felt in the lateral thigh.

ITS: An inflammatory condition of the iliotibial band. See Iliotibial Band Syndrome.

IVD: The gel-filled sac that is found between two vertebral segments. See Intervertebral Disc.

IVF Encroachment: A decrease in the overall size of the intervertebral foramen (the bony window through which the nerve roots passes) caused by enlargement of the superior facet or a degenerated disc. See Foraminal Stenosis.

Ivory Vertebra: A radiographic sign of uniformly increased radiopacity within a vertebral body. The most common cause is an osteoblastic metastasis. Other causes are Paget's disease, Hodgkin's lymphoma, degenerative sclerosis, and osteomyelitis.

J

Jackson Compression Test: A physical exam test. The patient is seated and rotates the head from side to side maximally. Pain on the side opposite the rotation suggests muscular strain, while pain on the same side suggests facet or nerve root involvement. The head is then laterally flexed with the ear brought toward the shoulder. This position is held while the examiner gives an axial compression force on the head. Exacerbation of the patient's axial pain complaints or radicular pain is a positive test. This maneuver is similar to a Spurling's sign, without the sudden compression. See Spurling's Sign.

Jackson's Lateral Compression Test: A physical examination maneuver used to "close-off" the foramen and compress the exiting nerve root. See Jackson Compression Test.

Jacobs Rods: Distraction and compression rods with hooks which are used for posterior fusion. These provide rigid surgical fusion and are used to correct scoliotic deformities.

JAMA: *Journal of the American Medical Association.*

Jamar Dynamometer: A brand name of grip-strength measuring devices often used to determine if a patient is giving maximum effort during functional capacities testing. The patient is asked to perform several sets of grip-strength measurements, and the coefficients of variation (CV) are calculated. If the CVs are above 15%, then it is thought that the patient is not giving maximal effort. This device can also be used to quantify the amount of force produced by the patient's hand while gripping. See Hand Dynamometer, Grip Dynamometer, Coefficient of Variation.

Janda: A neurologic retraining technique which involves repeated active movements in a variety of mechanical conditions (usually with proprioceptive feedback) in order to pattern the motor system.

Jansen's Test: A physical exam maneuver for osteoarthritis of the hip. The patient is asked to put one leg over the other with the ankle resting on the opposite knee. This maneuver tests external rotation of the hip and is reported to be restricted or cause pain in patients with osteoarthritis of the hip.

JCE: *Journal of Chiropractic Education.*

JCT: *Journal of Chiropractic Technique.*

JD: Doctor of Jurisprudence.

Jefferson Fracture: A comminuted fracture of the ring of the atlas. This is usually the result of an axial load or compression (direct blow on the vertex of the head). The occipital condyles act as a wedge and cause a bursting effect thus separating the ring of the atlas. There are usually four parts to this fracture. The fracture can be detected on an open-mouth view of the cervical spine as a bilateral displacement of the articular facet of the ring of the atlas. In most cases, this is a stable injury without neurologic involvement and can be treated with immobilization. Surgical fusion may be required. See Comminuted Fracture of the Ring of C1.

Jendrassik's Maneuver: A physical exam maneuver designed to increase the amplitude of a deep tendon reflex. If the patient is tested for a deep tendon reflex that is unobtainable, the patient is asked to interlock the fingers and pull the hands apart. The deep tendon reflex is then attempted while the patient is performing this maneuver. See Reinforcement Maneuver.

Jewett-Benjamin Cervical Brace: A cervicothoracic orthosis with contact points at the chin and occiput. This is used for stabilization of cervical flexion, extension, and lateral bending.

Jewett Brace: A three-point brace with two pads anteriorly over the sternum and pubis and one pad posteriorly over the thoracolumbar area. This system restricts flexion of the thoracic and lumbar spine. See Jewett Hyperextension, Hyperextension Brace, Three-Point Brace.

Jewett Contraflexion: A thoracolumbar orthosis which limits lumbar flexion.

Jewett Hyperextension: A three-point brace. See Jewett Brace.

JM: An abbreviation for *joint mobilization.*

JMPT: *Journal of Manipulative and Physiological Therapeutics.*

Job Analysis: A systematic evaluation of a specific work task. This might include the measurement of the biomechanical, cardiovascular, or metabolic demands of a job.

Job Site Analysis: An analysis of the patient's work area. This includes the components of performing a specific job, which include positioning of the patient, amount to be lifted, frequency of lifts, frequency of breaks, and tasks to be performed per unit of time. It is then determined how these influence job task performance. This is often used in an attempt to place a patient with restrictions back to work. See Job Site Evaluation, Job Site Visit, Job Task Analysis.

Job Site Evaluation: An analysis of the patient's work area. See Job Site Analysis.

Job Site Visit: Evaluating the job site to improve ergonomics or to determine if a patient can return to work. See Job Site Analysis.

Job Strength Index: A measurement usually included in a functional capacity evaluation which measures the maximum strength required to do the job divided by the strength the worker currently demonstrates. If the job strength index is very high (greater than 1) there may be a higher risk for injury (the job strength requirements are much greater than the worker's strength). If the job strength index is low (less than 0.5) the worker may be less likely to be injured because the strength exhibited in the test was greater than the strength required for the job. This was first investigated by Chaffin. See Job Strength Rating.

Job Strength Rating: A measurement usually included in a functional capacity evaluation which measures the maximum strength required to do the job divided by the strength the worker currently demonstrates. See Job Strength Index.

Job Task Analysis: Analysis of the components of performing a specific job through observation and measurement. See Job Site Analysis.

Joint Adjustment: The application of a force to a joint that takes it beyond its normal range of motion into the elastic range. See Manipulation.

Joint Auscultation: Listening over the TMJ with a stethoscope or electronic device to detect crepitus and popping sounds on joint movement. This is thought to correlate with disc involvement in TMJ pain disorders.

Joint Blockage: A chiropractic term which refers to an abnormality of spinal biomechanics involving a loss of normal movement of a vertebral motion segment. See Vertebral Subluxation Complex, Abnormal Spinal Segmental Motion, Osteopathic Lesions, Somatic Dysfunction, Articular Dysfunction.

Joint Manipulation: The application of a force to a joint that takes it beyond its normal range of motion into its elastic range. See Manipulation.

Joint Mobilization: Low-amplitude, low-velocity forces which are used to restore joint range of motion. See Mobilization.

Joint of Luschka: The joints which occur in the lower cervical spine from C2 through C7. See Uncinate Process.

Joint of Von Luschka: The joints which occur in the lower cervical spine from C2 through C7. See Uncovertebral Joint.

Joint Play Movements: Movements that are added into a joint during examination for the purpose of determining limitations or restrictions within the joint. These are usually distraction, compression, glide, and spin. These are movements necessary for full range of motion, but are not under direct voluntary control of the individual.

Jones Point: A tender point in a muscle which is considered a "monitoring" point. See Jones Tender Point.

Jones Strain–Counterstrain: A technique of treatment which is advocated for the treatment of acute and subacute muscular strain. See Strain–Counterstrain.

Jones Tender Point: A tender point in a muscle which is considered a "monitoring" point. It is thought that Jones points arise secondary to "strains" of the muscle spindle and neuromuscular reflex, which then translates into increased tone. A Jones point is treated by bringing the muscle into the "position of ease" or shortening the muscle for 90 seconds. The point is then reassessed or monitored throughout the procedure to see if it "extinguishes" (becomes much less painful or nontender) during or after treatment. See Tender Point, Jones Point.

Jugular Compression Test: A physical exam maneuver used to increase intrathecal pressure. Simultaneous pressure is applied to the internal and external jugular veins for approximately 2–3 minutes. A positive test is an increase in radicular symptoms. This test can be positive in patients with an HNP or an intraspinal neoplasm.

Jumper's Fracture: A thoracolumbar fracture caused by a fall or jump. This often involves the pedicles, facets, lamina, and vertebral body.

Jump Sign: A sudden contraction of muscle seen as a twitch in response to stimulation of a trigger point. See Twitch Response.

Juvenile AVM: An intradural arteriovenous malformation which is considered juvenile. See Type 3 AVM, AVM—Type 3.

Juvenile Rheumatoid Arthritis: A chronic inflammation of the synovial tissues which occurs in children and has many different etiologies. It is associated with sacroilitis, and cervical spine involvement occurs in 60–70% of patients. These spinal lesions are similar to the adult rheumatoid arthritis with the C2–3 segment being most commonly involved. Also, fusion of the facet joints and growth abnormalities are not uncommon.

Juvenile Scoliosis: Scoliosis that occurs between the ages of 3 and 10 years. See Scoliosis.

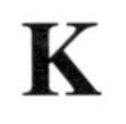

Kaneda Device: Instrumentation used for anterior interbody spinal fusion in which two rods are attached to the lateral vertebral bodies (one on each side). See Kaneda Rods.

Kaneda Rods: Instrumentation used for anterior interbody spinal fusion in which two rods are attached to the lateral vertebral bodies (one on each side). These rods attach to connecting plates in which two screws secure the plate to the appropriate vertebra. A vertebral body spreader can be used to assist with reduction, and the rods have four nuts each which are adjustable to allow for compression or distraction. See Kaneda Device, Kaneda SR.

Kaneda SR: This is a proprietary name for a Kaneda anterior spinal fixation system which utilizes smooth rods. See Kaneda Rods.

K-board: One of several different exercise boards designed to increase kinesthetic awareness. This is usually a small platform with different attachments on the bottom of the board. The patient stands on top of the board and performs exercises to increase kinesthetic awareness and proprioception. See Kinesthetic Board.

KC: A chiropractic adjusting table. See Knee-Chest Table.

Kelly Thermography: The measurement of skin temperature differences across the torso, head, and extremities. This is somewhat controversial, but some chiropractors use this as a means of evaluating subluxations and somatic lesions.

Kemp's Test: A physical exam maneuver which is essentially equivalent to a quadrant test. The patient is asked to extend and side bend to one side, testing the compression of the facet joint on that side. This test is used to determine possible facet joint pathology. In this position, when overpressure is applied, there is narrowing of the intervertebral foramen, so this test can also be positive in foraminal stenosis.

Kernig's Sign: A physical exam maneuver that is positive in patients with meningeal irritation. The patient lies supine with the hips and knees flexed. The knee is then extended pulling on the dura. A positive test is limited knee extension due to dural or meningeal irritation.

Ketoprofen: A nonsteroidal anti-inflammatory drug in the propionic acid class. See Orudis.

Key Grip: A grip used in manual medicine similar to gripping a door key. The thumb and second finger are used to grip the part being mobilized. For instance, this is a common grip used to mobilize the clavicle.

Key Lesion: An osteopathic or manual physical therapy term which refers to the biomechanical abnormality in the spine which should be the focus of treatment. It is thought that if this area is returned to normal biomechanics, the rest of the spine will also return to normal biomechanics.

Kibler-Fold: A physical examination technique in which the thumb and index finger are used to grasp the paravertebral skin and "roll" this tissue from inferior to superior. See Skin Rolling.

Kilian's Line: A ridge on the promontory of the sacrum.

Kinesiology: A chiropractic diagnostic technique based on the idea that the neuromuscular system can be accessed through specific neuromuscular pressure points. See Applied Kinesiology.

Kinesthesia: The perception of movement, weight, and position. This commonly refers specifically to the perception of joint angle.

Kinesthetic Board: One of several different boards designed to increase kinesthetic awareness. See K-board.

Kinetic Chain: The concept that all joints of the body are linked and that what occurs to one joint effects others. In the lumbar spine, SI joint dysfunction causing dysfunction in the lumbar spine would be an example. Another example would be a short leg causing the foot and ankle to supinate and invert to compensate, thus causing patellofemoral problems at the knee.

Kinetic Intersegmental Subluxation: A chiropractic term which refers to a hypomobile segment, a hypermobile segment, or a segment with aberrant motion.

Kissing Osteophytes: An inflammatory reaction seen in the lumbar and interspinous ligaments with degenerative joint disease characterized by bridging osteophytes between the spinous processes. See Baastrup Disease.

KJ: An abbreviation for *knee jerk*. Another way to say patellar tendon reflex. See Patellar Tendon Reflex, Knee Jerk.

Klippel-Feil Syndrome: A syndrome of osseus malformations of the cervical spine most commonly associated with a "short" neck. This syndrome is also characterized by congenital fusion of two or more cervical vertebrae. C2–3 is the most commonly fused level. See Congenital Short Neck Syndrome.

Knee-Chest Table: A chiropractic adjusting table in which the patient is in a quadruped position. Gonstead adjusting techniques are used. It apparently provides a mechanical advantage to the manipulator when adjusting the thoracic and lumbar spines. There is no support for the chest, abdomen, and pelvis so that the manipulation allows free movement of the surrounding spinal column in an anterior direction. See KC.

Knee Jerk: Another way to say patellar tendon reflex. See Patellar Tendon Reflex.

Knife Edge: The type of hand position used for manipulation in which the fifth metacarpal contacts the body.

Knight Brace: A type of TLSO which offers some control of the upper lumbar spine in flexion and extension as well as side bending. It likely does not provide solid control of lumbar rotation. The brace has two lateral and two posterior supports. See Chair Back Brace, Macausland Brace.

Knuckle to Shoulder: A type of lift tested during a functional capacity evaluation. The patient is asked to lift from just below waist height to shoulder height.

Kostuik-Harrington Device: Instrumentation used for anterior interbody fusion which is a modified version of the classic posterior Harrington rod. See Kostuik Rods.

Kostuik Rods: Instrumentation used for anterior interbody fusion which is a modified version of the classic posterior Harrington rod. Screws are inserted into the vertebral bodies laterally, and a Harrington distraction rod is placed through the screw holes and distracted in the usual fashion. C-washers are used to lock the rod in place, and a second heavier Harrington compression rod is then placed posterior to the first rod. This system can be used for distraction, compression, or stabilization. See Kostuik-Harrington Device.

Krag Fixator: A type of pedicle screw fixation used for a posterior spinal fusion. See Pedicle Screw Fixation, Vermont Spinal Fixator.

Kummell's Disease: Delayed posttraumatic vertebral collapse. This is a rarely reported, poorly documented, and poorly understood phenomenon. There is an acute traumatic event followed by the development of vertebral collapse after the traumatic event.

Kypholordotic Posture: A standing posture that combines a thoracic kyphosis with an excessive lumbar lordosis. There is an increase in the lumbosacral angle with an increase in anterior pelvic tilt and hip flexion.

Kyphoscoliosis: A type of structural scoliosis which has a kyphotic appearance caused by a posterior rib cage on one side.

Kyphosis: A curve in which the apex points posteriorly. The normal thoracic kyphosis is balanced out by the cervical and lumbar lordosis (opposite curves). The shape of the thoracic kyphosis can be changed by moving the pelvis or protracting/retracting the shoulders. See Hyperkyphosis, Hypokyphosis, Kyphotic Posture.

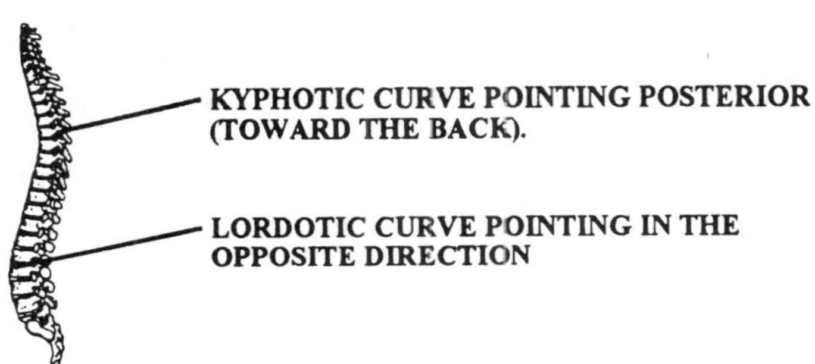

Kyphotic Posture: The head forward, rounded shoulders, "humpback" posture commonly seen in elderly women. This can also be seen in younger patients who have had trauma to the spine. There is an increased thoracic curve, protracted scapulae (rounded shoulders), and a forward head. There is often fatigue of the thoracic erector spinae and rhomboid muscles. Thoracic outlet syndrome can sometimes result as well as cervical posture syndromes. The tight structures are the pectorals, lats, and serratus anterior. The thoracic erector spinae, rhomboids, and middle and lower trapezii are often stretched and weak. See Forward Head Position, Kyphosis, Round Back Posture.

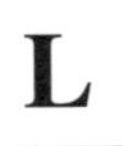

L: (1) An abbreviation for *left.* (2) An abbreviation in the chiropractic PGF listing system in which a spinous process is off to the left with the patient in the prone position. (3) An abbreviation for *lumbar.*

L1: An abbreviation for the first lumbar vertebra or first lumbar nerve root.

L1–2: An abbreviation for the intervertebral disc between the first lumbar vertebral body and the second lumbar vertebral body. Also, this denotes the L1–L2 motion segment.

L1–S1 Lordosis Angle: The angle formed by lines drawn through the top surface of L1 and the top surface of the sacrum. This is one method of measurement of the lumbar lordosis.

L2: An abbreviation for the second lumbar vertebra or nerve root.

L2–3: An abbreviation for the intervertebral disc between the second lumbar vertebra and the third lumbar vertebra. This also denotes the L2–3 motion segment.

L3: An abbreviation for the third lumbar vertebra or third lumbar nerve root.

L3–4: An abbreviation for the intervertebral disc space between the third lumbar vertebra and the fourth lumbar vertebra. This also denotes the L3–4 motion segment.

L4: An abbreviation for the fourth lumbar vertebra or fourth lumbar nerve root.

L4–5: An abbreviation for the intervertebral disc between the fourth lumbar vertebra and the fifth lumbar vertebra. This also denotes the L4–5 motion segment.

L4 Nerve Root: The fourth lumbar nerve root that exits between L4 and L5 and supplies various muscles in the lower extremity including quadriceps, iliopsoas, tibialis anterior, and gluteus medius. It supplies sensation to the medial calf. See L4 Root, Nerve Root—L4.

L4 Root: The fourth lumbar nerve root. See L4 Nerve Root.

L5: An abbreviation for the fifth lumbar vertebra or fifth lumbar nerve root.

L5 Nerve Root: This lumbar nerve root exits between L5 and S1. This nerve root supplies numerous muscles including the tibialis anterior, hamstrings, and gluteus maximus. The classic description of its sensory territory is the big toe. See L5 Root, Nerve Root—L5.

L5 SENSORY DISTRIBUTION

L5 Root: This lumbar nerve root exits between L5 and S1. See L5 Nerve Root, Nerve Root—L5.

L5–S1: The intervertebral disc between the fifth lumbar vertebra and the first sacral vertebra. This also denotes the L5–S1 motion segment. The majority of lumbar range of motion occurs at the L5–S1 segment.

la: A chiropractic abbreviation for *lamina.*

Labyrinthitis: Inflammation of the semicircular canals (labyrinth) in the inner ear. Significant vertigo is the most common symptom, and nystagmus can be seen clinically. It is usually a self-limited condition which is viral in origin. This can be confused with a perilymphatic fistula or a perilymph fistula which can be caused by a whiplash injury. See Vestibulitis.

Laguerre's Test: A physical exam maneuver which attempts to differentiate hip pain from lumbosacral pain. The patient lies in the supine position with the hip and knee flexed. The hip is then abducted and externally rotated. This is said to force the head of the femur against the anterior capsule of the hip joint. If pain in the hip is noted, the test is positive for the hip joint. If pain in the SI area is noted, this test is positive for pain in the low back.

Lamina: The upper portion of the neural arch which projects from the pedicles toward the midline. The lamina meet and fuse together in the midline forming the "roof" of the neural arch. The word is derived from the Latin *lamina*, meaning leaf or plate. The inferior lateral corner and inferior border of the lamina become the inferior articular process. The superior articular processes take their origin from the junction of the lamina and pedicle. See Vertebral Lamina.

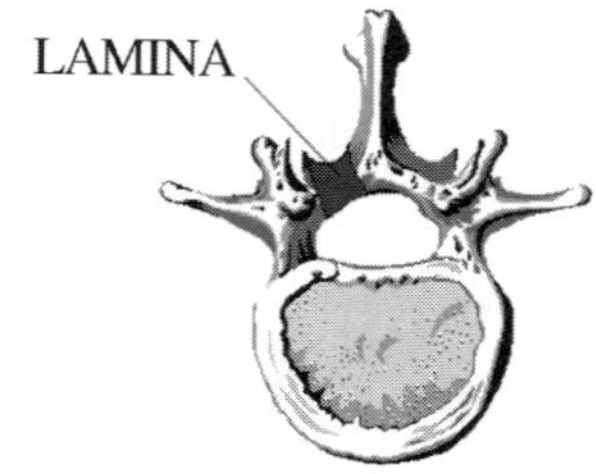

Laminar Fracture: A stable fracture of the lamina at any level of the spine which occurs most frequently in the mid to lower cervical spine with C5 and C6 being the most common levels. This type of fracture is best visualized on lateral x-rays. CT scanning may be necessary to demonstrate a fracture line.

Laminar Hooks: Hook-shaped attachments used to apply compression or distraction force with rodding systems such as Harrington, Cotrel-Dubousset, or Edwards. The curved attachment fits underneath the lamina and can be positioned to provide compression or distraction.

Laminectomy: A surgical technique in which the lamina and spinous process are removed to decompress the spinal canal or intervertebral foramen. This affords more of a decompressive effect than a laminotomy. This procedure is usually performed to "unroof" spinal stenosis and reduce the compression on the spinal cord and/or nerve roots. The ligamentum flavum is removed as well. A fat graft can be placed along the area where the lamina was removed. See Destabilizing Laminectomy, Total Laminectomy.

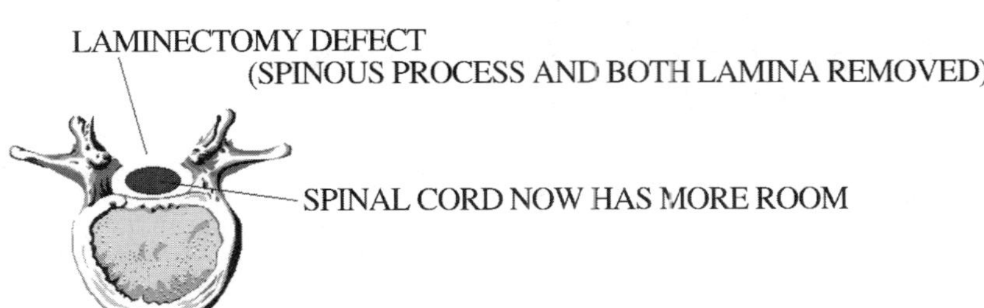

Laminoforaminotomy: A laminectomy with a foraminotomy. See Laminectomy, Foraminotomy.

Laminoplasty: The replacement of bone at the site of a previous laminectomy. The purpose of this procedure is to re-establish structural support and protection of the spinal cord. A bone graft can be placed by one of six different surgical procedures. This procedure is commonly used in children and in patients with ossification of the posterior longitudinal ligament to prevent progressive deformity of the spine. See OPLL.

Laminotomy: A surgical technique in which only a portion of the lamina is removed to decompress the intervertebral foramen. This can be performed through a smaller incision using microsurgical techniques. Extruded disc material is also commonly removed.

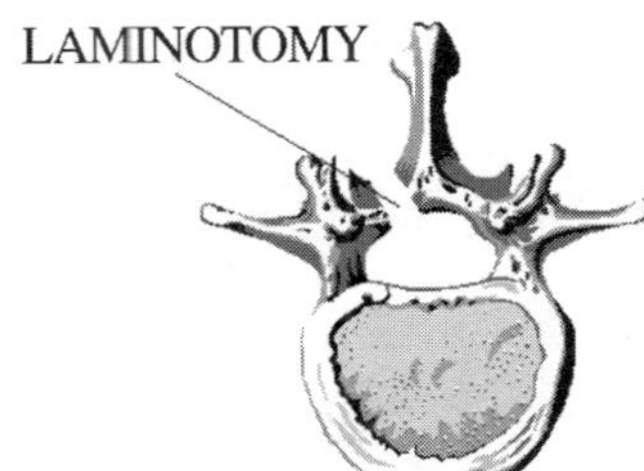

Lancinating Pain: Sharp or cutting pain.

LAO: An abbreviation for *left anterior oblique*.

Lap Belt Injury: A ligamentous or bony injury caused by a sudden flexion injury. The most common etiology is a motor vehicle accident with only a lap belt. These are less common since shoulder harnesses were mandated. They commonly occur in the upper lumbar spine. There may be an associated vertebral compression fracture. This can include ligamentous injuries to the supraspinous and interspinous ligaments as well as the facet capsules.

Lap Seat Belt Fracture: A fracture of the thoracolumbar spine which is caused by a flexion/distraction force. The fracture can restult from an MVA in which the patient was wearing an old style lap belt. See Chance Fracture, Seat Belt Fracture, Lap Belt Injury.

Large Mixed Nerve SEPs: Electrical potentials measured over the proximal part of a peripheral nerve, the spinal cord, and on the scalp after stimulation of a large mixed motor/sensory peripheral nerve. The most common nerve stimulated is the posterior tibial and peroneal nerves in the lower extremity and the median and ulnar nerves in the upper extremities. This is used as a diagnostic test for myelopathy. This technique is also used commonly in interoperative monitoring. See Somatosensory Evoked Potentials.

Larmor Frequency: The frequency at which hydrogen nuclei precess (or wobble) when a large external magnetic field is applied during magnetic resonance imaging (MRI). This is dependent on the strength of the magnetic field applied.

Lasegue Differential Sign: A physical exam maneuver in which the patient lies supine with the legs fully extended. The examiner performs a straight leg raising maneuver on the affected leg and notes the angle at which radicular pain is reproduced. The examiner then flexes the knee and thigh relieving the stretch on the sciatic nerve and nerve roots. The sign is said to be positive if the pressure is relieved. This can be helpful in differentiating hip pain from radicular pain.

Lasegue Rebound Test: A physical exam maneuver. The patient is in the supine position with both legs extended, and the examiner performs a straight leg raise. The leg is elevated to the point at which pain is produced. The extremity is then let go without warning. If the test causes a marked increase in low back pain, radicular symptoms, or muscle spasm, the test is considered positive. A positive test indicates disc involvement.

Lasegue Sitting Test: A physical examination maneuver. The patient is seated with legs hanging over the edge of the examination table. The examiner then fully extends one leg while checking for circulation, examining the skin, or checking for other foot and ankle abnormalities. A positive test is reproduction of radicular symptoms. This test is often used to double check a supine straight leg raising maneuver. However, some would argue that this is a different maneuver because the patient may be sensitized in a slump position to any dural or nerve root stretch. Also, in the seated position the pelvis is usually in a derotated position. See Seated Straight-Leg Raising Test.

Lasegue Test: A classic physical exam test for sciatica in which the patient lies supine with both legs extended. The hip and knee are flexed to approximately 90° with no pain elicited. The knee is then extended by the examiner with the hip in approximately 90° of flexion. If radicular symptoms are reproduced, a disc lesion or radiculopathy is suspected. See SLR.

Laser Therapy: Use of a laser for its superficial heating effects. There are many claims that laser light in some way effects overall cell metabolism and healing but there are no well-documented studies to support this theory.

Lat: An abbreviation for *lateral*.

Latent Trigger Point: A focus of hyperirritability within a muscle or its surrounding fascia that is nontender. This area is, however, diffusely tender to palpation. This is differentiated from an active trigger point in that an active trigger point is spontaneously tender. See Trigger Point.

Lateral: An x-ray that is taken from the side. See Lateral X-ray Film.

Lateral Bending: Bending to one side. See Lateral Flexion, Side Flexion.

Lateral Break: A chiropractic adjusting technique for the neck. The thrust does not rotate the neck; rather, the thrust is applied across the neck. See Cervical Break

Lateral Collis: An abnormal posture in which one shoulder is tilted or held high. This is often associated with cervical dystonia.

Lateral Deviation: A physical exam finding where the patient's spine is laterally flexed to one side in standing. See List.

Lateral Femoral Cutaneous Nerve: A nerve formed by the second and third lumbar roots. It becomes superficial at the ASIS and divides into two branches as it descends. The posterior branch provides sensation to the superior buttocks. The anterior branch passes through the fasciae lata in a small fibrous canal and provides sensation to the outer surface of the thigh. Entrapment of the anterior branch is associated with meralgia paresthetica. A tight ITB or tensor fascia lata may irritate this nerve and cause lateral thigh tingling or numbness. Also, it should be noted that this distribution of pain has been reported in SI dysfunction.

Lateral Flexion: Bending to one side. This is a coupled movement that involves both lateral bending and rotation. See Lateral Bending, Left Inferior Subluxation, Side Bending Lateroflexion, Flexion Right, Flexion Left.

Lateral Flexion Malposition: A chiropractic term which refers to a vertebra which is noted to be laterally flexed to the right or left on static testing. This is in relation to the adjacent vertebrae. Due to the orientation of the facets, the side that is inferior rotates posteriorly. The spinous is noted to be deviated to the left or right. See Right Inferior Subluxation.

Lateral Fusion: A type of surgical fusion of two vertebral segments which involves placing bone grafts laterally on the decorticated surfaces of the facet joints, transverse processes, and pars interarticularis.

Lateral Hemivertebra: The incomplete development of one side of a vertebra. See Hemivertebra.

Lateral Ischial Tuberosity: A pelvic dysfunction in which one ischial tuberosity is noted to be displaced laterally. There is increased tension in the sacrotuberous and sacrospinous ligaments which can cause referred pain down the back of the leg. The upper SI and symphysis pubis experience compressive forces while the lower SI and symphysis pubis experience tensile forces.

Lateralisthesis: A chiropractic term which refers to a vertebral body which has moved laterally in relation to the one above and the one below. This can be either to the right or to the left. See Left Lateral Subluxation, Right Lateral Subluxation.

Lateral Masses of the Atlas: The largest and most bulky portions of the atlas which support the head.

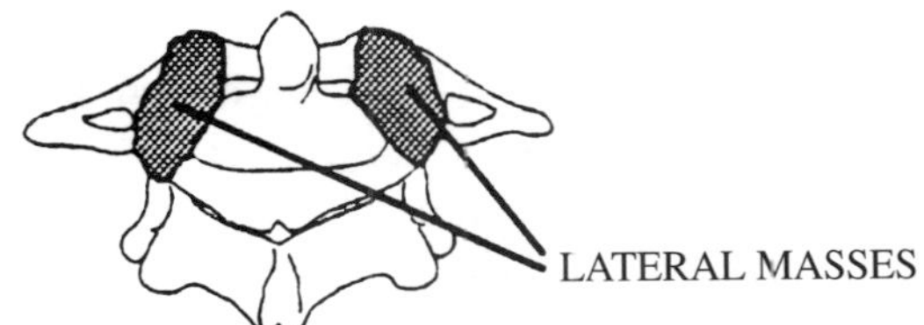

Lateral Pterygoid Muscle: A muscle that arises from the sphenoid bone and lateral pterygoid plate and inserts on the neck of the mandible, articular capsule of the TMJ, and disc of the TMJ. This muscle functions to open the jaw, protrude the mandible, and move the mandible from side to side. The myofascial pain referral pattern is to the TMJ and maxilla. Dysfunction in this muscle can result in decreased incisal distance.

Lateral Recess: A cone-shaped space on both sides of the vertebral canal opposite each of the pedicles. Bony hypertrophy in this area can lead to lateral recess stenosis and compromise of the exiting nerve root. See Radicular Canal, Nerve Root Canal.

Lateral Recess Stenosis: A decrease in size of the lateral recess, which is the area bounded by the pedicle, the superior articular facet, and the posterior lateral surface of the vertebral body and intervertebral disc. Bony hypertrophy of the superior facet, posterolateral osteophytes, or a far lateral disc herniation can cause nerve root entrapment. See Bony Compression. See Lateral Stenosis.

Lateral Sacral Crest: The tubercles which lie lateral to the sacral foramina. The upper two tubercles comprise the sacral tuberosity. This is the attachment site of the posterior sacroiliac ligament. The lower tubercles are anchors for the dorsal sacroiliac ligament and the sacrotuberous ligament.

Lateral Shift: A McKenzie physical therapy term used to denote a list to one side. It is thought that with lateral shifting extension alone will not reduce the nuclear protrusion until the shift is corrected. Once the shift is corrected, an extension program is added to maintain that correction.

Lateral Stenosis: A subcategory of lateral recess stenosis in which the nerve root is compressed as it exits the neural foramen. The nerve root is compressed because of hypertrophy of the superior articular facet or migration of the facet upward. See Lateral Recess Stenosis.

Lateral Subluxation: An asymmetric erosion of the lateral masses of C1 or C2. This can result in a lateral subluxation of C1 with respect to C2. The clinical finding is usually pain. This is often also associated with a rotational subluxation. On AP views of the upper cervical spine, if the lateral mass of C1 is displaced more than 2 mm lateral to the mass of C2, a lateral subluxation is suspected.

Lateral Wedge Fracture: A compression fracture which involves lateral collapse of the vertebrae. Therefore, wedging is seen when looking in the frontal plane. There may be associated injury of the facet on the same side. The lamina or pedicle can also be involved as well as fractures of the transverse processes. This can be associated with an iliopsoas injury and may be accompanied by a retro-peritoneal hemorrhage.

Lateral X-ray Film: An x-ray that is taken from the side.

LATERAL X-RAY VIEW

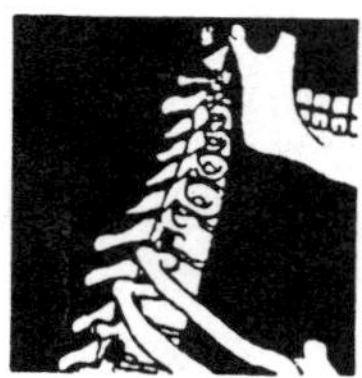

Laterodental Space: The spaces just lateral to the dens.

Lateroflexion: Bending to the right or left. See Side Bending, Lateral Flexion, Flexion Right, Flexion Left.

Latissimus Dorsi Muscle: A muscle arising from the spines of the lower six thoracic vertebrae, thoracolumbar fasciae, and posterior iliac crest and inserting on the intertubercular sulcus of the humerus. It is responsible for adducting, extending, and internally rotating the arm as well as stabilizing the scapula at the inferior angle. It is also an important muscle in spinal support and connects the low back to the upper extremities, acting as the link in the kinetic chain between the upper extremities and low back. Strengthening programs for low back pain often include strengthening of the latissimus dorsi. The myofascial referral pattern is to the inferior angle of the scapula, back of the shoulder, medial arm, and ulnar aspect of the hand. See Lats.

Lats: An abbreviation for *latissimus dorsi muscle.*

Laxity: A term that usually refers to excess movement in a joint or tissue. With respect to the spine, this often refers to an unstable vertebral segment or one that "moves too much."

LB: An abbreviation for *low back.*

LBD: An abbreviation for *low back disease* and *low back disorder.*

LBP: An abbreviation for *low back pain.*

LC: An abbreviation for *lower cervical.*

LCUT: An abbreviation for *lower cervical upper thoracic.*

L-D-C Spine: An abbreviation for lumbar-dorsal-cervical spines. This can be translated into lumbar-thoracic-cervical spines.

LDH: An extrusion of the nucleus pulposus through the anterior annular fibers. See Lumbar Disc Herniation, HNP.

Left Anterior Oblique: An x-ray term in which the patient is positioned facing the x-ray cartridge with the left shoulder forward and the right shoulder back. The patient is positioned obliquely so that the x-ray beam passes through the left posterior portion first and the right anterior portion last.

Left Anterior Sacral Torsion: An osteopathic or manual physical therapy term that denotes a left-on-left sacral torsion. See Left Forward Sacral Torsion.

Left Anterior Sacrum: An osteopathic or manual physical therapy term which refers to a sacrum in which the left sacral base is found to be anterior. See Unilteral Sacral Flexion—Left, Left Superior Sacral Shear.

Left Backward Sacral Torsion: An osteopathic or manual physical therapy term that denotes a left-on-right sacral torsion. There is a left-facing sacrum on a right oblique axis. The right sacral base is anterior and the left ILA is posterior and inferior. L5 is unable to extend on the sacrum and thus sacral-respiratory motion is inhibited. With lumbar extension, the right sacral base becomes more anterior.

Left-Facing Sacrum: An osteopathic or manual physical therapy term which describes a sacral torsion along an oblique sacral axis (from one sacral base to the opposite ILA). See Forward Sacral Torsion, Backward Sacral Torsion, Left-on-Right Sacral Torsion, Left-on-Left Sacral Torsion.

Left Forward Sacral Torsion: An osteopathic or manual physical therapy term that denotes a left-on-left sacral torsion. This is a left-facing sacrum on a left oblique axis and thought secondary to a tight right piriformis. The right sacral base is anterior in neutral or flexion and on lumbar extension corrects. The left inferior lateral angle is posterior and inferior. See Left Anterior Sacral Torsion.

Left Inferior Subluxation: A chiropractic term. This is a laterally flexed vertebra to the left with rotation to the left due to the orientation of the facet joints. See Lateral Flexion, LI.

Left Lateral: An x-ray which is taken with the patient's left side against the x-ray cartridge and the right side toward the x-ray beam. The beam then passes from right to left.

Left Lateral Subluxation: A chiropractic term which denotes a vertebral segment which has moved laterally to the left relative to the segment above and below. See Lateralisthesis.

Left-on-Left Sacral Torsion: An osteopathic or manual physical therapy term which describes a sacral torsion along an oblique sacral axis (from one sacral base to the opposite ILA). See Left Forward Sacral Torsion, Left-Facing Sacrum.

Left-on-Right Sacral Torsion: An osteopathic or manual physical therapy term which describes a sacral torsion found in lumbar backward bending. See Backward Sacral Torsion, Left-Facing Sacrum.

Left Posterior Oblique: An x-ray term in which the patient is positioned obliquely with the left side posterior and the right side anterior. The x-ray beam travels obliquely through the patient striking the right side first and then passing to the left side. The patient is facing away from the x-ray cartridge with the left shoulder touching the cartridge and the right shoulder forward away from the cartridge.

Left Posterior Subluxation: A chiropractic term which refers to a vertebra which is rotated to the left

(left facing or the left side of the vertebra has rotated posteriorly). Due to the orientation of the facets, the posterior side tends to move inferior. See Rotation Malposition, LP.

Left Superior Sacral Shear: An osteopathic or manual physical therapy term which refers to a sacrum in which the left sacral base is found in flexion. See Unilteral Sacral Flexion—Left.

Left Unilateral Sacral Flexion: An osteopathic or manual physical therapy term which refers to a sacrum in which the left sacral base is found in flexion. See Unilteral Sacral Flexion—Left, Left Superior Sacral Shear, Left Anterior Sacrum, Left Anterior Sacrum.

Leg Extension—Quadruped: A lumbar stabilization exercise. See Quadruped Leg Extension.

Leg Length Discrepancy: A difference in length between the lower extremities that has been postulated as a cause of low back pain. Most of the population has a leg length discrepancy. Leg length discrepancies can occur because of a congenitally short femur or tibia. It has also been postulated that they can occur secondary to SI joint problems. They are also thought to occur because of excess supination or pronation at the foot and ankle. Many chiropractors and manual therapists use leg length compared side to side to determine the effectiveness of their treatments. Also, it is thought that an anteriorly rotated ilium is associated with a short leg. See LLD, Short Leg Syndrome.

Leg Length Inequality: A difference in length between the lower extremities. See LLD, LLI.

Lesion: Used in the context of manual medicine, a lesion refers to an area of restriction of movement or a change in the position of one vertebrae in relation to another which is abnormal.

Levator Scapulae: A muscle that arises from the transverse processes of the atlas and axis and the transverse processes of C3 and C4 and inserts on the medial border of the scapula. This muscle is largely postural and also elevates and rotates the scapula downward as a secondary action. Innervation is C3–C4 and frequently the dorsal scapular nerve. The myofascial pain referral pattern is to the upper trapezius area, medial border of the scapula, and sometimes posterior shoulder.

Levoconvex: A radiology term used to describe a scoliosis. The apex of the curve points to the left.

Levo-scoliosis: A scoliotic curve with the convexity pointing to the left.

Lewin Punch Test: A physical examination maneuver which is performed with the patient standing. The examiner firmly percusses the buttock with a clenched fist on the affected side. If the punch produces referred pain in the back, the test is scored as positive. If punching on the opposite side does not produce pain, a disc lesion is suspected.

Lewin Snuff Test: A physical examination maneuver in which the patient is exposed to an aromatic substance and sneezing is induced. The test is positive if sneezing elicits an exacerbation of spinal or radicular pain. The test is positive in patients with disc lesions or dural irritation.

Lewin's Sign: The patient is asked to stand and asked to bring his knees into extension. Increased pain in the low back or leg will cause the patient to be unable to flex his knees if there is positive nerve root tension signs.

Lewin's Supine Test: A physical examination maneuver in which the patient is supine with both legs fully extended. The examiner firmly applies a downward pressure to the lower extremities while the patient is directed to perform a sit-up without using the upper extremities. The test is graded as positive if the patient is unable to perform this maneuver. It is thought that a positive test indicates lumbar arthritis, lumbar fibrosis, a degenerative disc with protrusion, sacroiliac or lumbosacral arthritis, or sciatica. However, this a nonspecific test that also can be positive in with patients with poor abdominal muscle tone or strength.

Lhermitte's Sign: A classic physical finding in cervical radiculopathy. The patient is usually seated with the head and neck in neutral position. The head and cervical spine are then flexed forward toward the patient's chest. A positive test is reproduction of sharp, electric, radiating pain or paresthesia along the spine and into one or more extremities.

LI: A chiropractic term which refers to a vertebra in which the mamillary or transverse process is laterally flexed left and inferior. See Left Inferior Subluxation.

Libman's Sign: A physical exam maneuver in which the patient's mastoid process is palpated deeply to determine response to pain. This is reportedly a test for nonorganic signs or symptom magnification.

Lidocaine: An amino amide which is commonly used for anesthetic infiltration. It has a rapid onset, moderate duration of action, and is relatively potent. Injectable solutions of 0.5%, 1.0%, 1.5%, and 2.0% are used for topical anesthesia, peripheral nerve blocks, and epidural anesthesia respectively. Also, 5% lidocaine with 7.5% glucose solution can be used for spinal anesthesia. The duration of action is 1–3 hours; however, the addition of epinephrine will significantly prolong the duration of action. See Xylocaine.

Lido Lift: A brand name for a computerized isometric lift station. See Lift Station.

Lieque Acupoint: An acupuncture point used for the treatment of headaches and neck pain that is located on the radial styloid process.

Lift Station: A mechanical or computerized device used to measure isometric lifting force. The measurements are taken in various positions such as floor lifts, waist lifts, and above shoulder lifts. This equipment is commonly used in a functional capacity evaluation to define lifting capabilities. See Lido Lift.

Ligament of Bougery: A ligament connecting the base of the transverse process to the mamillary process below. See Bougery Ligament.

Ligamentous Laxity: A loosening of the spinal ligaments which may be caused by degenerative disc disease or by acute trauma. This can lead to clinical instability (excess motion at one level).

Ligamentum Flavum: Literally, yellow ligament. A ligament which is adhered to the posterior surface of the spinal canal and is highly elastic owing to its high elastin content. This ligament can become less elastic with age and can buckle into the spinal canal, causing stenosis with extension. This process is called pseudohypertrophy of the ligamentum flavum, because the ligament does not typically enlarge.

Light Work: An NIOSH work category which involves frequently lifting up to 20 pounds and/or carrying up to 10 pounds. This job category also involves walking or standing to a significant degree.

Limbus Vertebra: A defect in the anterior ring apophysis of the vertebral body adjacent to the end plate. This is usually seen on lateral radiographs and appears as a chip off the corner. See Chip Fracture.

Limited Bone Scan: A bone scan of only one region of the body. See Bone Scan.

Lindner's Sign: A physical exam test where the chin is brought to the chest to screen for dural irritation. See Soto-Hall Sign.

Linea Splendens: A thickening of the ventral pia mater that completely envelops the entire length of the anterior spinal artery and its vein. The structure maintains the anterior position of the artery to the ventral median fissure.

Line of Drive: The direction of thrust during a manipulation or a mobilization. See LOD.

Lioresal: A muscle relaxant and antispasticity drug used most commonly in patients with spasticity due to spinal cord injuries. See Baclofen.

Lipping: An overgrowth of bone in response to injury. See Osteophyte.

List: A physical exam finding in which the patient's spine is bent to one side in standing. This suggests a herniated disc or nerve root tension. See Lateral Deviation.

Listing—Dynamic: A chiropractic term describing abnormal movement that is characteristic of one vertebra in relation to its adjacent segments. These usually are described as restrictions in flexion, extension, lateral flexion (right or left), and rotation (right or left). See Dynamic Listing, Fixation.

Listing—Static: A chiropractic term describing the spatial orientation of one vertebra in relation to its adjacent segments. This is defined as a malposition and is typically seen on x-ray. Vertebral malpositions can be seen in flexion, extension, lateral flexion (right or left), and rotation (right or left). See Static Listing.

LLD: A difference in length between the lower extremities that has been postulated as a cause of low back pain. See Leg Length Discrepancy.

LLI: A difference in length between the lower extremities. See LLD, Leg Length Inequality.

LMN: An abbreviation for *lower motor neuron.*

LMT: Licensed Massage Therapist.

L [number] L: A chiropractic term which denotes the lumbar segment number given is situated with the left transverse process posterior. This would mean that this segment is left facing. For example, an L4L would mean that the L4 segment has its transverse process posterior on the left or that the L4 segment is left facing.

L [number] R: A chiropractic notation which denotes the transverse process of the lumbar segment named is situated with the right transverse process posterior. This would be equivalent to a right-facing lumbar segment at that level. For example, an L3R would mean that the transverse process of L3 is posterior on the right or that this segment is right facing.

Localized Degenerative Disc Disease: Degenerative disc disease that occurs at one level. See Degenerative Disc Disease.

Localized Hypertonus: Increased local muscle tone due to irritation. See Spasm.

Local Twitch Response: A sudden contraction of muscle seen as a twitch in response to stimulation of a trigger point. See Twitch Response, Jump Sign.

LOD: The direction of thrust during a manipulation or a mobilization. See Line of Drive.

Lodine: A nonsteroidal anti-inflammatory in the pyranocarboxylic acid group. It has analgesic and anti-inflammatory properties. As with all nonsteroidals, GI side effects are possible. Renal and hepatic side effects are also not uncommon. There are drug interactions with antacids, aspirin, warfarin, phenytoin, glyburide, diuretics, cyclosporin, digoxin, lithium, and methotrexate. The recommended adult dosage for acute pain relief is 200–400 mg every 6–8 hours, not to exceed a total daily dose of 1,200 mg. For patients weighing less than 60 kg, the total daily dosage should not exceed 20 mg per kg. The drug can also be given two to three times a day for the treatment of osteoarthritis. It is available in 200-mg, 300-mg, and 400-mg capsules and tablets. See Etodolac.

Loganbasic: A chirporactic technique which utilizes sustained contact with low force. This technique is used by about 30% of all U.S. chiropractors. See Nonforce Technique.

Loma Linda Activity Sort: A test of perceived abilities sometimes performed as part of a functional capacity evaluation. The patient is asked to sort a deck of cards with different activities (similar to a West Tool Sort which uses cards with tools) as to his/her ability to perform the activity. The test is perfomed to obtain a score of perceived disability that can be compared with standardized percentile scores for age and sex.

Also, it is often performed to determine validity of testing (whether the patient is malingering or magnifying symptoms). There are cards with similar activity levels which need to be sorted into the same catagories by the patient for the test to be valid. See West Tool Sort.

Long C-curve: A type of scoliosis that usually extends the length of the thoracic and lumbar regions, thus the designation "long." There is usually a high shoulder on the convex side of the curve and a high pelvis on the concave side. This type of scoliosis is thus uncompensated.

Longissimus Cervicis: A muscle taking its origin from the transverse processes of T1 through T4 and inserting into the transverse processes of C2 through C6. It is responsible for extending the vertebral column and bending the head to the same side. Note that it travels from thoracic transverse processes to cervical transverse processes. Innervation is the dorsal primary rami of the spinal nerves.

Longissimus Thoracis: A muscle arising from the transverse processes of the lumbar vertebrae and inserting on the tips of the transverse processes of all thoracic vertebrae and the lower 9–10 ribs. It is responsible for extending the vertebral column and bending it to the same side while drawing the ribs inferiorly. Innervation is the dorsal primary rami of spinal nerves. Myofascial pain referral pattern is to the upper or lower buttocks.

Long Lever Technique: A nonspecific type of chiropractic manipulation. See Long Lever Thrust.

Long Lever Thrust: A nonspecific type of chiropractic manipulation in which a body part is used as a lever arm to direct forces to a region of the spine. A side posture manipulation or "million dollar roll" would be one example. See Long Lever Technique.

Long-Sit Test: A manual medicine test for an ilial rotation. This involves having the patient bridge then lower the buttocks to the table. The legs are then grasped around the ankles and extended. The leg length is noted and then the patient is asked to sit with the legs extended. The leg lengths are then again noted. If one leg becomes longer, the SI joint on that side is hypomobile, which suggests an SI joint dysfunction. An anteriorly rotated ilium will increase leg length more than a posteriorly rotated ilium. Some consider this an unreliable test owing to the many variables involved.

Long Thoracic Corset: A type of TLSO which is used to stabilize the thoracic spine. It restricts flexion/extension and lateral bending. This type of orthosis provides the least amount of control over the thoracic spine of all the thoracic orthoses.

Long Two-Poster Orthosis: A cervical orthosis which also extends down to the upper thoracic spine. This is more effective in limiting cervical range of motion than a Philadelphia collar, four-poster collar, or Thomas collar. It does limit cervical range of motion at all three axes. See Guillford Collar, Duke Collar.

Longus Capitis: A muscle arising from the transverse processes of T1 through T4 and inserting on the mastoid process. It is responsible for extending the head and bending it to the same side or rotating the face to the same side. Innervation is the dorsal primary rami of the spinal nerves of T1 through T4. This muscle also serves a function as a long stabilizer of the cervical spine.

Loose Packed Joint Position: The point in the range of motion at which the joint surfaces are the least congruent and the supporting structures are the most lax. For the facet joints, this would be in spinal neutral.

Lorazepam: A benzodiazepine used for the management of anxiety disorders or for the short-term relief of symptoms of anxiety or anxiety associated with depressive symptoms. See Ativan.

Lorcet: A narcotic pain reliever containing either 5 mg of hydrocodone and 500 mg of acetaminophen (5/500) or 10 mg of hydrocodone and 650 mg of acetaminophen (10/650). Physical addiction is possible. The usual dosage is one tablet every 4–6 hours with the total 24-hour dose not to exceed six tablets.

Lorcet-HD: Lorcet in capsule form (instead of tablet) which contains 5 mg of hydrocodone and 500 mg of acetaminophen. This is equivalent to Lortab 5.0. The usual dosage is one tablet every 4–6 hours.

Lordoscoliosis: Lordosis associated with a scoliosis. A lateral curvature of the spine associated with increased anterior curvature of the spine. See Scoliosis, Lordosis.

Lordosis: The normal curve of the lumbar spine which is maintained to balance the thoracic kyphosis. The shape of the lumbar lordosis can be changed by tilting the pelvis forward or backwards. The apex of the curve points anteriorly. See Lumbar Lordosis, Lordoscoliosis.

Lordotic: Of or pertaining to lordosis.

Lordotic Posture: A posture characterized by an increase in the lumbosacral angle, an increased lumbar lordosis, an increased anterior tilting of the pelvis, and hip flexion.

Lortab: A brand name for a hydrocodone and acetaminophen narcotic pain reliever. There are varying strengths of hydrocodone from 2.5 mg to 7.5 mg combined with 500 mg of acetaminophen. This is a narcotic analgesic that can cause CNS depression and addiction. Common dosages are 2.5/500, 5.0/500, and 7.5/500 as 1–2 tablets every 4–6 hours.

Loss of Joint Play: Joint play is usually taken to mean the viscoelastic properties or "give" of a joint. See Somatic Dysfunction, Viscoelastic.

Lou Gehrig Disease: A commonly fatal neurologic disorder with an unknown etiology. See ALS, Amyotrophic Lateral Sclerosis.

Low Back Index: A grading system for determining the severity of patients with low back pain. The grading system is between 1.0 and 4.0. Low is between 1.0 and 1.6, moderate between 1.7 and 3.2, and high severity between 3.3 and 4.0.

Lower Abdominals: The most inferior portion of the rectus femoris. Weakness here is thought to be associated with poor pelvic stability and low back pain.

Lower Abdominal Progression: Test maneuvers designed to determine the strength of the lower abdominals. More and more stress is added to the lower abdominals by changing the involvement of the lower extremities. For instance, one test involves having the patient in a supine position with the hips at 90° and knees at 90°. The patient is then asked to lower the hips and lower extremities down to the ground while keeping the lumbar spine flat against the table or in neutral position. If the patient is able to perform this maneuver completely, then there is 4/5 lower abdominal strength. This tests the strength of the external obliques and lower rectus abdominis. See Double Leg Lowering.

Lower Cervical Spine: The C3 through C7 vertebral segments exclusive of the C1 and C2 segments.

Lower Half Headache: A headache primarily in the lower face which is thought to be vascular in origin. This can also be confused with "atypical facial" neuralgia, sphenopalatine ganglion neuralgia, and vidian neuralgia.

Lower Trunk Rotation: A physical therapy exercise used to develop rotational coordination between the spinal musculature (intrinsic) and the abdominal musculature (extrinsic). The patient starts in the hook-lying position and drops the legs to one side in a slow, controlled manner. The legs are then returned to the upright position slowly and using proper muscular sequencing. As an advanced exercise, the legs can be crossed.

Low-velocity Thrust: A type of manipulation in which a slow manipulation or mobilization is applied to a joint. There is usually pre-stress placed on a joint so that this low-velocity maneuver gaps the joint and creates cavitation.

LP: A chiropractic term which refers to a vertebra which has rotated toward the left. The transverse process or mamillary process is noted to be deep on the right in prone testing. See Left Posterior Subluxation.

LPN: Licensed Practical Nurse.

LPO: An abbreviation for *left posterior oblique*.

L-rod: Spinal instrumentation which involves wires that encircle the lamina and are tied to a contoured, L-shaped stainless steel rod. See Luque Rods.

L–S Series: A series of x-rays of the lumbar spine which includes an anterorposterior view, a lateral view, two oblique views, and often a coned view of L5–S1. See Lumbosacral Series.

L-S: An abbreviation for *lumbosacral*.

L/S Strain: An acute injury to the musculature and ligamentous structures of the low back. See Lumbar Strain.

Lucent Cleft Sign: A radiographic sign which can be seen after whiplash injury. See Vacuum Cleft Sign.

Lumbago: An ICD-9 diagnosis code for a dull, aching pain in the lumbar region. It can also refer to myofascial pain of the lumbar spine. See Myofascial Pain.

Lumbalgia: A nonspecific term for low back pain.

Lumbar: Of or pertaining to the low back. The lumbar spine has five vertebrae stacked on top of the sacrum. Most of the movement in this region occurs at L5–S1 and L4–L5.

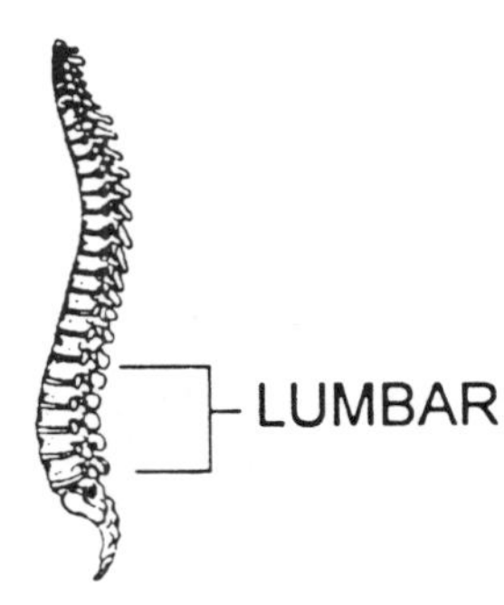

Lumbar Artery: A pair of arteries that take their origin from the posterior aorta from L1 through L4. At L5, the lumbar artery arises from the median sacral artery. The lumbar artery passes posteriorly around the vertebral bodies in the concavity located in the lateral surface of the vertebral body. It is covered by the tendinous arch of the psoas muscle. As the artery reaches the intervertebral foramen, it divides into several branches. The lateral branches pass through the psoas and quadratus lumborum and supply the abdominal wall. The others pass along with the ventral ramus and dorsal ramus of the spinal nerve supplying the paravertebral muscles innervated by those nerves. There is a posteriorly directed branch which passes below the transverse process and runs perpendicular to the lateral border of the pars interarticularis to enter the erector spinae musculature. The posterior branches also supply the facet joints, lamina, and spinous processes. The medially directed branches have three off-shoots: the anterior spinal canal branch, the posterior spinal canal branch, and the radicular branch. The anterior spinal canal branch forms an arterial arcade by sending ascending and descending branches to communicate with the lumbar arteries above and below. These arcades exist along the floor of the vertebral canal. The posterior branches form a similar arcade on the roof of the vertebral canal along the lamina and ligamentum flavum.

Lumbar Contusion: Bruising from a direct blow to the lumbar spine musculature. This results in capillary rupture, bleeding, edema, and a local inflammatory response.

Lumbar Corset: A soft, pliable low back support brace with or without hard metal stays.

Lumbar Curve: A scoliosis with its apex between L1 and L4.

Lumbar Disc Disorder with Myelopathy: An ICD-9 diagnosis code which usually refers to a large centrally herniated lumbar disc causing pressure on the lower spinal cord, conus medullaris, or cauda equina. See Conus Medullaris Syndrome, Cauda Equina Syndrome, Myelopathy.

Lumbar Disc Herniation: An extrusion of the nucleus pulposus through the anterior annular fibers. See LDH, HNP.

Lumbar Disc Syndrome: The symptom complex associated with a herniated disc or HNP. This is low back pain associated with radiating pain in a dermatomal distribution.

Lumbar Gravity Line: An x-ray sign which is used to determine overall standing posture. A lateral lumbar view is performed in standing. The center of the third vertebral body is located by drawing intersecting diagonal lines from opposing corner to opposing corner. A vertical line is then drawn from this point downward. The center of gravity of the trunk apparently passes through the center of the third lumbar body and should intersect the sacral base. If the line is anterior to the sacrum by more than 1 cm, shearing stresses increase across the facet joints. A posterior shift in the gravity line may indicate increased weight bearing on the posterior elements/facet joints. See Ferguson's Weight Bearing Line, Ferguson's Gravitational Line.

Lumbar Instability: A radiographic evaluation for lumbar instability due to trauma or degenerative disease. See Van Akkerveeken's Measurement of Lumbar Instability.

Lumbarization: A congenital variation of normal lumbar spine anatomy in which S1 is mobile and the S1–S2 interspace contains an intervertebral disc. This makes the S1–S2 segment the first mobile segment rather than the usual L5–S1.

Lumbar Lordosis: The normal curvature of the spine in the lumbar region with the convexity of the curve facing anteriorly. This is maintained to balance the thoracic kyphosis and distribute compressive forces. See Lordosis.

Lumbar Lordotic Angle: The angle on lateral x-rays between the top of L2 and the bottom of L5 which is used to measure the lumbar lordosis.

Lumbar Nerve Block: A local anesthetic block of the lumbar nerve roots as they exit from the foramen. The anesthesia is placed outside the epidural space. This differs from a selective nerve root block, which places anesthetic into the epidural space. A block at this level multiple distal muscles and large peripheral areas of sensation. See Somatic Lumbar Nerve Block.

Lumbar Plexus: A nerve plexus located in the lumbar region which is made up of the T12 through L4 anterior primary rami. It lies anterior to the upper lumbar transverse processes and deep to the psoas musculature. The iliohypogastric nerve, the ilioinguinal nerve, the genitofemoral nerve, the lateral femoral cutaneous nerve, and the accessory obturator nerve originate from the lumbar plexus. Also, the nerves to the quadratus lumborum, psoas major, psoas minor, and iliacus muscles originate from the lumbar plexus. See Lumbosacral Plexus.

Lumbar Puncture: The introduction of a needle into the subarachnoid space for the purpose of sampling CSF for diagnosis, measuring CSF pressure, injecting medications such as anesthetics or steroids, or injecting contrast material such as for a myleogram. See Spinal Tap.

Lumbar Radiculopathy: An ICD-9 diagnosis code which usually refers to a lumbar or S1 radiculopathy caused by an HNP. See Lumbosacral Neuropathy and Radiculopathy, Radiculopathy.

Lumbar Roll: A side-lying chiropractic adjusting technique. Force is applied simultaneously to the shoulder and pelvis. The shoulder is thrust in one direction while the pelvis is usually thrust in the opposite direction. This is a long lever, nonspecific manipulation.

Lumbar Sprain/Strain: An acute injury to the musculature and ligamentous structures of the low back.

This is usually a self-limited problem that resolves in days to weeks. This is also somewhat of an overused term for nonspecific diagnoses for a number of specific lumbar problems. See Lumbar Strain.

Lumbar Spring Test: The introduction of a PA mobilization to each lumbar segment to test for hypo- or hypermobility. Pressure is usually planed over the spinous process but springing can be performed over the transverse processes to check for rotational hyper- or hypomobility.

Lumbar Stabilization: A rehabilitation program used to stabilize the lumbar spine through the pelvis that involves neuromuscular retraining, flexibility, and strengthening. See Dynamic Lumbar Stabilization.

Lumbar Strain: An acute injury to the musculature and ligamentous structures of the low back. This is usually a self-limited problem that resolves in days to weeks. L/S strains which do not resolve within six weeks may represent other pathology including annular tears. See L/S Strain, Lumbar Sprain/Strain.

Lumbar Sympathetic Block: A block commonly used in patients with lower extremity reflex sympathetic dystrophy. The lumbar sympathetic chain in the lower thoracic, L1, L2 area is infiltrated with anesthetic or a sympathetic blocking agent. See Sympathetic Block—Lumbar.

Lumbar Triangle: An anatomic triangle located just above the ilium. The borders are the latissimus dorsi, the external oblique, and the ilium. See Petit's Triangle.

Lumbocostal: Referring to the lumbar region and ribs.

Lumbodorsal: Referring to the thoracic and lumbar spine.

Lumbodorsal Fascia: A thick sheet of connective tissue that covers the superficial musculature of the lumbar spine. See Thoracodorsal Fascia.

Lumbolumbar Lordotic Angle: A radiographic measurement of the lumbar lordosis measured on a standing lateral film. A line is drawn parallel to the superior end plate of L2 and another line parallel to the inferior end plate of L5. The angle between these two lines is measured.

Lumbopelvic Rhythm: A descriptive term based on the concept that the lumbar spine flexes forward first in forward bending and then is followed by the pelvis rotating forward. Those two separate coordinated movements allow the patient to bend over and touch the floor. The gluteal muscles are extremely important in lumbopelvic rhythm as they provide most of the force in re-extension (lifting things from the floor).

Lumbopelvic Support: A pelvic belt used in SI joint syndrome where hypermobility is suspected. See SI Belt.

Lumbosacral: Referring to the lumbar and sacral portions of the spine.

Lumbosacral Agenesis: An unusual congenital vertebral malformation characterized by vertebropelvic instability. There is failure of formation of part of the lumbar spine and sacrum. This causes an imbalance in muscular function. There is also malformation of the ventral neural elements causing lower leg atrophy and joint deformities.

Lumbosacral and Thoracic Neuropathy and Radiculopathy: An ICD-9 diagnosis code which usually refers to a lumbar or S1 radiculopathy caused by an HNP.

Lumbosacral Angle: A radiographic measurement of the angle between the superior end plate of L2 and the base of the sacrum. This is usually measured with a standing lateral x-ray film. See Lumbosacral Lordotic Angle.

Lumbosacral Corset: A type of TLSO (brace that extends from under the shoulders to the pelvis) which is made of fabric and provides minimal support to the lumbar spine. See Corset, Lumbosacral Orthosis.

Lumbosacral Curve: A scoliosis with its apex at L5 or below.

Lumbosacral Disc: Another term for the L5–S1 disc.

Lumbosacral Dysfunction: This term refers to anything from garden variety low back pain to something as specific as biomechanical abnormalities in the L5–S1 segment.

Lumbosacral Facet: Another term for the L5–S1 facet joint.

Lumbosacral Instability: Ligamentous instability seen at L5–S1, usually demonstrated on flexion–extension views of the lumbar spine. See Instability.

Lumbosacral Joint: Referring to the area where the sacrum and the iliac bones form a joint. See Sacroiliac Joint.

Lumbosacral Lordotic Angle: A radiographic measurement of the angle between the superior end plate of L2 and the base of the sacrum. This is usually measured with a standing lateral x-ray film. See Lumbosacral Angle.

Lumbosacral Neuropathy and Radiculopathy: An ICD-9 diagnosis code which usually refers to a lumbar or S1 radiculopathy caused by an HNP. See Lumbar Radiculopathy, Radiculopathy.

Lumbosacral Orthosis: Similar to a TLSO but shorter. This is used to stabilize the lumbar region and usually refers to either a hard or soft brace. See Lumbosacral Corset.

Lumbosacral Plexus: Referring to a combination of the lumbar and sacral plexuses. See Lumbar Plexus, Sacral Plexus.

Lumbosacral Scoliosis: A scoliosis with its apex at L5 or below.

Lumbosacral Series: A series of x-rays of the lumbar spine which includes an anterior-posterior view, a lateral view, two oblique views, and often a coned view of L5–S1. See L-S Series.

Lumbosacral Sprain/Strain: An injury to the musculature of the low back and sacral regions. See Acute Low Back Strain.

Lumbosacral Strain: An injury to the musculature of the low back and sacral regions. See Lumbosacral Sprain/Strain.

Luque Fixation: Posterior segmental fixation with a wire that encircles the lamina in combination with a metal rod. The wire enters the spinal canal—and has inherent risks by doing so—but forms a sturdy attachment. This system is primarily used to correct neuromuscular scoliosis. See Pedicle Screw Fixation.

Luque Fixator: A type of pedicle screw fixation used for posterior spinal fusion.

Luque Rods: Spinal instrumentation which involves wires that encircle the lamina and which are tied to a contoured, L-shaped stainless steel rod. The rod is bent back on itself forming a loop with L-shaped ends which oppose each other. This portion is anchored to the spinous process or to the pelvis. This type of instrumentation is used for the correction of scoliosis, the treatment of fractures, and for clinical instability. See L-rod.

Luschka's Joint: The joints which occur in the lower cervical spine from C2 through C7. See Uncovertebral Joint.

Luxated Joint: Complete dislocation of the joint, i.e., no contact between the joint surfaces. See Subluxation.

Luxation: From an orthopaedic standpoint, abnormal joint movement beyond normal range of motion (an incomplete dislocation). See Subluxation.

LVN: Licensed Vocational Nurse.

Lymphoma: A malignant tumor which usually presents as a systemic disease with skeletal manifestations but can occur as an isolated bony tumor. There is some controversy as to whether this tumor is primary or metastatic in the spine. It should be noted that lymphoma is the most common malignancy found in the epidural space and primary lymphomas within the epidural space have been encountered. However, most lymphomas in the epidural space are thought to be due to paraspinal lymph nodes. Plain radiographs show some bony erosion or may be completely abnormal. Myelography or CT myelography is extremely reliable. MRI can be helpful. Surgical decompression usually involves laminectomy, and neurologic compromise is not uncommon. See Reticulum Cell Sarcoma.

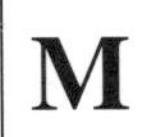

m: An abbreviation for *mamillary process*.

Macausland Brace: A lumbar support brace which gives excellent control in flexion and extension. It is less effective in side bending because of the lack of lateral uprights. It is not as effective in controlling rotation as other devices that can potentially be used. See Chair Back Brace.

MacNab's Line: A radiographic sign used to detect superior articular process facet imbrication (subluxation). In effect, this line is used to detect overriding facet joints and significant degenerative disease. A lateral lumbar view is used, and a line is drawn parallel to the inferior end plate. The relationship of this line to the superior articular process below is assessed. The line should lie above the tip of the adjacent superior articular process of the level below.

Magerl External Spinal Fixator: Instrumentation used for a posterior spinal fusion using pedicle screws. This is an external fixator which is adjustable in three dimensions. See Magerl Fixator, Pedicle Screw Fixation.

Magerl Fixator: A type of pedicle screw fixation used for posterior spinal fusion. See Magerl External Spinal Fixator.

Magnetic Cortical Stimulation: A method of monitoring the integrity of the corticospinal tract and motor pathways during spinal surgery. See Motor Evoked Potential.

Magnetic Resonance Imaging: An imaging technique which utilizes magnetic fields to obtain detailed pictures of both soft tissue and bony anatomy. See MRI.

Magnified Illness Behavior: A nonspecific term implying unconscious magnification of symptomatology out of proportion to pathology. See Symptom Magnification Syndrome.

Magnuson's Test: A physical exam test used to determine if the patient is malingering. The site at which the patient reports pain is marked. The patient is then distracted and the back examination is resumed. If the site is no longer tender, the patient could be malingering.

Maitland: A manipulative physical therapy technique developed by Geoffrey Maitland. See Maitland Technique.

Maitland Certified: A certification program most prevalent in the UK and Australia which credentials physical therapists in Maitland mobilization techniques. See Maitland Technique.

Maitland Technique: A manipulative physical therapy technique developed by Geoffrey Maitland which concentrates on establishing normal segmental spinal motion through the use of mobilization. Unlike other techniques, vertebral position is not addressed. See Maitland.

Major Curve: A term used to designate the larger of two scoliotic curves. This is usually a structural scoliosis.

Major Depression: An ICD-9 diagnosis involving depressed mood and/or loss of interest in life and/or loss of pleasure in normal, everyday activities for at least two weeks. See Depression, Major.

Malformation Retro-medullaire: An AV fistula where the nidus is the nerve root sleeve dura. See Dural AV Fistula.

Malgaigne Fracture: The most common fracture of the pelvis, which results from a double vertical shearing injury. This is an unstable, through and through fracture of one portion of the pelvic ring and is defined as a one-sided double vertical fracture of the superior pubic ramus and ischiopubic ramus, with fracture or dislocation of the SI joint.

Malignant Multiple Myeloma: A malignant tumor which occurs in the spine. This is relatively uncommon, occurring in 2–3 patients per 100,000. Spinal lesions are usually metastatic in a progressive systemic disease and are usually fatal within 2–3 years. The five-year survival rate is 18%. Reccurrence is not uncommon after many years of disease-free survival, and this is detected using serum protein immunoelectrophoresis. The treatment of choice is usually radiation, but surgical treatment has been advocated either to prevent vertebral body collapse or stabilize vertebral body collapse once instability has occurred. This tumor is one of a continuum of B cell lymphoproliferative diseases.

Malingerer: A medicolegal term for one who consciously and willfully misrepresents illness or symptoms in order to escape work duties and/or for financial compensation. True malingering is thought to be rare. Compare with symptom magnification syndrome. See Factitious Disorder, Malingering.

Malingering: A medicolegal term for one who consciously and willfully misrepresents illness or symptoms in order to escape work duties and/or for financial compensation. True malingering is thought to be rare. Compare with symptom magnification syndrome. See Factitious Disorder, Malingerer.

Malleo-Loc Brace: The brand name for a thermoplastic and Velcro ankle brace which provides excellent ankle support. A variety of ankle braces can be used in patients that have dynamic ankle instability due to motor weakness.

Malposition: A chiropractic term denoting abnormal or anomalous vertebral position. A malposition can be in flexion, extension, lateral flexion (right or left), or in rotation (right or left). A malposition is a static finding. For instance, a malposition is found and named without considering abnormal movement. See Static Intersegmental Subluxation, Static Vertebral Malposition.

Mamillary Process: A small, smooth bump on the posterior edge of each superior articular process. This lies just above and slightly medially to the accessory process. This name is derived from the Latin for "small breast" because of its appearance.

Mandibular Pain Dysfunction Syndrome: Pain emanating from the temporomandibular joint. See TMJ Dysfunction, Arthrosis Temporomandibularis, Temporomandibular Joint Arthrosis, TMJ Myofascial Pain, Tempormandibular Dysfunction.

Manipulation: The application of a force to a joint that takes it beyond its normal range of motion into its elastic range. The most common types of manipulation are chiropractic and osteopathic. Many physical therapists also utilize manipulation. The mechanism of action is unknown but is thought to include reflex muscle inhibition, the reduction of subluxations, increasing directional joint range of motion, or the reduction of "meniscoids." See adj, Adjustment, Grade 5 Mobilization, Dynamic Thrust, High-velocity Thrusting, Joint Adjustment, Joint Manipulation.

Manipulation under Anesthesia: Manipulation of the spine with the patient under general anesthesia. This is usually performed by chiropractors in conjunction with an M.D. or D.O. team and is used only in well-screened patients. The goal is to "reduce" a disc herniation.

Mannkopf's Sign: A physical exam test for symptom magnification. The patient's pulse is taken prior to deep palpation of a very painful area. This painful palpation should increase the pulse approximately 10 beats per minute if the patient is in extreme pain. If palpation does not increase the heart rate, then the patient is exaggerating his symptoms.

Manual Lymph Drainage: The application of deep pressure to the skin to allow lymphatic pathways to drain.

Manual Materials Handling: A type of industrial work which involves lifting and moving objects as the main occupational task. See MMH.

Manual Muscle Test—Grade 1: A measure of muscle strength where the muscle being tested is unable to move a joint through any part of its range of motion. See Grade 1 Manual Muscle Test.

Manual Muscle Test—Grade 2: A measure of muscle strength where the muscle being tested is able to move a joint against gravity through only part of its available range of motion. See Grade 2 Manual Muscle Test.

Manual Muscle Test—Grade 3: A measure of muscle strength where the muscle being tested is able to move a joint against gravity (without resistance) through its full range of motion. See Grade 3 Manual Muscle Test.

Manual Muscle Test—Grade 4: A measure of muscle strength where the muscle being tested is able to move a joint (against resistance) through its full range of motion. See Grade 4 Manual Muscle Test.

Manual Muscle Test—Grade 5: Normal muscle strength.

Manual Muscle Testing: Physical exam testing used to grade muscle strength. The most common scale is graded 0–5, with a 5 being normal muscle strength and a 4/5 considered complete range of motion against gravity with some resistance. Various muscle groups can be isolated and tested and compared side to side for relative strength, looking for specific areas of weakness. This can be helpful in designing a rehabilitation program focused on those specific areas of weakness. See Highet's Scale.

Manual Physical Therapist: A physical therapist that concentrates on a hands-on approach to treatment. This includes mobilization of the spine as described by Maitland or Paris, Norwegian manual therapy, muscle energy technique, osteopathic manipulative therapy, strain-counterstrain, and other techniques. See Manual Therapy.

Manual Physical Therapy: Physical therapy which concentrates on a hands-on approach to treatment. See Manual Therapy.

Manual Therapy: Physical therapy which concentrates on a hands-on approach to treatment. This includes mobilization of the spine as described by Maitland or Paris, Norwegian manual therapy, muscle energy techniques, osteopathic manipulative therapy, strain-counterstrain, and multiple types of chiropractic manipulation and techniques. See Manual Physical Therapy, Manual Physical Therapist.

Manual Traction: This is axial distraction that is applied by manual means (i.e., hands). See Traction.

Manual TX: Physical therapy which concentrates on a hands-on approach to treatment. See Manual Physical Therapy.

Marcaine: An amino amide anesthetic which has a significantly prolonged duration of action relative to traditional amino amides. See Bupivacaine.

March Test: A common physical exam test used to detect SI joint dysfunction (abnormal SI joint movement). See Gillet's Test.

Marfan Syndrome: A connective tissue disease usually seen in tall men (also occurs in women). With respect to the spine, there is an associated scoliosis.

Marginal Syndesmophyte: A vertically oriented calcification adjacent to the intervertebral disc or vertebra. See Syndesmophyte.

Marie-Strumpell Disease: Also known as bamboo spine because of its bamboo shoot-like appearance on x-rays. See Ankylosing Spondylitis, AS, Von Bechterew Disease, Rheumatoid Spondylitis, Pelvospondylitis Ossificans.

Massage: Deep or light pressure applied to muscles and/or fascia for the purpose of muscle relaxation, facial release, or increasing local blood flow. See Myofascial Release, Myotherapy, Ischemic Compression, Trigger Point, Therapeutic Massage.

Materials Handling Activity: A measure of the four physical requirements for work: lift, carry, push, and pull. This can be included within a functional capacity evaluation. See FCE.

Maximum Cervical Compression Test: A test very similar to a Spurling's sign. The patient is seated comfortably with the head and neck in neutral position. The patient is then asked to actively rotate the head and hyperextend the neck toward the side of the radicular complaints. Reproduction of these complaints suggests significant foraminal encroachment. This test can be performed with flexion and rotation as well. See Spurling's Sign.

Maximum Effort: A determination made during testing that is used to decide if a patient is giving a true maximum effort. See Maximum Voluntary Effort.

Maximum Medical Improvement: A term used in worker's compensation to denote when the patient has received maximum benefit from ongoing medical care. See MMI.

Maximum Voluntary Effort: A determination made during testing that is used to decide if a patient is giving a true maximum effort. This is often used to rule out malingering or symptom magnification. It is usually defined as three or more calculated coefficients of variation above the cut point. This means that the patient has performed ten separate trials of a measurable activity. The coeffiecent of variation is then determined for each trial. More than two trials with a coeffiencent of variation greater than 15% would mean that the patient is not giving maximum voluntary effort. See Maximum Effort, MVE.

MC: An abbreviation for *mid-cervical.*

McGill-Melzack Pain Questionnaire: One of numerous pain questionnaires that provides a relatively rapid way of objectively measuring pain experience.

McGregor's Line: A radiographic sign used to detect vertical subluxation of the upper cervical spine on lateral radiographs. A line is drawn from the hard palate to the posterior lip of the foramen magnum. If the odontoid is greater than 4.5 mm above this line, a vertical subluxation is suspected.

McKenzie Exercises: A system of low back rehabilitation designed by Robin McKenzie of New Zealand. Extension is emphasized in parts of the program to combat biomechanical creep into forward flexion. However, flexion is also used in many of the exercises. Also, the program is based on the idea that specific movements (including movements to the side) will centralize radiating low back pain. Movements that cause low back pain to radiate down an extremity are avoided. The correction of lateral shifts and lists is emphasized. See Dysfunction Syndrome, Derangement Syndrome, Postural Syndrome.

McKenzie Extension: A system of low back rehabilitation designed by Robin McKenzie of New Zealand. See McKenzie Exercises.

McKenzie Lumbar Roll: A proprietary name for a series of lumbar rolls first advocated by McKenzie. This includes a full-sized lumbar roll, which is a cylindrical low back brace used for maintaining the lumbar lordosis while sitting. This also includes a D-section lumbar roll, which is commonly placed on a seat back in the lumbar lordosis.

Mechanical Interface: The nervous system interfaces with the surrounding connective tissue at a "mechanical interface." See Adverse Neural Tension, Adverse Mechanical Tension, MI.

Mechanical Low Back Pain: Low back pain secondary to muscle overload caused by shunting of work from the gluteal region to the low back. This is also used as a general nonspecific term that encompasses multiple low back diagnoses.

Mechanical Muscle Energy Technique: A type of muscle energy technique in which the musculature is fired to pull the segment or joint back into alignment. To do this, the origin and insertion are reversed, and the patient is asked to contract the muscle or musculature which will pull the segment back into alignment. See Muscle Energy Technique.

Mechanical Muscle Stimulation: Deep or light pressure applied to muscles and or fascia for the purpose of muscle relaxation, facial release, or increasing local blood flow. See Massage.

Meclizine: An antihistamine used most commonly for diseases affecting the vestibular system and for dizziness. See Antivert.

med: An abbreviation for *medial.*

Medial Branch: The branch of the dorsal ramus which supplies sensation to the facet joints. The medial branches of L1–L4 run across the top of their respective transverse processes and pierce the intertransverse ligament at the base of the transverse process. The nerve then runs along the transverse process near the junction of the transverse process and the superior articular process. It then travels medially around the base of the superior articular process and is covered by the mamillo-accessory ligament. It then courses over the lamina where it divides into branches that supply the multifidi, the interspinous muscles and ligaments, and the two facet joints. The medial branch supplies the facet joints above and below its position. There is apparently also some innervation of the facet joint from the dorsal ramus ventrally. The L5 medial branch has a similar course, but crosses the ala of the sacrum instead of the transverse process. It supplies the facet joint of L5 before traveling to the multifidi. Note that the medial branch supplies only the muscles that attach to the spinous process and lamina of the lumbar vertebra innervated by that segment.

Medial Branch Block: The injection of anesthetic and usually steroids to block the medial branch of the sinuvertebral nerve (innervation of the facet joint). This is usually performed to determine if the facet joint is the pain generator. Each facet joint is supplied by two nerves, the medial branch above and the medial branch below. The L1 through L4 medial branches are located at the roots of the lumbar transverse processes. The L5 dorsal ramus (medial branch for the L5 segment) is located at the ala of the sacrum. Under fluoroscopy, the needle is directed ventrally and medially toward the target. An oblique lateral approach is commonly used, and the needle is introduced until the transverse process is contacted. The needle is then readjusted to aim at the root of the transverse process or the ala of the sacrum at L5. Anesthetic is then injected. See Cryoanalgesia, Dorsal Rhizotomy.

Medial Ischial Tuberosity: A pelvic dysfunction in which one ischial tuberosity is noted to be displaced medially. The sacrotuberous and sacrospinous ligaments are noted to be lax. The lower SI joint will be under compression while the superior SI joint will be in tension.

Median Crest of the Sacrum: The midline depression which occurs posteriorly on the sacrum and ends inferiorly in the sacral hiatus. The upper portion of the crest is the origin of the aponeurotic fibers from the latissimus dorsi. The crest is punctuated by three or four tubercles, which are the remnants of the spinous processes of the sacral vertebra.

Medical Exercise Therapy: A philosophy in exercise prescription which includes specific positioning and strength training for a specific area, a functional exercise stimulus, and various amounts of unloading to bring the affected body part through a pain-free strengthening program. An assessment is first done to find the "weak link" in the system. The idea is that normal weight training often exposes that weak link to tissue overload and thus increases symptoms. Unweighting systems as well as positioning are utilized to allow that body part to work through a pain-free range of motion. There are three phases of MET, the first being termed the "restitutional phase." In this phase the primary goals are elimination of symptoms and maximizing the oxygen delivery to the tissues for healing. The second phase is the "protectional phase." This is a phase of increasing tolerance and stamina of the target tissue to functional stresses during ADLs. The third phase is the "advanced" or "upper border phase." In this phase the tolerance and stamina of tissue is increased to higher-level athletic or work place stresses. A Norwegian brand of exercise equipment called SABA is common in medical exercise therapy programs. SABA uses an incline sled in conjunction with pulleys. See MET, SABA, Gravity Unloading, Unloading Therapy.

Medium Work: A NIOSH work category which involves frequently lifting up to 50 pounds and/or carrying up to 25 pounds.

Medrol: A brand of methylprednisolone tablets. This is a synthetic glucocorticoid (steroid). This has been used clinically to decrease the inflammation associated with acute radiculopathy, ankylosing spondylitis, and other anti-inflammatory conditions. For contraindications and drug interactions refer to Steroid. Medrol tablets are available in 2-mg, 4-mg, 8-mg, 16-mg, 24-mg, and 32-mg tablets. The common dosage is once a day, and steroid tapers are commonly used. See Steroid.

Medrol Dosepak: A brand of methylprednisolone tablets. It comes in a package of 21 tablets. See Methylprednisolone, Medrol.

Med-X: A brand of isotonic conditioning and testing equipment for the cervical, thoracic, and lumbar spine.

Mehta Angle: The angle between the rib and the vertebra in the thoracic spine that is used to predict the possibility of progression in infantile scoliosis (rib–angle difference). See Rib Vertebral Angle Difference.

Melorheostois: A rare bone dysplasia which *rarely* affects the spine and ribs. It usually affects only one side of the body and more commonly affects the extremities. The presenting symptom is pain exaggerated by activity, and, on x-ray, there is a characteristic hyperostosis resembling melted wax that has dripped down the side of a candle.

Menière's Disease: A disorder of unknown etiology which is characterized by vertigo, nausea, vomiting, and tinnitus. This is caused by a dilatation of the membranous chamber of the semicircular canals in the inner ear and is associated with unilateral hearing loss. Treatment is usually palliative and involves medications to help the nausea, vomiting, and vertigo. Common treatments include meclizine and scopolamine patches.

Meninges: The coverings of the brain and spinal cord which include the dura, the arachnoid, and the pia mater.

Meningioma: A benign tumor of the central nervous system which is composed of cells that line the arachnoid mater and originate from the dura. The mass effect can cause neurologic signs and symptoms. Treatment involves surgical excision if there is neurologic compromise.

Meningitis: An inflammation of the membranes covering the spinal cord. This can be caused by a bacterial, fungal, or viral infection. Symptoms include headache, malaise, nausea, fever, stiff neck, sore throat, photophobia, and vomiting. The condition is usually rapidly progressive.

Meningocele: A protrusion of the meninges through a defect in the neural arch of the vertebral body. The sac-like protrusion contains the dura, pia, and arachnoid, but not neural tissue. This is in direct contrast to a myelomeningocele, which contains everything in a meningocele, as well as neural tissue. See Spina Bifida.

Meniscoid: A meniscus-like body which is thought to become trapped in the facet joint and cause acute facet locking. It is thought that manipulation releases this entrapped meniscoid from the facet joint and allows normal motion. However, there has been some controversy as to whether meniscoids exist. See Cuneiform Synovial Fold.

Mennell's Sign: A physical examination maneuver in which the patient is standing and the examiner places his/her thumbs over the patient's PSISs. The examiner then slides one thumb upward and inward and then downward and outward. The sign is positive if tenderness is increased in either direction. If the pain is significant in the outward and downward movement, a gluteal strain is suspected. If tenderness is elicited when sliding inward and upward, a strain of the superior SI ligaments is suspected.

MENS: An electrical modality used to decrease pain and spasm. See Microcurrent Electrical Stimulation, TENS, Interferential E-stim.

MEP: A method of monitoring the integrity of the corticospinal tract and motor pathways during spinal surgery. See Motor Evoked Potential.

Mepivacaine: An amino amide–type of anesthetic similar to lidocaine. There is a relatively rapid onset of action with a moderate duration of action. This is used for infiltration, peripheral nerve blocks, and epidural anesthesia in concentrations from 0.5% to 2.0%. Mepivacaine is not effective as a topical anesthetic, which is one difference from lidocaine. In adults, Mepivacaine is less toxic than lidocaine. Mepivacaine provides a longer duration of anesthesia than lidocaine when used without epinephrine.

Meralgia Paresthetica: A lesion of the anterior branch of the lateral cutaneous nerve of the thigh (lateral anterior femoral cutaneous nerve). A sensory neuritis with symptoms of tingling, burning, and sensory loss in the outer surface of the thigh. The long superficial course of the lateral anterior femoral cutaneous nerve exposes it to trauma, especially as the anterior branch passes through the fasciae latae. Etiology can include hyperextension of the hip, direct pressure through tight belts, significant weight gain or loss, and other factors. Involvement is usually unilateral. This disorder is more common in men than women. Common treatments include allowing time to pass (the syndrome is usually self-limited); removal of all factors that would place direct or indirect pressure on the nerve; nonsteroidals; steroid bursts; splitting the fascia at the point of emergence; or treating the associated SI dysfunction.

Meric Technique: A chiropractic technique that involves a system of analysis and adjusting in which the body is divided into zones. This technique is used by just under one fourth of U.S. chiropractors.

Merick Maneuver: A chiropractic adjusting technique which uses a slow-acceleration and low-amplitude thrust.

Meridian Therapy: The application of manual pressure to acupuncture meridians for the purpose of decreasing pain. See Acupressure.

Meschan Angle: A radiographic method for measuring the degree of spondylolisthesis. Unlike the more common Meyerding grading system, this involves intersecting angles. See Meyerding Method.

Mesodermal Pain: Pain derived from the mesodermal tissues. This is used to describe pain that is radiating to a specific distribution, but does not originate from the nerve roots or radiate in a specific dermatomal pattern. Mesodermal pain can be caused by injury to the ligamentous and muscular structures. The referred pain patterns of trigger points are a type of mesodermal pain. See Cloward Areas, Splanchnic Pain.

MET: (1) An abbreviation for *metabolic unit*, a unit of physical exertion. (2) A philosophy in exercise prescription which includes specific positioning and strength training for a specific area, a functional exercise stimulus, and various amounts of unloading to bring the affected body part through a painless strengthening program. See Medical Exercise Therapy. (3) A system of evaluation and treatment based on correcting joint position by affecting changes in neuromuscular reflexes and muscle tone. See Muscle Energy Technique.

Metabolic Unit: A unit of physical exertion. See MET Level, MET.

MET Level: A unit of physical exertion often used by exercise physiologists. For instance, an activity requiring 5.0 METs requires much more energy and exertion than an activity requiring 2.0 METs. See Metabolic Unit, MET.

Methocarbamol: A muscle relaxant which decreases muscle tone by causing sedation. See Robaxin.

Methylprednisolone: A long-acting, injectable steroid. The brand name is Depo-Medrol. This is one of the more common substances injected into joints and bursas to decrease inflammation. It is a depot preparation that is commonly used in spinal blocks and epidurals. It is also used in the acute management of spinal cord injury. See Depo-Medrol.

Metrecom: A proprietary name for an electronic device that measures range of motion.

Metrizamide: A water-soluble x-ray contrast medium used commonly for myelography and CT-myelography. This is absorbed from the CSF approximately 6 hours postinjection and excreted by the kidneys. Anaphylactic reactions to this dye are possible. See Amipaque.

Mexiletine: An antiarrhythmic (heart) drug used occasionally for severe, intractable chronic pain. This drug is contraindicated in patients with cardiogenic shock or pre-existing second- or third-degree AV blocks. This drug may raise liver function tests and can also cause a worsening of a pre-existing arrhythmia. It should be used with caution in patients with hypotension and severe congestive heart failure because there is potential for aggravating these conditions. Patients with liver disease or decreased liver function should also avoid this drug as mexiletine is metabolized in the liver. When given with phenytoin, there can be a lowering of mexiletine drug levels. It is contraindicated for use with cimetidine. Use of magnesium hydroxide or theophylline will also alter drug levels. In drug studies, there was a 41% chance of upper GI distress. CNS disturbances such as tremor, light-headedness and coordination difficulties were reported in 10–12% of patients. One common dosage scheme is 150 mg a day to start, increasing by 150-mg increments every 3 days until 600 mg a day is reached. The maintenance level is 600 mg a day. If no significant decrease in pain complaints is noted, the drug should be discontinued immediately. Caution should be used when prescribing this drug because of the risk of side effects. See Mexitil.

while moving the patient through specific maneuvers. Through this technique, manual therapists determine which segments or joints are fixated (not moving correctly). See Intersegmental Range of Motion Palpation.

Motion Restriction: An osteopathic or manual physical therapy term which refers to the direction a spinal segment cannot move. The motion restriction of a segment is the direction in which it is treated with direct treatment.

Motion Segment: A unit made up of two adjacent vertebrae that move against one another. The spine consists of many stacked motion segments. These motion segments taken together allow for spinal movement as a whole.

Motor Deficit: A term that describes loss of motor strength often with decreased deep tendon reflex. This can be seen with injury to several levels of the nervous system, including radiculopathy, myelopathy, or peripheral nerve injury.

Motor Evoked Potential: A method of monitoring the integrity of the corticospinal tract and motor pathways during spinal surgery. The motor cortex is stimulated by an electromagnetic pulse, and the impulse is then recorded distally. Motor evoked potentials can be performed using an electrical stimulator placed over the vertex of the head or using a transcranial magnetic stimulator delivering an electromagnetic pulse. The distal pick-up site is usually the tibialis anterior. See MEP, Magnetic Cortical Stimulation, Transcranial Magnetic Stimulation.

Motorized Traction: The application of traction (axial distraction) with a motorized device. This traction force is higher than can be applied manually (with hands) and is intermittent. See Traction.

Motor Nerve: A peripheral nerve which contains only motor fibers.

Motor Unit Recruitment: A finding noted during a needle EMG exam. The patient is asked to contract the muscle being tested. As each motor unit (a group of motor fibers innervated by the same nerve fiber) fires, it can be seen on the screen. The rate and order of this firing is the motor unit recruitment.

Motrin: A nonsteroidal anti-inflammatory drug which is in the propionic acid class. See Ibuprofen, Advil.

Movement Dysfunction: An osteopathic or manual physical therapy term in which the dysfunction is named for the direction in which a segment will not move. For instance, an extension dysfunction would denote a segment that cannot extend. This is in contrast to a positional dysfunction. In this case, the "positional dysfunction" would be a flexed segment. This means that the segment exists in the flexed state.

Movement Imbalance: A shift in the point about which a rigid body rotates away from the normal. This can be caused by muscle imbalance, fascial tightness, or problems in the joint capsule. This term is often used by therapists who focus on treating muscle imbalances.

Movement Patterning: The use of repetitive movements to repattern the motor cortex. The emphasis is on developing proper muscular coordination, and often proprioceptive feedback (such as touching) is given during the movement. See Feldenkrais, Alexander Technique, Aston Patterning.

MP: A chiropractic term which refers to palpating either the spinal segments or an SI joint while moving the patient through specific maneuvers. See Motion Palpation.

mp: An abbreviation for *mamillary process.*

MPE: An abbreviation for *motion palpation exam.* See Motion Palpation.

MPS: Pain emanating from the muscles which often radiates to other areas of the body. This is commonly associated with trigger points, tender points, and other phenomena described by Travell and Simons. See Myofascial Pain Syndrome, Trigger Point, Myofascial Trigger Point.

MRI: An imaging technique which uses magnetic fields to obtain detailed pictures of both soft tissue and bony anatomy. This technique can be very effective in diagnosing HNP, tumors, vascular abnormalities, and, lately, a host of diagnoses caused by bony encroachment. It can be enhanced by the use of gadolinium, which helps visualize vascularized scar tissue more clearly. Most lumbar MRIs include T1 weighted sagittal cuts (fat is bright), T2 weighted sagittal cuts (water is bright), and proton density weighted sagittal cuts (better for anatomy). Axial images are also often included. See Magnetic Resonance Imaging.

THREE DIFFERENT IMAGE TYPES IN MRI:

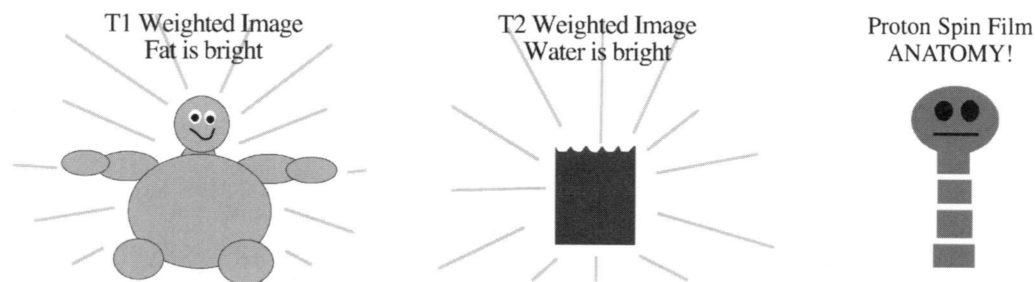

MS: A central nervous system disorder which affects the brain stem and spinal cord, as well as the brain and sometimes peripheral nerves. See Multiple Sclerosis.

MSPT: Master of Science of Physical Therapy.

MSW: Master of Social Work.

MT: An abbreviation for *mid-thoracic.*

MUAP: An abbreviation for *motor unit action potential.* The electrical potential seen on an EMG screen when a motor unit (a collection of muscle fibers innervated by the same axon) fires. MUAPs can become abnormal when there is nerve damage (denervation) or in disease processes that involve the nerves or muscles.

Multifidi Strain: An injury which tears fibers of the multifidus muscle. The multifidi are intersegmental muscles that provide segmental stabilization. There is decreased range of motion to the opposite side of the strain with a list to the same side. The gait is antalgic, and there may be tenderness in the deeply placed multifidi musculature.

Multilevel Disc Desiccation: This is usually noted on MRI with decreased T2 signal intensity within the nucleus pulposus indicating decreased hydration of the disc and disc degeneration. See Degenerative Disc Disease.

Multiple Sclerosis: A central nervous system disorder which commonly affects the brain stem, brain, and spinal cord as well as the peripheral nerves. Sclerotic plaques (white matter lesions) are seen on MRI; these represent areas of axonal demyelination. Multiple neurologic signs and symptoms are found which do not appear to localize to a common site in the CNS. These include loss of vision in one or both eyes, vertigo, numbness, burning sensations or paresthesias, incontinence, double vision, speech disturbances, lack of coordination, or paralysis. Remission is common and can be either partial or complete. Some patients experience multiple attacks and remissions. There is a chronic progressive form which can lead to severe disability and death. Death usually occurs from the complications of disability. Many patients are fully functional 10 years after the first attack, and approximately 25% are fully functional 30 years after the first attack. Treatment can be difficult, and an effective treatment or cure has not yet been established. See MS.

Multisegmental Mobility: The mobility of many segments taken as a whole.

Muscle Contraction Headache: A headache caused by cervical myofascial pain. See Tension Headache.

Muscle Dominance: When the action of one of a synergistic pair of muscles exceeds the action of its synergist. This distorts the motion of that joint or motion segment and contributes to the disuse of the synergists. Effectively, this means that one muscle is abnormally stronger than the other muscles that also control a given movement. This is thought to cause muscle imbalance and problems within the joint. This terminology is used by physical therapists who work on muscle imbalances.

Muscle Energy Technique: A system of evaluation and treatment based on correcting joint position by effecting changes in neuromuscular reflexes and muscle tone. Specific maneuvers are used to decrease the "gamma gain" within the muscle spindle causing the muscle to relax and lengthen. It is thought that this muscle relaxation causes dysfunctional joints to return to their functional positions. Muscle energy techniques use very light isometric contractions countered with very light resistance, held commonly for six seconds. This treatment approach has become very popular with manual physical therapists and traditionally was used and developed by osteopaths. See MET, Direct Technique, Mechanical Muscle Energy Technique, MM Energy, Neuromuscular Mobilization, Posimetric Relaxation, Postfacilitation Stretch, Postisometric Relaxation.

Muscle Hypertrophy: An increase in the cross-sectional size of a structure. See Hypertrophy.

Muscle Setting Exercise: Isometric exercise against a very small amount of resistance. This describes general static muscle contractions used to maintain mobility between muscle fibers and decrease muscle spasm and pain.

Muscle Spasm: Increased local muscle tone due to irritation. See Localized Hypertonus, Spasm, Muscular Splinting.

Muscle Spindle: A receptor which reports on the length of muscle and adjusts length by setting muscle tone. These spindles lie parallel to the muscle fibers and can be attached to skeletal muscle or the muscle tendon. Two types of fibers are inside the spindle: a nuclear bag fiber and a chain fiber. In different muscles the ratio of these types of fibers vary. In the center of the spindle there is a receptor called an annulospiral receptor with "flower spray receptors" on each side. The annular spiral endings discharge rapidly and respond to even small changes in muscle length. The flower spray endings compensate for this by firing only when larger changes in muscle length have occurred. There are also fine, intrafusal fibers which alter the sensitivity of the spindle. These are affected by gamma efferent supply to the intrafusal fibers. Conscious activity in the cortex may modify the gamma gain and thus influence muscle tone. It has also been postulated that muscle energy techniques can affect the gamma gain and thus affect muscle tone.

Muscle Stim: An electrical modality used to decrease pain and spasm. See Interferential E-stim, Muscle Stim Unit, Muscle Stimulation, Muscle Stimulator.

Muscle Stimulation: An electrical modality used to decrease pain and spasm. See Interferential E-stim, Muscle Stimulation, Muscle Stimulator.

Muscle Stimulator: An electrical device used to decrease pain and spasm. See Interferential E-stim, Muscle Stimulation, Muscle Stimulator.

Muscle Stim Unit: An electrical device used to decrease pain and spasm. See Interferential E-stim, Muscle Stimulation, Muscle Stim.

Muscle Stretch Reflex: A physical exam maneuver that checks the integrity of the "wiring" of the muscle being tested. See Deep Tendon Reflex, DTR.

Muscular Antalgia: Muscular spasm which causes an alteration in gait or an antalgic gait. For instance, a spasm in the right quadratus lumborum would cause the right hip to ride high during gait and likely prevent weight bearing on the left hip, as this would stress the right quadratus lumborum. This is also used as a chiropractic radiographic term which refers to the spine being pulled to one side by muscular spasm. For instance, spasm of the right iliopsoas would cause the L2, L3, and L4 vertebral bodies to be pulled toward that side as the muscle shortened.

Muscular Splinting: Increased local muscle tone due to irritation. See Localized Hypertonus, Spasm, Muscle Spasm.

MVE: The amount of effort put forth during testing. Coefficients of variation are usually taken to determine if the patient is putting forth a maximum voluntary effort. See Maximum Voluntary Effort.

Myalgia: Pain emanating from the muscles. This can signify point tenderness within a muscle (i.e., tender points) or diffuse pain due to systemic disease.

Myalgic Encephalomyelitis: A somewhat controversial diagnosis. See Chronic Fatigue Syndrome.

Myelitis: Literally, an inflammation of the spinal cord. This usually causes symptoms similar to that of a spinal cord lesion. The most common of these illnesses is transverse myelitis.

Myelodysplasia: A group of disorders which includes meningocele, myelomeningocele, and rachischisis. All of these disorders involve defects of the neural tube. See Spina Bifida, Spinal Dysraphism.

Myelogram: The injection of a radiographic contrast medium into the subarachnoid space through a lumbar puncture. This effectively outlines the spinal cord and spinal nerve roots on an x-ray series. This was used to make the diagnosis of HNP, central canal stenosis, or foraminal stenosis before CAT-scan and MRI were available. Currently, this procedure has been all but replaced by CT-myelogram. See CT-Myelogram, Myelography.

Myelographic Column: The column of dye seen on a myelogram. Indentations in this column can be associated with a herniated disc, tumors, stenosis, and other mass lesions. See Contrast Column.

Myelography: The injection of a radiographic contrast medium into the subarachnoid space through a lumbar puncture. See Myelogram.

Myelomeningocele: A sac-like protrusion through a defect in the neural arch. In this particular case, the sac-like protrusion contains abnormal spinal cord or CNS tissue. See Spina Bifida.

Myelopathy: A term which refers to dysfunction of the spinal cord. A common cause is central canal stenosis due to osteophytes, facet hypertrophy, or pseudohypertrophy of the ligamentum flavum or a large central HNP. The most common symptom in cervical myelopathy is difficulty ambulating and weakness in the lower extremities. Long tract signs and a sensory level can be present. In lumbar myelopathy, the patient often complains that he is able to ambulate without symptoms when bent over a shopping cart or in a flexed position, but has symptoms with ambulation in the extended, upright position. See Central Canal Stenosis, Intervertebral Disc Disorder with Myelopathy, Lumbar Disc Disorder with Myelopathy.

Myelopathy—Cervical: A clinical syndrome that involves impingement of the cervical spinal cord. See Cervical Myelopathy.

Myeloradiculitis: Myelopathy with inflammation of the spinal nerve roots.

Myeloradiculopathy: A myelopathy which also affects spinal nerve roots.

Myodysneuria: A chiropractic term which refers to painful paraspinal muscle spasm.

Myofascial Pain: Pain emanating from the muscles and fascial structures. The most common finding is "tender spots" within the musculature. Trigger points can also be found (discrete areas which refer pain or symptoms to another location). See Lumbago, Myositis, Tension Myalgia, Trigger Point.

Myofascial Pain Syndrome: Pain emanating from the muscles which often radiates to other areas of the body. This is commonly associated with trigger points, tender points, and other phenomena described by Travell and Simons. See Trigger Point, Myofascial Trigger Point, MPS, Myofascitis.

Myofascial Release: Very deep tissue massage or manipulation for the purpose of lengthening tight fascial planes or tissues. See Massage, Ischemic Compression, Trigger Point, Soft Tissue Mobilization.

Myofascial Restriction: Decreased movement of one fascial plane on another.

Myofascial Trigger Point: Classically, a taut palpable band in muscle that is painful to touch and refers pain in a characteristic distribution to another (often adjacent) body area. See Trigger Point.

Myofascitis: A term synonymous with myofascial pain. Literally inflammation in the muscles and fascial covering of the muscles. This can also be associated with trigger points. See Myofascial Pain Syndrome.

Myofibrosis: A term described by Travell which denotes replacement of muscle tissue by fibrous tissue.

Myogenic Scoliosis: A lateral curvature of the spine due to a primary disease of muscle such as muscular dystrophy.

Myogenic TOS: Thoracic outlet syndrome that is caused by muscular tightness. For instance, two common sites of entrapment of the brachial plexus are the scalenes and pectoralis minor. See Thoracic Outlet Syndrome.

Myopathic Scoliosis: Scoliosis caused by a myelopathy. For instance, scoliosis is often associated with muscular dystrophy and caused by chronic severe muscular weakness in the muscles that otherwise support the spinal column.

Myositis: A nonspecific term referring to inflammation within the muscles. This usually refers to myofascial pain. See Myofascial Pain.

Myotatic Reflex: A physical exam maneuver that checks the integrity of the "wiring" of the muscle being tested. See Deep Tendon Reflex, DTR.

Myotendinoses: A painful area within a muscle with increased tension.

Myotherapy: The application of progressively stronger pressure on a trigger point. This pressure causes ischemia within that portion of the muscle followed by a hyperemic response on the release of pressure. This is thought to "release" the trigger point. See Shiatsu, Myotherapy, Acupressure, Massage, Ischemic Compression.

N

N: An abbreviation for *negative*.

N: An abbreviation for *nerve*.

N: An abbreviation for *normal*.

N&T: An abbreviation for *numbness and tingling*.

Nabumetone: A nonsteroidal anti-inflammatory drug that exhibits anti-inflammatory, analgesic, and antipyretic properties. See Relafen.

Nachlas' Knee Flexion Sign: A physical exam maneuver in which the knee is passively flexed with the patient in the prone postion. A positive sign is if the patient experiences pain in the low back or along the femoral nerve. It is thought to be positive in patients with femoral nerve irritation or radiculopathy of L2, L3, or L4. See Femoral Nerve Stretch Test.

NACM: National Association of Chiropractic Medicine.

Naffziger's Syndrome: Compression of the neurovascular bundle (usually irritation of nerves) in the shoulder girdle area between the first rib and clavicle, by a cervical rib, at the second and third ribs, between the anterior and middle scalenes or underneath the pectoralis minor and clavipectoral fascia. See Thoracic Outlet Syndrome.

Naffziger's Test: Compression of the jugular veins bilaterally to increase cerebral spinal fluid pressure. If there is irritation of the nerve roots or dura, this is reported to increase low back pain or extremity symptoms.

Nagele's Pelvis: A congenital pelvic deformity in which there is complete ankylosis of the SI joint on one side and deformity within the pelvis itself. This is caused by a distorted development of the pelvis and its associated innominate bone.

Nalfon: A nonsteroidal anti-inflammatory drug in the benzeneacetic acid class. It possesses anti-inflammatory, analgesic, and antipyretic properties. As with all nonsteroidal anti-inflammatory drugs, there is a risk of GI side effects, as well as renal and hepatic side effects. There are drug interactions with aspirin, phenobarbital, hydantoin, sulfonamides, sulfonylureas, and Coumadin. Recommended dosage is 200 mg every 4–6 hours, up to 300–600 mg three or four times a day. It is available in 200-mg, 300-mg, and 600-mg pulvules and tablets. See Fenoprofen.

Naprosyn: A nonsteroidal anti-inflammatory drug in the phenylpropionic acid class. The drug interacts with oral anticoagulants and probenecid. Common dosages range between 250 mg and 500 mg taken twice a day. It is available in 250-mg, 375-mg, and 500-mg tablets. See Naproxen Sodium, Anaprox, Aleve.

Naproxen Sodium: A nonsteroidal anti-inflammatory drug in the phenylpropionic acid class. See Anaprox, Naprosyn, Aleve.

Narrowing: A radiographic term which usually refers to narrowing of the intervertebral disc space. With disc degeneration, the disc begins to loose its ability to hold onto water, and the size of the disc space decreases on x-ray. This can be seen on x-rays. This also can indicate a herniated disc in that the herniated material has squirted out of confines of the annulus, and the overall height of the disc is decreased. Narrowing can refer to stenosis (foraminal, central, canal, or lateral recess). See Disc Space Narrowing.

Nash-Moe System: A system for quantifying the degree of rotation in scoliosis. See Pedicle Migration.

Nautilus: A brand name of exercise equipment which uses a cam to alter the resistance during the range of motion.

NC: A clinical symptom complex associated with lumbar central canal stenosis. See Neurogenic Claudication.

NCA: National Chiropractic Association.

NCM: Nurse Case Manager.

NCS: Nerve conduction studies. See EMG/Nerve Conduction Study.

NCV: Nerve conduction velocity. See EMG/Nerve Conduction Study.

Neck Clock: A home exercise. See Cervical Clock.

Neck Pain: An ICD-9 diagnosis which is extremely nonspecific. Obviously, neck pain can have multiple causes.

Neck Retraction: A physical therapy stretch designed to stretch the suboccipital musculature. See Chin Tuck.

Neoplasm: Abnormal growth of tissue, which is another term for cancer.

Neri's Bowing Sign: In this test, the patient moves into forward flexion while standing. If the knee on the affected side automatically moves into flexion, nerve root tension is suspected.

Nerve Block: The injection of local anesthetic into an area which surrounds a nerve for the purpose of causing a local conduction block (stopping nerve transmission). This is usually performed as a diagnostic or therapeutic procedure for neurogenic (nerve) pain.

Nerve Conduction Velocity: A test used to determine the function of the peripheral nerves and nerve roots. See EMG/Nerve Conduction Study.

Nerve Release: A concept first developed by Maitland and then developed further by Butler. The idea is that the nervous system must be mobile to allow movement of the vertebral column and limbs. See Adverse Neural Tension, ANT.

Nerve Root: A collection of nerve fibers that exits the spinal cord through the bony window of the foramen. There are two nerve roots that join together to form a spinal nerve. These are the dorsal and ventral nerve roots, also known as the dorsal and ventral rami. See Radicular Pain, Spinal Nerve Root.

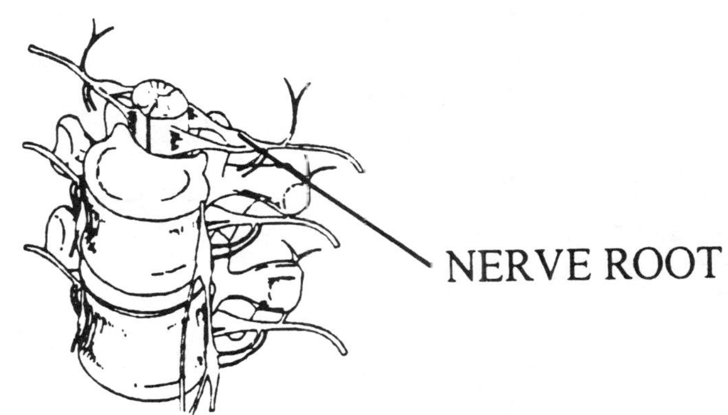

Nerve Root and Plexus Disorders: An ICD-9 diagnosis code which usually refers to radiculopathy. See Radiculopathy.

Nerve Root Anomaly—Type 1: A nerve root anomaly with an aberrant course. See Type 1 Nerve Root Anomaly, Anomaly—Type 1.

Nerve Root Anomaly—Type 2: A nerve root anomaly where the number of roots in an intervertebral foramen is variable. See Type 2 Nerve Root Anomaly, Anomaly—Type 2.

Nerve Root Anomaly—Type 3: A nerve root anomaly in which there are extra dural connections. See Anomaly—Type 3, Type 3 Nerve Root Anomaly.

Nerve Root Block: Injection of corticosteroids (anti-inflammatories) and a local anesthetic onto the nerve root sleeve surrounding a nerve root. See Selective Nerve Root Block.

Nerve Root Canal: The "window" through which the spinal nerve root exits. The roof of the canal is formed by the superior articular process, the superior margin of the lamina, the ligamentum flavum, and the pars interarticularis. The floor is formed by the intervertebral disc and the posterior vertebral body. The lateral wall is composed of the pedicle while the medial wall is formed by the dural sac. See Lateral Recess.

Nerve Root Compression: Pressure on a nerve root due to a herniated disc or bony encroachment such as foraminal stenosis or lateral recess stenosis. This is to be differentiated from a chemical radiculitis where inflammation around the nerve root is suspected. See Radiculopathy.

Nerve Root Compromise: Pressure on a nerve root due to a herniated disc or bony structures within the neural foramen. This can be a cause of radiculopathy. See Radiculopathy.

Nerve Root Decompression: The surgical release of pressure from a nerve root. This procedure is performed with most spinal surgeries performed to treat radiculopathy. Bone spurs, disc material, and tumors can be removed to allow normal nerve function. A laminotomy, laminectomy, or foraminotomy can be performed.

Nerve Root Filling: During a myelogram, dye is injected into the subarachnoid space and outlines the nerve roots. If there is pressure on a nerve root, that nerve root will not fill with dye. See Filling—Nerve Root, Filling Defect.

Nerve Root L4: The fourth lumbar nerve root that exits between L4 and L5 and supplies various muscles in the lower extremity including quadriceps, iliopsoas, tibialis anterior, and gluteus medius. It supplies sensation to the medial calf. See L4 Root, L4 Nerve Root.

Nerve Root L5: This lumbar nerve root exits between L5 and S1. This nerve root supplies numerous muscles including the tibialis anterior, hamstrings, and gluteus maximus. The classic description of its sensory territory is the big toe. See L5 Root, L5 Nerve Root.

Nerve Root—S1: The first sacral nerve root that exits between L5 and S1. This nerve root supplies various muscles including the gastrocsoleus. See S1 Nerve Root.

Nerve Root Sheath: The covering of the nerve root that is continuous with the dura. See Periradicular Sheath.

Nerve Root Tension Sign: A physical exam maneuver traditionally used to detect a lumbar radiculopathy (pinched nerve in the back, herniated disc, etc.). See Straight-Leg Raising Maneuver.

Nerve Root Tethering: When a nerve root is stretched over an immobile object. For instance, a nerve root can be tethered on a ruptured intervertebral disc. When that nerve root is stretched (such as with a straight-leg raising maneuver), compression is placed on the nerve root, and numbness or paresthesias are experienced. See Straight-Leg Raise.

Nerve Tension Sign: See Straight-Leg Raise.

Nerve Tension Test: A physical exam test that screens for nerve root dysfunction. In the spine, this is usually synonymous with a straight-leg raising test. The leg is raised with the knee extended and the patient lying supine. If the test is positive, numbness or tingling radiates into the leg in a specific nerve root distribution. See Straight-Leg Raise.

Network Chiropractic: An integration of chiropractic techniques which utilizes light touch or taps to relieve spinal tension to clear the body of central nervous system interference. Changes in the sequence or timing of adjustments are determined by objective changes such as leg length. This technique is reported to "release" spinal imprints or facilitation caused by physical, emotional, or chemical stress.

Neural Arch: The arch of bone which attaches to the back portion of the vertebral body and surrounds the neural elements that pass through the spinal canal. The neural arch is made up of the pedicles and lamina.

Neural Arch Fracture: A fracture of the bony elements posterior to the posterior longitudinal ligament. These can occur during flexion, rotation, or axial loading in extension (hangman's fracture of C2). These fractures may be overlooked on x-ray, and CT scan can be helpful in identification. There may be associated fractures of the transverse processes or associated spondylolisthesis at the lower lumbar levels. They are considered unstable fractures and require external immobilization or internal fixation.

Neural Element Impingement: Nerve root impingement. See Radiculopathy.

Neural Foramina: The space through which the nerve root and nerve root sheath must pass to exit the spinal canal. See Foramen.

Neuralgia: Pain in the distribution of a nerve or nerve root.

Neuralgic Amyotrophy: An ICD-9 diagnosis code (brachial plexopathy or neuropathy) for dysfunction of the brachial plexus of unknown etiology. This is thought to be caused by viral, immunologic, or toxic factors. There is weakness in the arm, accompanied by sensory loss and diminished reflexes which occurs over several days. The upper portion of the brachial plexus is the most commonly affected, meaning that the musculature of the shoulder and upper arm is commonly involved while the hand is spared. The condition is usually unilateral and is usually self-limited over several months to years. This diagnosis is commonly confused with a cervical radiculopathy.

Neural Mobilization: "Freeing up" the nervous system through stretching and mobilization. The nervous system must be mobile to allow movement of the vertebral column and limbs. See Dural Mobilization, Adverse Neural Tension.

Neurapraxia: The temporary loss of nerve function caused by compression of a peripheral nerve with no structural damage to the axon. There may be local damage to the myelin sheath. Complete nerve recovery is expected. See Neurapraxic.

Neurapraxic: The temporary loss of nerve function. See Neurapraxia.

Neuraxis: A term denoting the brain stem and spinal cord.

Neurectomy: The surgical removal of a nerve, usually performed to relieve chronic neuropathic pain.

Neuritis: Inflammation or irritation of a nerve. When used in the context of spine medicine this can have several meanings. One meaning would equate this with a radiculopathy or radiculitis. It can also be used to refer to thoracic outlet syndrome.

Neurofibroma: A tumor which is relatively common in the spinal cord, accounting for approximately one-quarter of spinal tumors. Most of these tumors are intradural, about 10% are exclusively extradural, and another 10% are both intra- and extradural. They are usually solitary tumors, but it is possible to see multiple lesions, and they usually arise from the spinal nerve root. They are often hourglass-shaped or dumbbell-shaped, and excision is indicated to avoid significant cord compression. Whenever an extradural tumor is encountered, intradural exploration should be performed since they are more commonly intradural.

Neurofibromatosis: An inherited disorder that affects nerve roots, cranial nerves, and peripheral nerves. Scoliosis is associated with this disease approximately 50% of the time. This is the so-called elephant man's disease.

Neuroforaminal Compromise: Any decrease in the size of the foramen with pressure on the nerve root. See Foraminal Stenosis, Radiculopathy.

Neurogenic Claudication: A clinical symptom complex associated with lumbar central canal stenosis. The patient reports that walking causes lower extremity pain and that walking in a flexed posture ("shopping cart posture") is more comfortable. This is usually differentiated from vascular claudication because the patient can exercise with the lower extremities in a flexed position often without difficulty (such as riding a bicycle). With vascular claudication this would be expected to cause symptoms. See NC, Spinal Claudication.

Neurogenic Motor Evoked Potential: A method of monitoring the integrity of the corticospinal tract and motor pathways during spinal surgery. See NMEP, Motor Evoked Potential, MEP.

Neurogenic Recruitment: The recruitment of a muscle the extent to which a nerve can activate that muscle.

Neurogenic Scoliosis: A lateral curvature of the spine due to a primary disease of the nervous system, such as ALS.

Neurogenic TOS: A rare thoracic outlet syndrome involving severe compression of the neurovascular bundle versus minor irritation. The compression causes denervation of the corresponding muscle groups and/or venous or arterial blockage. This is a surgical emergency which usually requires a scalenectomy or first rib resection. See Thoracic Outlet Syndrome, Neurovascular Thoracic Outlet Syndrome.

Neurologically Intact: A normal neurologic exam. With respect to the spine, this implies that no signs of radiculopathy or myelopathy were found.

Neurologist: A physician who specializes in treating disorders of the nervous system and has completed an AMA-approved specialty training program in neurology.

Neurology: The study of the nervous system.

Neuromuscular Massage: A soft tissue mobilization technique based on the work of Stanley Lief. See Neuromuscular Therapy.

Neuromuscular Mobilization: A system of evaluation and treatment based on correcting joint position by effecting changes in neuromuscular reflexes and muscle tone. See Muscle Energy Technique.

Neuromuscular Re-education: A type of massage therapy. This also can refer to proprioceptive neuromuscular facilitation (PNF) work. However, this term is often used in reference to standard deep tissue massage. See NR.

Neuromuscular Technique: A soft tissue mobilization technique based on the work of Stanley Lief. See Neuromuscular Therapy.

Neuromuscular Therapy: A soft tissue mobilization technique based on the work of Stanley Lief. The therapy is based on the belief that adhesions and hardening of the muscle fibers can block nervous impulses through impingement and irritation of the nervous structures as they pass through the musculature. There is also heavy emphasis on removing any "function-interfering factors" such as tensions, contractions, adhesions, or spasms. The "neuromuscular" lesion is thought to be associated with congestion of the local connective tissues, disturbance of the acid–base balance of connective tissues, fibrous infiltration (adhesions), and chronic muscular contractions. Fatigue, exhaustion, bad posture, local trauma, systemic toxemia, dietetic deficiencies, and psychosomatic causes can bring about these muscular tensions. See NMT, Neuromuscular Re-education, Neuromuscular Technique.

Neurontomesis: An injury which involves a through-and-through separation of a nerve. Conduction through the nerve is almost immediately disrupted. Spontaneous recovery is uncommon. See Neurotomesis.

Neuropathic Scoliosis: Scoliosis caused by neuromuscular disease such as muscular dystrophy. See Neurogenic Scoliosis.

Neuropathy: Dysfunction of a nerve due to loss of the myelin sheath, axonal damage, or a local conduction block.

Neuropathy and Radiculopathy: An ICD-9 code roughly equivalent to radiculopathy. See Radiculopathy, Neuropathy.

Neurosurgeon: A physician who specializes in surgery of the brain and nervous system and who has completed an AMA-approved specialty training program in neurosurgery.

Neurosurgery: Surgery of the brain and nervous system.

Neurotension Signs: Physical exam signs used to detect abnormal nerve root or peripheral nerve tension causing nerve irritation or dysfunction. For instance, a straight-leg raising maneuver would be an example of a neurotension sign. See Adverse Neural Tension.

Neurothlipsis: Pressure on a nerve which is direct or indirect. One example would be pressure on the nerve root in the intervertebral foramen causing vascular congestion of the perineural tissues.

Neurotomesis: An injury which involves a through-and-through separation of a nerve. Conduction through the nerve is almost immediately disrupted. Spontaneous recovery is uncommon. See Neurontomesis.

Neurovascular Thoracic Outlet Syndrome: Thoracic outlet syndrome involving severe compression of the neurovascular bundle versus minor irritation. See Neurogenic TOS.

Neutral Group: An osteopathic or manual physical therapy term which refers to a type 1 dysfunction. This is a spinal curvature which is found in neutral but disappears in flexion or extension. Neutral groups are usually seen in combination with type 2 osteopathic lesions in which the type 2 lesion is a transition from one curve to the next.

Nifedipine: A calcium channel blocker commonly used for angina, but also used for patients with migraine headaches and reflex sympathetic dystrophy. This drug selectively inhibits calcium ion influx across the cell membranes of vascular smooth muscle. This drug is contraindicated in patients with excessive hypotension, severe obstructive coronary artery disease, beta blocker withdrawal, and congestive heart failure. Blood pressure must be monitored to avoid hypotension when starting the drug. This drug may also increase LFTs. There are drug interactions with beta blockers, long-acting nitrates, digitalis, anticoagulants, and cimetidine. Procardia, a trademark name of nifedipine, is supplied in 10-mg and 20-mg capsules taken three times a day. The XL form can be taken once a day and is supplied in 30- , 60- , and 90-mg tablets. See Procardia, Procardia XL, Adalat, Adalat CC.

NIH: National Institutes of Health.

Nimmo Point: A chiropractic term which is roughly equivalent to a trigger point. These areas may be associated with the subluxation complex. See Trigger Point.

Nimmo Technique: The technique used to resolve Nimmo points or trigger points. Pressure from the thumb, elbow, or a "Nimmo tee" is applied to these areas to reduce pain and edema. This is a similar concept to the one of trigger points made popular by Janet Travell. This technique is used by approximately 40% of U.S. chiropractors. See Tonus Receptor Technique, Nimmo Point.

NIOSH: National Institute for Occupational Safety and Health.

NMEP: A method of monitoring the integrity of the corticospinal tract and motor pathways during spinal surgery. See Motor Evoked Potential, Neurogenic Motor Evoked Potential, MEP.

NMT: A soft tissue mobilization technique based on the work of Stanley Lief. See Neuromuscular Therapy, Neuromuscular Technique, Neuromuscular Massage.

Nociceptors: Free nerve endings within the peripheral nervous system which are responsible for the perception of pain.

Nonanatomic Sensory Loss: Reported loss of sensation by the patient on neurologic exam that clearly does not correspond to any known dermatomal pattern. Note that many *different* dermatomal maps have been published by various neuroanatomists. Also, there is some person-to-person variation in normal dermatomal patterns (up to 10%). See Dermatome, Nondermatomal Sensory Loss.

Nonarticular Rheumatism: A term which is roughly equivalent to diffuse systemic myofacial pain. See Fibromyalgia.

Noncapsular Pattern: This is usually limited movement in a single direction while all other movement directions are relatively unrestricted. This commonly occurs when muscles are tight. See Capsular Pattern.

Noncontained Herniation: A term which is roughly equivalent to diffuse systemic myofascial pain. See Disc Extrusion, Disc Sequestration.

Nondermatomal Sensory Loss: Reported loss of sensation by the patient on neurologic exam that clearly does not correspond to any known dermatomal pattern. See Nonanatomic Sensory Loss, Waddell's Test.

Nondominant Hand: The hand opposite the dominant hand. See Dominant Hand.

Nonforce Technique: A chiropractic term which refers to a light adjusting force being administered to correct a spinal subluxation. Examples would be activator therapy, toftness technique, SOT, trigger point, or loganbasic.

Nonmaterial Handling Activity: The nonspecific physical tasks of sitting, standing, walking, stooping, kneeling, crouching, reaching, handling, fingering, feeling, climbing, balancing, and driving. Job-specific nonmaterial handling activities may include keyboard use, tool use, fine motor coordination, and other job-specific work activities.

Nonneutral Dysfunction: See Type 2 Dysfunction.

Nonorganic Pain Behaviors: Pain behaviors which are secondary to symptom magnification and psychological issues and not to organic pathology. It should be cautioned that a thorough investigation of the patient's problem needs to be performed before this term should be used.

Nonorganic Signs: This term applies to any test used to identify magnified illness behavior or malingering. See Waddell's Test.

Nonspondylitic Spondylolisthesis: A slippage of one vertebra on another without a fracture in the pars interarticularis. This usually refers to a degenerative spondylolisthesis which is caused by degenerative facet joints and not a fracture in the neural arch.

Nonstructural Curve: A lateral curvature of the spine which is secondary to soft tissue imbalance and not to bony changes (structural). See Nonstructural Scoliosis, Adaptive Scoliosis, Adaptive Curve, Adaptive Rotoscoliosis.

Nonstructural Scoliosis: A lateral curvature of the spine which is secondary to soft tissue imbalance and not to bony changes (structural). This is defined by a curve that corrects on forward flexion or recumbent side bending x-rays. The curve can be superimposed on a structural scoliosis and, in this instance, may not appear to correct completely on dynamic testing. By definition, this curve is adaptive in nature or due to another structure. See Nonstructural Curve, Adaptive Scoliosis, Adaptive Curve, Adaptive Rotoscoliosis.

Norgesic: A mild-to-moderate analgesic used for musculoskeletal disorders. This compound contains 25 mg of orphenadrine, 285 mg of aspirin, and 30 mg of caffeine. Orphenadrine is a centrally acting compound which blocks reticular formation input and affects crossed extensor reflexes. This medication should not be used in patients with glaucoma, pyloric or duodenal obstruction, achalasia, prostatic hypertrophy, or obstructions at the bladder neck. This medication is also contraindicated in patients with myasthenia gravis and patients known to be sensitive to aspirin or caffeine. Common adult dosage is one to two tablets 3–4 times daily. Usage more than 2 days a week may cause rebound headache.

Norgesic Forte: A double strength form of Norgesic, an analgesic used for musculoskeletal disorders. See Norgesic.

Nortriptyline: A tricyclic antidepressant which is also used for chronic pain. It probably acts by interfering with the transport, release, and storage of catecholamines. As with all tricyclics, this drug should be given with caution to patients with cardiovascular disease. This drug has a tendency to prolong conduction time through the AV node and has anticholinergic side effects. Cimetidine interacts with this drug by significantly increasing the plasma concentrations. It is contraindicated for use with reserpine. The drug is supplied in 10-mg, 25-mg, 50-mg, and 75-mg capsules. When used for chronic pain it is usually given in the evening (10–25 mg). Since nortriptyline is more stimulating than other tricyclic antidepressants, it can be tolerated during the day by some patients. The antidepressant dose is usually 25 mg three or four times a day. Dosage should begin at a low level and increase as required. Dosage above 150 mg a day is not recommended. See Pamelor.

NR: An abbreviation for *neuromuscular re-education*. See Neuromuscular Re-education.

NRC: An abbreviation for *nerve root compression*. See Nerve Root Compression.

NRLSr: An osteopathic or manual physical therapy term which refers to a segment with a type 1 dysfunction as per Fryette's laws. This denotes a segment which is rotated to the left and side bent to the right in neutral (as opposed to flexion or extension). Neutral dysfunctions tend to occur in groups.

NRrSL: An osteopathic or manual physical therapy term which refers to a segment which is rotated to the right and side bent to the left in neutral (as opposed to flexion or extension). This is a type 1 dysfunction which follows Fryette's first law. Neutral dysfunctions tend to occur in groups.

NS: An abbreviation for *no show*.

NSAID: An abbreviation for *nonsteroidal anti-inflammatory drug*. Included in this drug category are Advil, Aleve, Nuprin, Motrin, aspirin, Feldene, Relefen, DanPro, Voltaren, Cataflam, Naprosyn, and Dolobid.

Nuchal Area: The area of the posterior occiput below the perinuchal line.

Nuchal Ligament: A triangularly shaped, band-like ligament which runs from the posterior border of the occiput to the spine of C7 in the midline. This structure also attaches to the posterior tubercle of the atlas, the spinous processes of the cervical vertebra, and the interspinous ligaments. Some believe that it has a major proprioceptive role in conjunction with the cervical erector spinae musculature. From an evolutionary standpoint, it serves to provide atlanto-occipital extension as the lower cervical spine is brought into flexion. This would presumably allow a quadruped to graze by thrusting the mouth forward. The nuchal ligament is often tight along with the suboccipital musculature after a subacute to chronic whiplash injury, contributing to the head-forward chin-out posture.

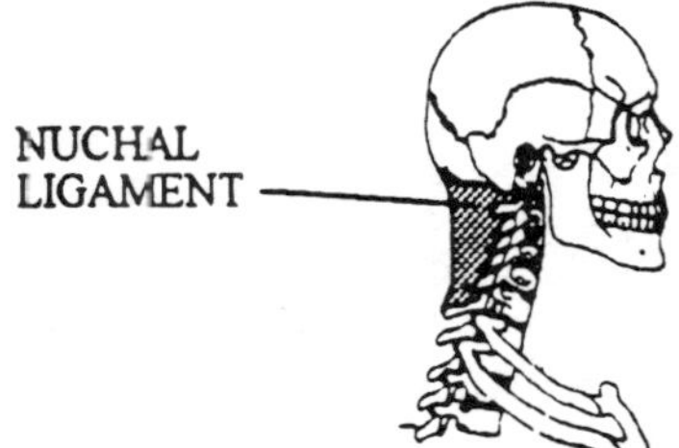

Nuchal Rigidity: Stiff neck. A physical exam sign associated with meningitis.

Nuclear Protrusion: An extrusion of the nucleus pulposus through the anterior annular fibers. See Disc Bulge, HNP.

Nucleogram: An x-ray following the injection of radiographic constast into the nucleus of the disc. See Discogram and Nucleometry.

Nucleometry: The x-ray or CT scan examination of the nucleus of the disc during a discogram. Since dye is injected into the disc, the nucleus of the disc will have a characteristic oval appearance with rounded edges. Extravasation (leaking) of the dye or nuclear clefts indicates an abnormal annulus or disc. See Nucleogram.

Nucleus Pulposus: The inner gel-like portion of the intervertebral disc. This structure holds water in younger individuals; with age, it loses water, thus causing disc degeneration and dehydration. This is the portion of the disc that "herniates" through the annulus in a disc herniation. It consists of proteoglycans and a collagen meshwork.

Nutated Sacrum: An osteopathic or manual physical therapy term which refers to a sacrum which is flexed or "nodded" forward. This usually occurs in patients with excessive lumbar lordosis. The patient usually lacks full lumbar flexion (forward bending) due to limited sacral extension. The ILAs are more prominent bilaterally. See Bilateral Sacral Extension.

Nutation: Derived from a Latin term meaning "nodding." In the lumbar spine, nutation usually describes the ilium or the sacrum. If the ilium is nutated, it is rotated anteriorly or flexed. With respect to the sacrum, nutation refers to a flexed sacrum or one that is bending forward. The sacrum normally nutates with lumbar extension and counter nutates with lumbar flexion.

Nutrient Foramina: The one or more large holes located on the posterior surface of the vertebral body. These foramina allow the nutrient arteries and basal vertebral veins to penetrate the vertebral body.

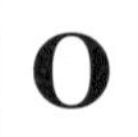

O: An abbreviation for *objective*.

OA: An abbreviation for *osteoarthritis*.

OA: Occipito-atlantal joint. This designation is often used in the osteopathic or manual physical therapy community rather than AO. See AO, Occipital-Atlantal Joint.

OA Joint: A joint between the skull and the atlas (C1). See Occipital-Atlantal Joint.

O-beam: A movable 4 × 4 beam placed on foam. See Oscillating Beam.

Ober's Test: A physical exam test for ITB tightness. The patient is in a side lying position while the hip and leg are brought back into extension while testing for tightness in the ITB by looking for a hip which stays abducted. It can be positive in patients with trochanteric bursitis or SI joint syndrome. See Iliotibial Band, Iliotibial Band Syndrome.

Objective: A finding that is observed by the examiner and not dependent on patient report.

Objective Discography: A term used to describe patient pain response during discography. After the dye has been injected into the disc and the patient has reported a pain response, a local anesthetic is injected and the patient is asked to rate his pain. If the pain is almost completely or completely abolished by the anesthetic, this is considered objective evidence that the patient's pain complaints are emanating from the disc. This is the same as an R2 response. See R2 Response.

Oblique Axis of the Sacrum: An axis of sacral motion described in osteopathic literature. This is movement about an axis that travels from one superior portion of the SI joint to the opposite inferior portion of the SI joint. This is the axis of motion associated with sacral torsions. This axis can best be described with a matchbook. If one holds a matchbook by diagonally opposite corners, the motion that takes place when the matchbook is tipped by a finger simulates the motion of the sacrum on an oblique axis.

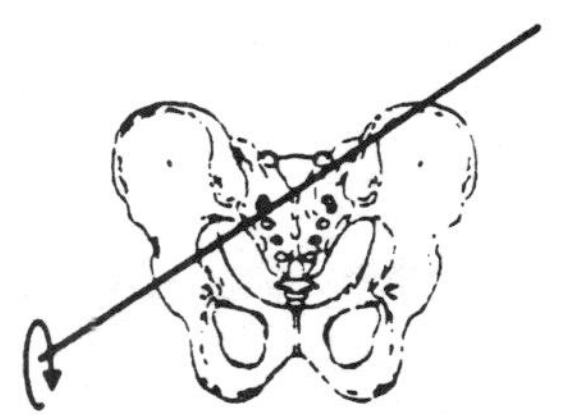

OBLIQUE AXIS OF SACRAL MOTION

Oblique: One of several views usually obtained in a cervical spine or lumbar spine series. These radiographs are commonly used to evaluate the pars interarticularis, which is disrupted in spondylolysis. A screening is performed for a positive "Scottie dog sign." This view can also be used to find some of the rare tumors affecting the pedicle. Also, obliques can be helpful in evaluating foraminal size and status of the facet joints. See Scottie Dog Sign.

Obturator Muscles: A pair of muscles that consist of the obturator externus and internus. They are both external rotators of the hip. The obturator internus passes through the lesser sciatic foramen and has a bursa between it and the lesser sciatic notch. The externus is supplied by the obturator nerve (L3–L4), and the internus is supplied by the nerve to obturator internus and superior gemellus (L5–S2).

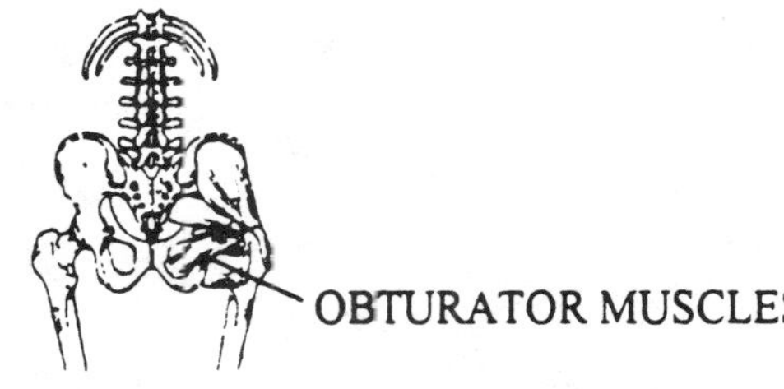

Oc: An abbreviation for *occiput.*

Oc-A: A chiropractic abbreviation for *occiput anterior.*

occ: An abbreviation for *occasional* and *occiput.*

Occ Doc: Medical slang for an occupational medicine physician.

Occipital: Referring to the back of the head.

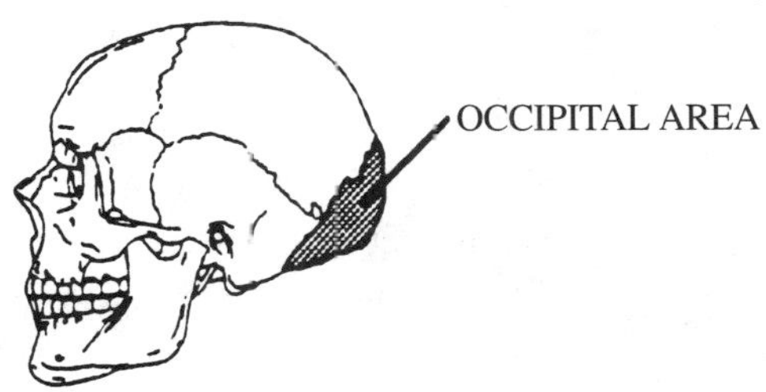

Occipital-Atlantal Instability: Excess motion in the joint between the occipital condyle of the skull and the atlas. On flexion extension views, this is defined as greater than 1 mm of C0–C1 translation. This is between the base of the occiput and the top of the dens. An increase in this distance of more than 1 mm is believed to indicate instability. This assumes that the transverse ligament of the axis in intact. Also, axial rotation greater than 8° to one side is considered instability.

Occipital-Atlantal Joint: A joint between the skull and the atlas (C1), or the articulation between the occipital condyle of the skull and the superior articular surface of the atlas. See OA Joint.

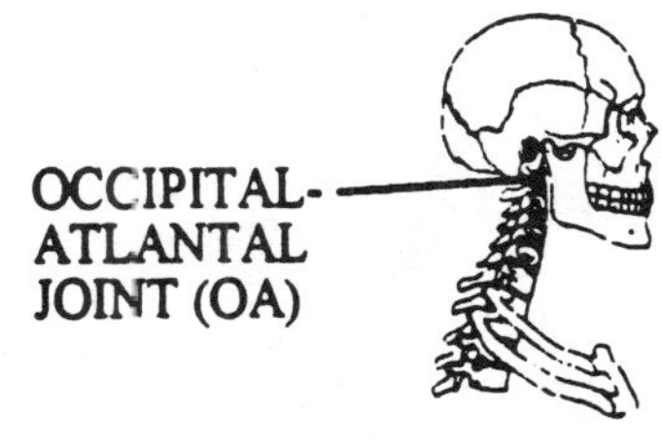

Occipital Condyle Fracture: A rare fracture of the occipital condyle. Type 1 is an impacted occipital condyle. Type 2 is a fracture associated with a basilar skull fracture. Type 3 is an evulsion fracture. Types 1 and 2 are caused by axial compression, and type 3 is caused by anterior-posterior translation and axial rotation. This fracture can be missed on plain x-rays, and it is suggested that CT scans with sagittal and coronal reconstructions be used for diagnosis.

Occipital Condyles: Bony prominences on the inferior of the occiput that articulate with the atlas. This makes up one part of the OA joint.

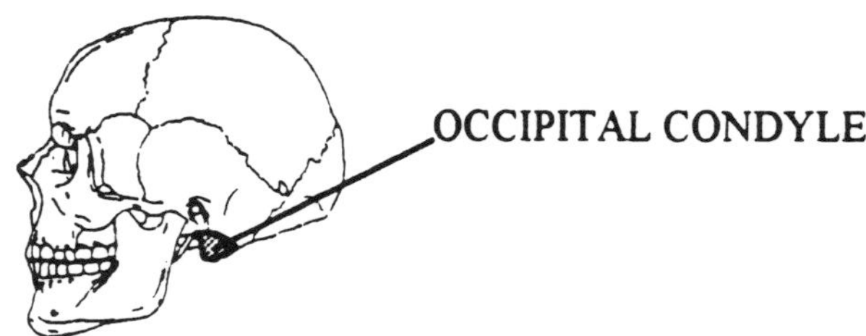

Occipital-Frontal Headaches: Pain which is usually described as starting at the base of the skull or in the back of the head and radiating to the forehead. See Frontal-Occipital Headaches.

Occipitalization of the Atlas: A congenital atlanto-occipital fusion. This is one of the more common anomalies of the upper cervical spine. This most often involves fusion of the anterior arch of the atlas to the anterior rim of the foramen magnum. Several adjacent vertebrae can also be involved. This malformation occurs frequently in conjunction with other malformations.

Occipital Neuralgia: A clinical syndrome involving irritation of either the greater occipital nerve or the lesser occipital nerve. More commonly, the greater occipital nerve is involved. The lesser occipital nerve syndrome tends to present with occipital headaches or tingling sensation which refers into the occipital area. See Greater Occipital Neuralgia.

Occipitoatlantoid Articulation: A joint between the skull and the atlas (C1). See OA Joint.

Occipitocervical Fusion: Fusion of the occipital condyles to the atlas.

Occipivot: A proprietary name for a self-mobilization device used to treat greater occipital nerve and lesser occipital nerve trigger areas to reduce headache pain. This also places pressure on the suboccipital area and can be helpful in the treatment of tension headaches.

Occiput-to-Wall Distance: A physical exam maneuver which tests flexion in the cervical spine. The patient stands with the heels and back against a wall. The chin is kept horizontal while the patient attempts to touch the wall with the occiput. The distance in centimeters is then measured from the wall to the occiput. This is often used to follow progressive loss of extension in the cervical spine.

Occlusion: Where the upper and lower teeth fit together.

Occulo-pelvic Reflex: A theory that altering the position of the head alters the posture of the pelvis. This also occurs in the reverse.

Occupational Medicine: A speciality of medicine which concerns itself with work-related diseases. This includes training in toxicology.

Occupational Medicine Physician: A doctor who is board certified in occupational medicine.

Ochronosis: A rare, hereditary metabolic disorder which is characterized by a defect in amino acid metabolism. Homogentisic acid is deposited in the tissues. This is a familial disorder which has a 2:1 male-to-female prevalence. There are bluish-brown pigmentations on the skin, cornea, sclera, and cartilage of the ears. The articular symptoms resemble ankylosing spondylitis (with less pain). There is progressive stiffness in the spine, hips, knees, and shoulders by age 40–50. There is a decreased lumbar lordosis and thoracic kyphosis as is seen with AS. On radiographs, multilevel disc calcification is seen with vacuum phenomena. There is ligament calcification and premature degenerative joint disease.

Oc-L: A chiropractic abbreviation for *occiput left.*

Oc-P: A chiropractic abbreviation for *occiput posterior.*

Oc-R: A chiropractic abbreviation for *occiput right.*

O'Donoghue Maneuver: A physical exam test that attempts to differentiate muscular from ligamentous injury. The patient is seated with the head and neck in neutral position. The examiner grasps the patient's head with both hands. The patient then attempts rotation against isometric resistance; pain production in this first stage of the test suggests strain of the activated musculature. If this test is negative, the examiner passively rotates the head and neck to one side to the limit of joint play. Pain reproduced here suggests ligamentous injury.

Odontoid Fracture: A fracture of the tooth-like process of C2. This accounts for 15–20% of all cervical fractures and can be complicated by neurologic deficit in up to 25% of cases. There are three types of fractures. Type 1 is a rare horizontal fracture through the body of the dens. Type 2 is a fracture of the neck of the dens at its junction with the vertebral body of C2. As a result of the poor blood supply to the odontoid, the type 2 fracture is difficult to treat even with halo fixation, and the nonunion rate is up to 33%. Type 3 fractures include the dens and extend into the body of C2. The integrity of the transverse ligament should be determined by MRI to rule out clinical instability. See Fractured Dens, Fractured Odontoid.

Odontoid Integrity Test: A test for the stability of the odontoid. The patient is in the supine position with the head supported by the examining table. The transverse process of C1 on the right is stabilized, and a shear force is imparted laterally on the left transverse process of C2 directed to the right. The opposite direction is then performed, and the examiner observes for excessive muscle guarding. If integrity is thought to be suspect, an open-mouth view and a cervical spine series may be helpful to rule out an odontoid fracture.

Odontoid Process: A tooth-like process which arises from the body of the axis. This acts as a pivot point for the rotation of C2 on C1. It articulates with C1 anteriorly and is separated from C1 by a bursa. It is contained posteriorly by the transverse ligament and forms the remainder of the atlantoaxial articulation. See Dens.

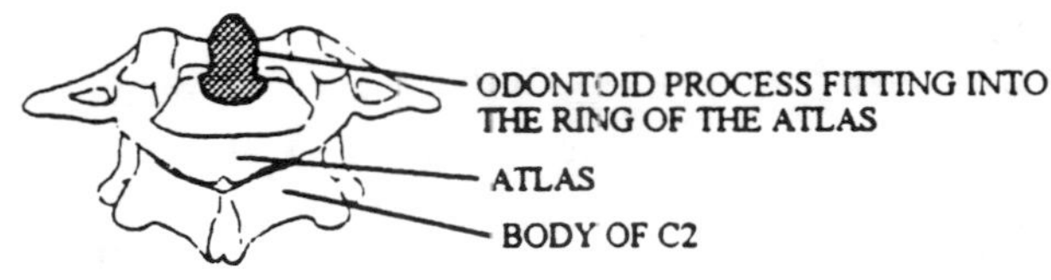

Odontoid Process Erosion: The x-ray appearance of the dens in patients with severe rheumatoid arthritis. There are large synovial erosions which appear as pieces taken out of the odontoid. This has also been called "whittling of the peg" due to the appearance of the odontoid.

Odontoid Process Fracture: A fracture of the tooth-like process of C2. See Odontoid Fracture.

Oldfeldt Protocol: An exercise regimen which involves strengthening the latissimus dorsi, abdominals, and erector spinae.

Omni: A name brand of metrizamide. See Omnipaque.

Omnipaque: A name brand of metrizamide. This is a water-soluble, nonionic contrast medium used for myelography and CT-myelography. See Omni.

OMT: The type of manipulation performed by most osteopaths and manual physical therapists. This usually refers to a low-velocity, low-to-medium–amplitude technique where a joint is carried through its full range of motion with the goal being to increase joint movement and function. This also refers to a variety of different techniques along a broad spectrum including craniosacral, combined treatment, muscle energy technique, and MFR. See Osteopathic Manipulative Therapy.

One-eyed Pedicle Sign: A radiographic sign seen with lytic metastases of the spine. There is unilateral destruction of one pedicle. On the AP view, only one pedicle is seen, giving rise to the name "one-eyed" pedicle. See Winking Owl Sign.

Ongley's Solution: A prolotherapy injection solution. See P2G.

Ongley's Technique: An injection technique used for prolotherapy that was made popular by Ongley and Dorman. A P2G solution (phenol and glycerin) is used and injections are given every 1–2 weeks. Osteopathic manipulation is also commonly used in conjunction with injections. See Prolotherapy, West Coast Method.

Open-Book Fracture: A complete separation of the symphysis pubis and disruption of one or both SI joints. See Sprung Pelvis.

Open-Book Pelvis: A complete separation of the symphysis pubis and disruption of one or both SI joints. See Sprung Pelvis.

Open-Book Test: A physical exam maneuver in which pressure is placed on the iliac crests with a downward and outward force with the patient lying supine. This maneuver should reproduce pain in the SI joint area. It predominantly stresses the anterior fibers of the SI joint and is usually positive in patients that have injured that portion of the joint. This may be positive in patients with outflare conditions.

Open Kinetic Chain: A combination of joints which act in linkage such that the terminal end is free and not fixed. An example of open kinetic chain exercise is knee extension where the foot is not fixed (seated quad sets).

OPLL: Ossification of the posterior longitudinal ligament. The deposition of calcium in the posterior longitudinal ligament which can lead to spinal stenosis. This disorder is primarily seen in Asian patients. See Ossification of the Posterior Longitudinal Ligament.

Oppenheimer Erosions: Erosion of the anterior lumbar vertebral body due to an abdominal aortic aneurysm. This is thought to be due to the increased transmission of the aortic pulsations which causes direct trauma to the anterior vertebral bodies.

Oppenheim Sign: An extensor reflex of the toes similar to a Babinski sign. This suggests upper motor neuron or corticospinal tract dysfunction. Heavy pressure is applied over the tibialis anterior as it is stroked from proximal to distal. A positive test is an extensor response in the toes and fanning similar to a Babinski response.

ORIF: An abbreviation for *open reduction internal fixation.*

Ortho-bionomy: A form of soft tissue mobilization which involves using gentle movements and shortened muscle positions to relax and balance muscles and ligaments. There is also a strong emphasis placed on re-educating the neuromuscular system. There are similarities among this technique, muscle energy technique, and Jones strain–counterstrain.

Orthopedics: Referring to the specialty of orthopedic surgery.

Orthopedic Spine: A subspecialty of orthopedic surgery devoted to the surgical management of disorders of the spine.

Orthopedic Surgeon: A physician who specializes in surgery of the bony skeleton, ligaments, tendons, and muscles.

Orthopedic Surgery: Surgery of the bony skeleton, tendons, ligaments, and muscles.

Orthotic: A custom-made shoe insert used to control pronation or supination in the forefoot. Orthotics are sometimes used to provide a heel lift or to control the pronation or supination which may be related to a functional or structural short leg. See Rigid Orthotic.

Orudis: A nonsteroidal anti-inflammatory drug in the propionic acid class. There are drug interactions with diuretics in that there is a greater risk of developing renal failure with the concomitant use of Orudis and these drugs. Toxicity can develop if taken in combination with methotrexate. The common dosage is 50 mg four times a day or 75 mg three times a day. In elderly patients or those with impaired renal function, the dose should be reduced by one half to one third. See Ketoprofen.

Oscillating Beam: A movable 4 × 4 beam placed on foam. The beam is usually between 15 and 20 feet long and used to aid in stabilization and balance programs. The patient is asked to walk on the beam while maintaining neutral spine posture. See O-beam.

Oscillations: Joint mobilizations of the spine which are applied with alternating pressure. Regular oscillations at two or three per second are applied for 1–2 minutes. The speed of the oscillations is varied for different treatment outcomes. For example, low-amplitude, high-speed oscillations are used to inhibit pain, while slower oscillations are used to relax muscle guarding. This is commonly used in the Paris and Maitland techniques. See Oscillatory Mobilization.

Oscillatory Mobilization: Joint mobilizations of the spine. See Oscillations.

Ossification of the Posterior Longitudinal Ligament: Deposition of calcium in the posterior longitudinal ligament which can cause compression on the anterior spinal artery (ischemic myelopathy) or compression on the spinal cord (myelopathy). This is seen more commonly in Asian patients. This is a progressive disease process with ongoing pathology seen in 25–80% of patients who have had operative decompression. The disorder can also be asymptomatic. See OPLL.

Osteitis Condensans Ilii: An isolated SI arthropathy. There is a heavy female predominance, especially in women of child-bearing age. There are chronic complaints of low back pain and stiffness. There is pain and tenderness over the SI joint with occasional radiation of pain into the lower extremity and groin region. ESR, CBC, RF, and HLA-B27 are negative. On x-ray, there are characteristic bilateral, dense, triangular-shaped areas of subchondral sclerosis in the iliacus near the lower posterior joint margin. This is known as hyperostosis triangularis ilii. The differential diagnosis includes ankylosing spondylitis. The etiology of this condition is controversial. See Hyperostosis Triangularis Ilii.

Osteitis Pubis: Pain in the area of the symphysis pubis, often seen in runners, is due to overuse or to direct trauma. This condition is also seen in patients who have undergone surgery near the symphysis pubis. Spasm can be seen in the adductor muscles of the thigh, and pain can be increased with resisted adduction. There is severe tenderness over the pubic symphysis. Erosions and later sclerosis are seen radiographically. Common treatments include ice then heat, anti-inflammatory medications, injection of corticosteroids, muscle balancing, and rest.

Osteoarthritis: The most common form of arthritis. This is a degenerative process that includes spondylosis and spurring of the vertebral bodies. Cartilage degeneration is the hallmark of this type of arthritis. The cause is obscure, but possibilities include changes in the synthesis of proteoglycans or their degradation, defects in synovial fluid and chondrocyte function, and cartilage fatigue and damage secondary to long-standing trauma or abrasion. The prevalence increases with age, with women over the age of 45 being most often affected with severe disease. Men have hip involvement more often, with women having more distal extremity involvement. See Spondylosis.

Osteoblastoma: A benign tumor of the spine which usually involves the posterior elements. This tumor usually occurs in the second or third decade of life, and the most common complaint is back pain. The pain is unrelated to physical activity and is most noticeable at night. Nonsteroidal anti-inflammatory drugs often provide significant relief. Even though this tumor is benign, it can produce significant spinal deformity. The most common deformity is scoliosis, and excision usually provides significant pain relief as well as resolution of the major deformity. Large spinal deformities may need to be corrected with excision and instrumentation.

Osteochondroma: A benign bony tumor of the spine which is the most common skeletal dysplasia. Vertebral involvement occurs in approximately 7% of all osteochondromas. Neurologic compromise is rarely seen. Sixty percent occur in the cervical spine, and 79% occur at or above T6. If neurologic compromise is seen, excision of the tumor usually restores function.

Osteogenic Scoliosis: An irreversible curvature of the spine with bony changes and a fixed rotation of the vertebrae. See Structural Scoliosis.

Osteoid Osteoma: A benign bony tumor which shows a predilection for spinal involvement and almost always involves the posterior elements. Patients usually present with this condition in their second or third decade of life. The most common complaint is back pain unrelated to activity and that is worse at night. Nonsteroidal anti-inflammatory drugs often produce dramatic relief of symptoms. Demonstration on radiographs can be difficult because by definition, this tumor is less than 2 cm in diameter and easily obscured by the overlapping shadows of the vertebral column. CT scan, however, usually demonstrates the lesion well, but thin-slice CT is suggested. The most sensitive imaging technique is a technetium bone scan. Radiographically, there is expansion of cortical bone, with a thin rim of reactive bone between the lesion and the surrounding soft tissue. This tumor can produce significant spinal deformity in the form of scoliosis. Surgical excision usually corrects the deformity and decreases pain. Instrumentation may need to be used in cases where there is large spinal deformity or when excessive excision of bone is necessary.

Osteomalacia: A softening of adult bone due to lack of calcium deposition. There are many causes, but most revolve around calcium, phosphorus, or vitamin D metabolism. Nonspecific radiographic changes show osteopenia, a course trabecular pattern, loss of cortical definition, pseudofractures, and bony deformity. The bony deformity is usually seen in weight-bearing bones. In the pelvis, inferior displacement of the sacrum produces a change in shape of the pelvic inlet.

Osteopath: Referring to an osteopathic physician (DO). See DO, Osteopathic Physician.

Osteopathia Stratia: A very rare clinical entity which involves linear bands of dense bone seen in the metaphyses and diaphyses of long bones. There is also a characteristic "sun burst" effect which represents dense bone formation in a fan-like pattern radiating from the acetabulum to the iliac crest.

Osteopathic Convention: The convention by which osteopathic dysfunctions are named. These rules define how osteopaths and many manual physical therapists name vertebral joint dysfunction. For instance, the barrier to movement is not named, but the displacement that barrier would cause is. Therefore, if the segment cannot move into flexion, it is named in extension. Also, the upper segment is always named in relation to the lower segment.

Osteopathic Lesions: A term which refers to an abnormality of spinal biomechanics involving a loss of normal movement of a vertebral motion segment. See Joint Blockage, Vertebral Subluxation Complex, Abnormal Spinal Segmental Motion, Somatic Dysfunction, Articular Dysfunction.

Osteopathic Manipulative Treatment: The type of manipulation performed by most osteopaths and manual physical therapists. See OMT.

Osteopathic Physician: A physican who has completed a graduate course of medical education at an AOA-approved college of osteopathic medicine. See DO, Osteopath.

Osteopenia: Decreased bone mass. See Osteoporosis, Radiolucency.

Osteophyte: An overgrowth of bone in response to injury. See Bone Spur.

Osteophytectomy: The surgical removal of an osteophyte that is causing central canal stenosis or foraminal stenosis. This is usually performed as a part of another procedure, such a discectomy and fusion or laminectomy and laminotomy.

Osteoporosis: Decreased density of normally mineralized bone that leads to mechanical failure and results in fractures from small amounts of trauma. There is a decreased capacity for bone repair, which reduces mechanical strength. Bone mass peaks between 30 and 35 years of age, and then begins to decrease. At menopause, the rate of decline increases tenfold. At the age of 70, bone loss rate in females parallels the bone loss rate in males. Fair-haired Northern Europeans tend to be more susceptible. Trabecular bone is preferentially affected. Vertebral fractures are commonly seen in a wedge pattern, crush pattern, and a biconcave fracture of the end plates. Type 1 osteoporosis is postmenopausal, and type 2 is senile. See Osteopenia.

Osteotomy: Literally, the cutting of bone. As a surgical procedure, this is performed to realign or correct joint deformity.

OT: Occupational Therapist.

OTJ: An abbreviation for *on the job*.

OTR: Registered Occupational Therapist.

Outer Annulus: The outermost portion of the outer covering of the disc (the annulus). This can be easily visualized on MRI studies. A complete tear of the outer annulus usually corresponds to a disc herniation. This portion of the annulus inserts into Sharpey's fibers, which insert into the vertebral body.

Outflare: An osteopathic or manual physical therapy term which usually refers to the ilium being externally rotated or turned out relative to the sacrum. This can occur if the articular surface of the sacrum is convex instead of the usual concave. However, this is one of the less common iliosacral dysfunctions. See Externally Rotated Innominate, Iliac Outflare.

OV: An abbreviation for *office visit*.

Oxaprozine: A nonsteroidal anti-inflammatory drug in the propanoic acid group. See DayPro.

Oxford Technique: This is the reverse of the DeLorme system. It was designed to decrease resistance as muscle fatigue develops. The maximum weight that the patient can lift at 10 repetitions is determined. The patient then performs 10 repetitions at that maximum, 10 repetitions at three-quarters of that maximum, and 10 repetitions at one-half of that maximum. The technique attempts to decrease the detrimental effects of muscle fatigue. A warm-up period is recommended. See DeLorme Technique.

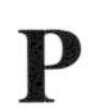

P

P: An abbreviation for *pain, plan, posterior,* and *procedure*.

P+: A notation made during discography that describes that the patient reported a reproduction of only part of their usual symptom complex.

P+/−: A notation made during discography that describes that the patient reported vague pain or pain that is clearly different from their usual symptom complex.

P++: A notation made during a provocative procedure such as a discogram that corresponds to a familiar pain response. See P2 Response.

P0: A notation made during discography that describes that the patient reported no pain response with injection or distension of the disc. See Discography.

P1 Response: A notation used during a discogram that corresponds to unfamiliar pain provoked by the test. See Discordant Pain Response.

P2G: A prolotherapy injection solution which contains 2.5% phenol, 25% glucose, 25% glycerin, and pyrogen-free water. This solution is commonly used with Ongley's technique. See P25G, Ongley's Solution, Phenol.

P25G: A prolotherapy injection solution. See P2G.

P2 Response: A notation made during a provocative procedure such as a discogram that corresponds to a familiar pain response. If the pain is familiar to the patient, it is believed that this disc is the source of the patient's pain. See P1 Response, R1 Response, R2 Response, Concordant Response, Discography, Pain Recreation, Subjective Discography.

PA: An x-ray which is taken with the patient's right side against the x-ray cartridge. An abbreviation for *posteroanterior*.

Pacinian Corpuscle: A receptor which is found in the periarticular connective tissue and is rapidly adapting. These receptors are primarily responsible for reporting the rate of acceleration of movement and delivering messages successively during motion. This has also been termed an acceleration receptor. It is also important in sensing vibration.

Paget's Disease: A metabolic disease of bone which affects the spine. Both osteoblasts (bone formation) and osteoclasts (bone breakdown) are hyperactive. This leads to excessive turnover of bone. There is a first phase of increased osteoclastic resorption of bone, a second phase of increased resorption balanced by increased formation, and finally a phase of "burn out" with little osteoclastic or osteoblastic activity. All three phases can be present simultaneously in the same bone. There is an increased urinary output of collagen breakdown metabolites such as hydroxyproline. Paget's disease affects about 3% of the middle-aged and elderly population. Sixty percent of patients have involvement of lumbar spine, 45% the thoracic spine and sacrum, with only about 15% in the cervical spine. There is no predilection for males or females. Two out of three patients with disease seen on x-ray are asymptomatic. A viral etiology is suspected. Bony pain is a common complaint but does not need to be present. There is skull enlargement and thickening, and secondary hearing loss can develop. Tinnitus, vertigo, headache, and other symptoms are not uncommon. X-ray shows a mosaic appearance and deformity in the lower extremities is common due to the weight-bearing stresses on softened bone. There can be an "arrow sign" which indicates an advancing resorption wedge. Malignancy in the form of sarcoma occurs in approximately 1% of patients.

Pain, Chronic: An ICD-9 diagnosis code for chronic pain. See Chronic Pain Syndrome.

Pain Clinic: A multidisciplinary team approach for treating patients with chronic pain. Education is emphasized, as well as physical conditioning, self-management techniques, decreasing narcotic dependence, and addressing psychological barriers to recovery. This is usually performed in a three or four week outpatient setting. See Chronic Pain Syndrome, IOP.

Pain Disorder Associated with Psychological Factors: A psychological disorder associated with pain that is not due to a diagnosed medical condition. This diagnosis is not used if the patient also meets the criteria for a somatization disorder.

Pain Drawing: The patient is presented with the outline of a body and asked to describe the distribution and type of pain by drawing on that figure. This is a method of quantifying pain.

Pain Generator: An anesthesia term which refers to an anatomic structure that is causing symptoms. The pain generator is usually located through diagnostic blocks and injections. For instance, if the SI joint is anesthetized and the patient's pain disappears, it is thought that the SI joint is the pain generator.

Pain, Psychogenic: An ICD-9 diagnosis code for somatoform disorder, chronic pain syndrome, symptom magnification syndrome, and somatization disorder. See those terms for more specific descriptions.

Pain Re-creation: A possible pain response during discography. See Concordant Pain Response, P2 Response.

Pain Scale: One method for quantifying pain. There are many different types of pain scales. The most common is a 0–10 scale, with 0 being no pain and 10 being suicidal pain.

Palato-occipital Line: A radiographic sign used to detect basilar impression. See Chamberlain's Line.

Palmer Diversified: A chiropractic technique where the primary manipulative force is the practitioner's hands. See Diversified Technique.

Palmer-Gonstead-Firth Listing System: The most common way to list or record chiropractic vertebral malpositions. See PGF Listing System.

Palmer Package: A number of chiropractic techniques which are taught at Palmer College of Chiropractic. There is a strong emphasis on correcting spinal subluxations and re-establishing the normal neurologic balance of the lumbar spine. See Palmer Technique.

Palmer Technique: A chiropractic technique that originated with Palmer College of Chiropractic. There is a strong emphasis on correcting spinal subluxations and establishing normal neurologic balance of the spine. Any additional therapies are only employed after the spinal subluxations have been resolved. This includes elements of diversified technique, Thompson technique, and Gonstead technique. See Palmer Package.

Palmer Upper Cervical Technique: A chiropractic technique that utilizes the x-ray analysis and adjusting techniques developed by B. J. Palmer to correct subluxations in the upper cervical spine (C1–C2). This technique is used by approximately one fourth of U.S. chiropractors. See HIO, Hole in One.

palp: An abbreviation for *palpable*, *palpated*, *palpate*, *palpatory*, and *palpation*.

Palpable Band: A palpable band of muscle fibers usually associated with a trigger point. This is an area which is usually linear in nature and runs along the course of muscle fibers during muscle palpation. See Trigger Point, Taut Band.

Pamelor: A tricyclic antidepressant which is also used for chronic pain. See Nortriptyline.

Pancake Vertebra: An extremely flat vertebral body associated with vertebral collapse. See Vertebra Plana.

Pantaloon Spica: A lumbar orthosis which immobilizes the thoracic and lumbar areas and extends down to usually one thigh. In this way, this immobilizes L5–S1 more effectively. However, there is some controversy as to whether this does provide additional stability. See TLSOT.

Paracervical Musculature: The paraspinal musculature of the cervical spine. See Paraspinal Musculature.

Paraflex: A muscle relaxant which contains 250 mg of chlorzoxazone. This drug acts at the spinal cord and subcortical level where it inhibits the reflex arcs involved in producing and maintaining skeletal muscle spasm and tone. It does have a sedative effect, so the concomitant use of alcohol or other CNS depressants is contraindicated. Usual adult dose is one caplet (250 mg) three or four times a day. Initial dosage can be up to two caplets two to four times a day, and doses of three caplets three or four times a day have also been given.

Paralumbar Musculature: The erector spinae musculature or long spinal extensors. This is the musculature that can be easily palpated during a physical exam on either side of the lumbar spinous processes.

Paramedian Herniated Disc: See Central HNP, Paramedian HNP.

Paramedian HNP: A herniation of the nucleus pulposus that occurs in the midline instead of the usual posterior and lateral direction. See Central HNP, Paramedian Herniated Disc.

Paraphysiological Space: The small amount of "space" between the elastic and anatomic barriers. This usually refers to the point beyond where vertebral movement stops passively during manipulation.

Paraspinal Musculature: The erector spinae musculature or long spinal extensors. This is the musculature that can be readily palpated on either side of the spinous processes during an exam. See Paraspinous Musculature, Paravertebral Musculature, Paracervical Musculature.

Paraspinal Tenderness: Tenderness in the muscle mass on either side of the spinous processes (the back muscles that can easily be palpated just under the surface of the skin).

Paraspinous Musculature: The erector spinae musculature or long spinal extensors. See Paraspinal Musculature.

Paraspinous Tenderness: Tenderness in the muscle mass on either side of the spinous processes (the back muscles that can easily be palpated just under the surface of the skin).

Paravertebral: Adjacent to the vertebral column.

Paravertebral Line: A vertical line formed by connecting the tips of the transverse processes.

Paravertebral Musculature: The erector spinae musculature or long spinal extensors. See Paraspinal Musculature.

Paravertebral Sympathetic Ganglia: A portion of the autonomic nervous system that consists of a chain of ganglia that lies on either side of the vertebral column. See Sympathetic Ganglia, Sympathetic Chain.

Paresthesia: An abnormal sensation which can be either spontaneous or evoked. This is similar to dysesthesia but is not painful.

Paroxetine Hydrochloride: An antidepressant with a chemical structure unrelated to the other selective serotonin reuptake inhibitor (SSRI) antidepressants (Zoloft and Prozac). See Paxil.

Pars: A slang term for the pars interarticularis. See Pars Interarticularis.

Pars Interarticularis: A term which means literally "the part between the articulations." This is the portion of the vertebra which lies between the superior facet joint and the inferior facet joint. This section of bone is fractured in a spondylolysis or spondylolisthesis. See Pars.

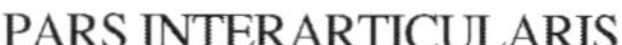

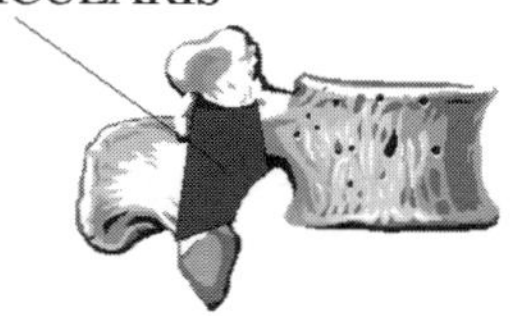

Pars Interarticularis Defect: A fracture or congenital defect in the bony portion connecting the facet joints. This is associated with spondylolysis and spondylolisthesis. A pars defect is usually noted on oblique x-rays as a collar on the Scottie dog or a decapitated Scottie dog. See Scottie Dog Sign, Spondylolysis.

Pars Lateralis: The area just lateral to the pelvic foramina in the sacrum. These are grooves that run laterally from the foramina and mark the passage of each of the ventral sacral roots. The origin of the piriformis muscle is on a ridge between each of the grooves.

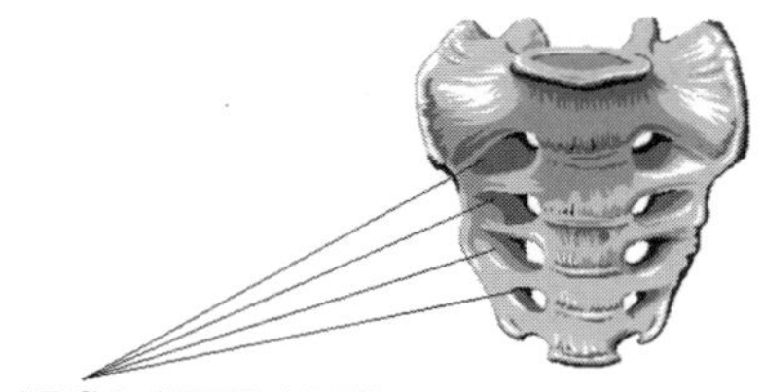

Partial Medial Facetectomy: The surgical removal of up to one-third of the medial aspect of the facet. This procedure is usually performed during a laminectomy in order to further decompress a spinal stenosis.

Partial Squats: A quadriceps–gluteal muscle strengthening excercise which involves partial (to a knee angle of less than 45°) knee bends. See Minisquats, Squats.

Pass: An abbreviation for *passive.*

Passion Fracture: A fractured rib caused by the compressive force of a hug. The fourth through ninth ribs are the most commonly fractured. The fracture site is frequently found at the lateral aspect of the rib. Fractures of the upper ribs are uncommon owing to the overlying supporting musculature. Fractures of the lower ribs are also uncommon (ten through twelve) due to the fact that they are usually free ribs and very mobile. See Bear Hug Fracture.

Passive Knee Flexion: A maneuver described by Cyriax which checks the mobility of the L3 nerve root. See PKB.

Passive Mobility: In the spine, passive range of motion is measured in flexion, extension, side bending, or rotation. See Passive Range of Motion.

Passive Mobility Testing: Passively taking the lumbar spine through various movements including flexion, extension, side bending, rotation, or side gliding to detect restricted movements.

Passive Neck Flexion: A physical exam maneuver first described by Brudzinski as one of the clinical signs of meningitis. See PNF.

Passive Range of Motion: In the spine, passive range of motion (ROM) is measured in flexion, extension, side bending, and rotation. This differs from active range of motion in that the patient uses no voluntary muscle contraction and must be taken through the ROM by the examiner. See PROM, Passive Mobility.

Passive Scapular Approximation Test: A physical exam maneuver in which the patient is standing with arms at the sides. The examiner approximates the scapulae by pushing the shoulders back into retraction. Pain in the scapular area suggests a compression syndrome of the T1 or T2 nerve roots.

Patellar Tendon Reflex: The reflex contraction of the quadriceps muscle with tapping of the patellar tendon. A normal reflex suggests that the motor portion of the L2–L4 nerve roots are functioning normally. A decreased reflex can be due to a herniated nucleus pulposus at L2–L4. An increased reflex can be due to an upper motor neuron lesion. See PTR.

Pathological Collapse: The collapse of vertebral body due to tumor and osteolytic destruction.

Pathological Fracture: Vertebral body collapse due to osteolytic destruction and neoplasm.

Pathological Reflex: A cutaneous reflex, which, if present, is abnormal. The classic example is a Babinski reflex, which implies upper motor neuron dysfunction.

Pathological Spondylolisthesis: Slippage of one vertebra onto another due to bony collapse caused by disease. See Type V Spondylolisthesis.

Patrick's Test: A test for SI joint syndrome which puts the hip into flexion, abduction, and external rotation. See FABER Test.

PA View: An x-ray which is taken with the patient's right side against the x-ray cartridge. See Posteroanterior View.

Paxil: An antidepressant with a chemical structure unrelated to the other selective serotonin reuptake inhibitor (SSRI) antidepressants (Zoloft and Prozac). This drug is contraindicated for use in patients taking MAO inhibitors. There are drug interactions with tryptophan, warfarin (Coumadin), cimetidine, phenobarbital, and phenytoin. Co-administration of Paxil with other SSRIs and many of the tricyclic antidepressants may decrease P_{450} enzyme activity. The tricyclics on this list are nortriptyline, amitriptyline, imipramine, and desipramine. In these instances, the patient may require lower doses of Paxil because the P_{450} enzyme is responsible for breaking down Paxil. There are also drug interactions with alcohol, lithium, digoxin, diazepam, and propranolol. The recommended initial dose is 20 mg a day. The dose range is 20–50 mg a day. Patients that respond to a 20-mg dose may benefit from 10-mg-a-day dose increases up to the maximum of 50 mg a day. Paxil is supplied in 20-mg and 30-mg tablets. See Paroxetine Hydrochloride.

PB: An abbreviation for *pelvic bench.*

PC: An abbreviation for *phone call.*

PDPR %: Patient describes pain reduction as ______ %.

PDR: *Physicians' Desk Reference.*

PE: An abbreviation for *physical examination.*

Peanut: A type of Swiss ball which is elongated to provide more lateral stability. See Swiss Ball.

Peanut Ball: A type of Swiss ball which is elongated to provide more lateral stability. See Swiss Ball.

pect. maj.: An abbreviation for *pectoralis major.*

pect. min.: An abbreviation for *pectoralis minor.*

Pectoralis Minor Syndrome: Compression of the neurovascular bundle by the pectoralis minor or clavipectoral fascia. The brachial plexus accompanied by the axillary vein and artery passes underneath the pectoralis minor. There can be compression of the neurovascular bundle between the pectoralis minor and rib cage, or the neurovascular bundle can be "caught" on the origin of the pec minor on the coracoid process. Symptoms are similar to those found with other thoracic outlet syndromes. There is also a myofascial referral pattern to the anterior shoulder. The hyperabduction test is usually employed for diagnosis. This involves abducting the arm and moving it behind the head. This puts the neurovascular bundle on stretch as it hooks underneath the coracoid process. Common treatments include myofascial release of the pec minor and or clavipectoral fascia, injection and stretch of the pec minor, postural exercises, correction of rib cage restrictions, correction of thoracic spine dysfunction, strengthening of the upper back musculature and scapular stabilizers, and adverse neural tension stretching. See Hyperabduction Syndrome, Thoracic Outlet Syndrome.

NERVE PASSING UNDER THE POINT WHERE THE PEC MINOR INSERTS INTO THE CORACOID PROCESS.

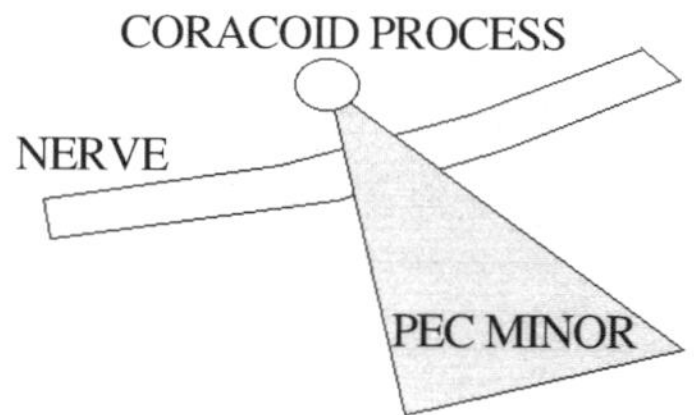

Pectus Carinatum: A prominent sternum produced by an anterior displacement of that bone. This is a congenital abnormality associated with Morquio's syndrome. See Pigeon Breast.

Pectus Excavatum: The most common deformity of the chest. There is a midline depression of the sternum which is seen on physical examination, as well as lateral x-rays of the chest. There is a posterior displacement of the sternum.

Pedicle: Pillars of bone which project from the back of the vertebral body which form the first part of the ring which surrounds the spinal canal. The pedicles originate from the upper portion of the vertebral body. The word is derived from the Latin *pediculus,* which means little foot. The neural arch seems to stand on the vertebral body with the pedicles as feet when the vertebra is viewed from above. The pedicles transmit both tension and bending forces that are channeled from the posterior elements. These forces are then transmitted to the vertebral bodies. Muscular action is also transmitted to the vertebral body through the pedicles, which act as levers because the musculature is attached to the posterior elements. See Vertebral Pedicle.

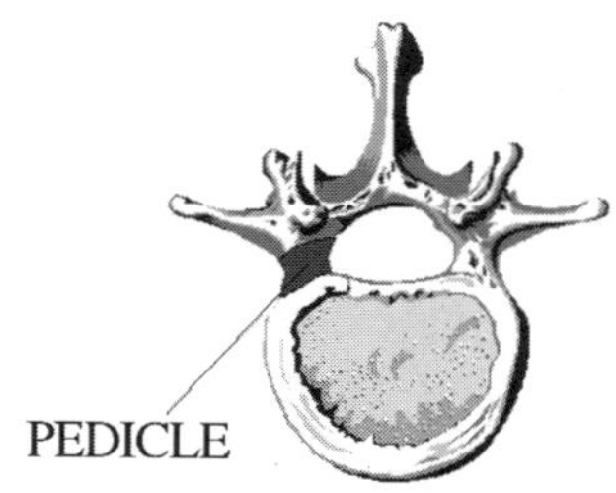

Pedicle Method: A radiographic method for determining the degree of rotation in scoliosis. The rotation of the pedicle on the convex side of the curve is graded between 0 and 4.

Pedicle Migration: One method of determining the degree of rotatory scoliosis by determining the degree the pedicle has migrated from its neutral position on AP radiography. See Nash-Moe Method.

Pedicle Screw Fixation: Instrumentation of the spine in which screws are placed through the pedicles, and then attached to connecting rods to completely immobilize a portion of the spine. This is done to increase the chances of bony fusion at the levels immobilized. It is also thought that use of pedicle screws forms a stronger attachment so that fewer segments must be immobilized to achieve fusion. Potential disadvantages include neurologic complications due to pedicle screws, as well as problems in the radiographic evaluation of fusion due to the internal fixation device obscuring the fusion mass. See Steffee Plates, Roy-Camille Plates, Luque Fixation, Magerl External Spinal Fixator, Dyck Fixator, Krag Fixator, Wiltse System, Wiltse Fixator.

Pedicle Screws: Screws which are drilled into the pedicle and attach many common posterior instrumentation systems to the spine. The pedicle is the strongest region of the vertebra with a cylinder of cortical bone surrounded by a small amount of cancellous bone. Therefore, this is an excellent place to attach instrumentation. Screws can be introduced safely through the center of the pedicle because the nerve roots lie below the pedicle. See Posterior Spinal Fusion.

Pedicular Stress Fracture: A rare stress fracture through the lumbar pedicle. This is due to posterior spinal fusion when hypermobile segments are created above or below the level of the fusion. The fact that one or more segments no longer move (are fused) causes the segments to move too much (become hypermobile).

Pelvic Alignment: The relation of the pelvic ring to the sacrum. This would include alignment of the sacrum on the ilium, the alignment of the sacrum within the two iliac articulations, and the alignment of the ilia to each other. See Pelvic Obliquity.

Pelvic Belt: An immobilization device used in SI joint syndrome where hypermobility is suspected. See SI Belt.

Pelvic Bench: A chiropractic table used for adjusting which is low to the ground and allows for easier side posture manipulation of the pelvis.

Pelvic Block: Paired wedges which are used primarily for positioning of the lumbosacral and sacroiliac joints by chiropractors. The idea is that these will produce a sustained stretch over time. They are placed in different positions in order to obtain different vectors of stretch.

Pelvic Bone: The ilium, ischium, and pubis named as one unit. See Innominate.

Pelvic Clock: An imaginary clock face superimposed over the pelvis for the purpose of patient education and instruction. When the patient is asked to move to 12 o'clock, the pelvis is derotated by contracting the abdominals and bringing the front of the pelvis superior. When the patient is asked to move to 6 o'clock, the pelvis is rotated forward and the anterior pelvis is brought downward. The patient can also perform lateral movements to 3 and 6 or diagonal movements 2, 4, 7, or 10. The anterior superior iliac spines can be monitored by the examiner or the patient for symmetry.

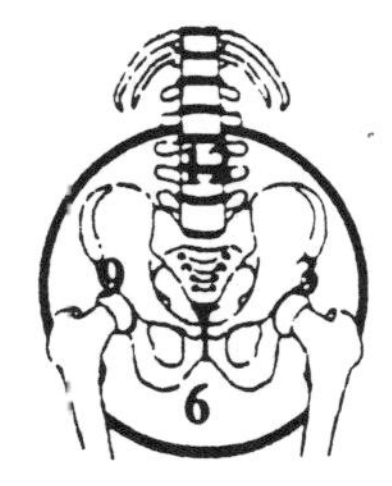

PELVIC CLOCK

Pelvic Floor Release: A myofascial release technique which is commonly used in association with treatment for SI joint dysfunction. There is a superficial release technique described around the coccyx and pubic symphysis; a deeper technique has also been described.

Pelvic Inlet: The large opening in the center of pelvic ring. See Inlet of the Pelvis.

Pelvic Lateral Tilt: A chiropractic term denoting a pelvis which is not level in the horizontal plane. For instance, one ASIS is higher or more superior than the other. This is associated with lateral flexion of the lumbar spine and an adducted hip on one side with an abducted hip on the other. From an osteopathic standpoint, this would be consistent with a pubic shear (upslip/downslip).

Pelvic Obliquity: An unlevel pelvic base. This is frequently seen with a leg length discrepancy and represents a pelvic tilt in the frontal plane. This can also refer to an SI joint dysfunction. See Pelvic Alignment.

Pelvic Ring: The circular structure formed by the two halves of the pelvis and the sacrum. This architecture provides strength to the pelvis with the sacrum acting as the keystone. There are articulations in the ring at the SI joints posteriorly and the symphysis pubis anteriorly.

Pelvic Rotation: A chiropractic term denoting a pelvic position in which one ASIS is anterior to the other. This is a rotation around the vertical (y) axis. This is also known as an internally or externally rotated innominate or ilium. From an osteopathic standpoint, this would be equivalent to an inflare or outflare of the ilium.

Pelvic Sling: A type of supportive bandage that may provide some compression across the pelvic ring to reduce open book fractures or fractures of the pubic symphysis.

Pelvic Stabilization: A rehabilitation program used to stabilize the lumbar spine through the pelvis that involves neuromuscular retraining, flexibility, and strengthening. See Dynamic Lumbar Stabilization.

Pelvic Tilt: Rotation of the entire pelvis such that the anterior pelvis is brought superior or inferior. This then increases (anterior tilt or anterior pelvis downward) or decreases (posterior tilt or anterior pelvis upward) the lumbar lordosis.

Pelvic Tilts: A physical therapy excercise in which the patient rotates the pelvis forward and backward to increase kinesthetic awareness of the pelvis or increase muscular coordination and recruitment.

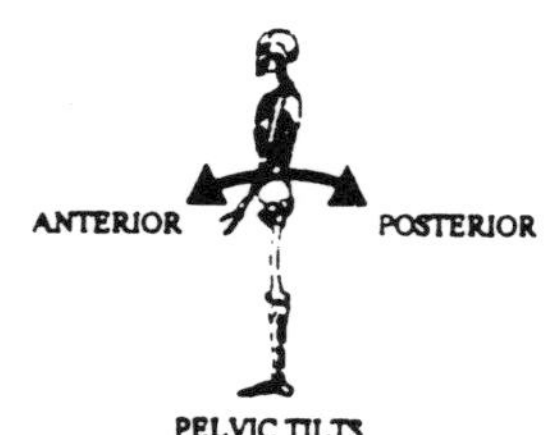

Pelvic Traction: A common way to deliver lumbar traction. See Traction.

Pelvis: The bony ring that surrounds the sacrum. The sacrum can be considered the keystone of the bony arch that provides support for the spine. The pelvic ring is mobile through the SI joints and pubic symphysis.

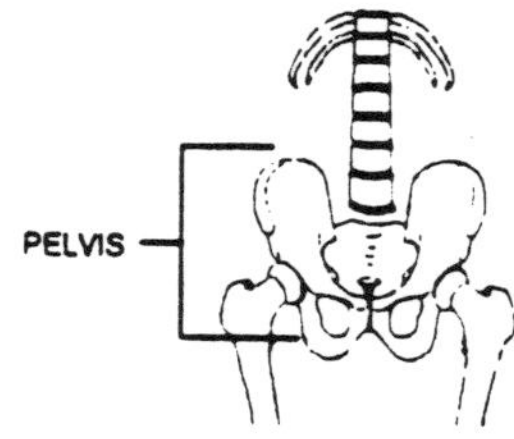

Pelvospondylitis Ossificans: An inflammatory disease of the spine which greatly restricts spinal movement. It is often associated with morning pain and occurs primarily in young adults. Also known as bamboo spine because of its bamboo shoot-like appearance on x-rays. See Rheumatoid Spondylitis, Ankylosing Spondylitis, AS, Von Bechterew Disease, Marie-Strumpell Disease.

Pencil-sharpened Spinous Process: A radiographic term which describes the tapered spinous processes most commonly seen in the cervical spine of patients with rheumatoid arthritis.

Penning Method: A method for determining segmental instability described by Penning in 1960. This method is considered less time-consuming than previous methods for determining the degree of segmental flexion/extension motion on flexion/extension films. The extension film is superimposed on the flexion film, with the C7 vertebral body exactly matching. A line is drawn along one of the edges of the flexion film onto the extension film. Next, C6 is superimposed and a second line is drawn. The angle between the lines is the degree of flexion/extension movement between C6 and C7. The range of motion between other vertebrae is then determined. Average values of segmental motion are based on the examination of 20 normal healthy adults.

PERC: The removal of bulging disc material percutaneously through a large-bore needle inserted into the disc space. See Percutaneous Discectomy, Percutaneous Nucleoectomy.

Perched Facets: A facet dislocation where the tip of the superior facet is resting on the tip of the inferior facet. There is a rupture of the facet capsule.

Percocet: A powerful narcotic pain reliever which contains 5 mg of oxycodone and 325 mg of acetaminophen. Oxycodone is a semisynthetic narcotic analgesic similar to morphine. This is used in moderate to moderately severe pain. The usual adult dosage is one tablet every 6 hours as needed for pain. See Percodan—Demi.

Percodan: A powerful narcotic pain reliever which contains 4.5 mg of oxycodone hydrochloride, 0.38 mg of oxycodone terephthalate, and 325 mg of aspirin. This drug is habit-forming. The usual adult dosage is one tablet every 6 hours as needed for pain. See Percocet.

Percodan—Demi: This is a similar formulation with oxycodone and aspirin, but contains only 2.25 mg of oxycodone. The usual adult dosage is one to two tablets every 6 hours. See Percocet, Percodan.

Percutaneous Discectomy: The removal of bulging disc material percutaneously through a large-bore needle inserted into the disc space. A posterior lateral approach is used, and the needle is placed into the disc using fluoroscopic (x-ray) guidance. The disc material is removed using laser, cutting, sucking, or laser appliances. See Percutaneous Microdiscectomy, PMD, PERC, PLD.

Percutaneous Disc Treatment: The removal of bulging disc material percutaneously through a large-bore needle inserted into the disc space. See Percutaneous Discectomy.

Percutaneous Microdiscectomy: The removal of bulging disc material percutaneously through a large-bore needle inserted into the disc space. See Percutaneous Discectomy.

Percutaneous Nucleoctomy: See Percutaneous Nucleoectomy.

Percutaneous Nucleoectomy: The removal of disc material through a large-bore needle in order to avoid soft tissue damage and postoperative adhesions around the nerve roots which can be complications of conventional surgeries. This involves reduction of interdiscal pressure due to fenestration of the anulus fibrosus and partial removal of the disc materials. It is thought that the reduction of interdiscal pressure results in a relief of irritation of the nerve root or pain receptors in the outer annulus. See Percutaneous Discectomy, Percutaneous Nucleotomy, PERC, PN.

Perianal Sensation: Sensation around the anus which is provided through the sacral nerve roots. Perianal sensation is often lost with spinal stenosis involving the conus medularis or cauda equina syndrome.

Periarthritis Calcarea: The deposition of hydroxyapatite crystals in multiple locations. See Hydroxyapatite Deposition Disease.

Perilymphatic Fistula: An abnormal communication between the semicircular canals. This has been reported to occur following whiplash injuries. It is usually associated with hearing loss, with or without vertigo. An ENG or AEBR can be helpful in evaluating this disease process.

Perineural Fibrosis: Scarring around nerve roots which can occur after a surgical procedure. If the scarring constricts the nerve roots, a "post or failed laminectomy syndrome" can occur. This term can also be used to describe restrictions around peripheral nerves. See Epidural Fibrosis, Adhesive Arachnoiditis, Root Sleeve Fibrosis.

Periosteal Pain Points: Points along the periosteal attachments of muscle to bone (entheses) which are noted to be tender with specific muscle overload or joint dysfunction. For instance, pain on the coccyx may be due to gluteus maximus, piriformis, or levator ani overload. Periosteal acupuncture has also been described in which acupuncture points are deemed to be along periosteal attachments. See PPP.

Periosteal Trigger Point: An isolated point of tenderness where a tendon or aponeurosis inserts onto the periosteum. In the lumbar spine, this is most common at the PSIS, but can be identified over the spinous processes, sacrum, or pelvic brim. These areas are often injected with anesthetic and corticosteroids and are common sites for prolotherapy.

Periosteoradial Reflex: A physical exam maneuver that tests the integrity of the C6 nerve root. See Brachioradialis Reflex.

Periph: An abbreviation for *peripheral.*

Peripheral Neuropathy: A generalized "slowing" of the peripheral nervous system which usually presents with decreased sensation in a stocking and glove distribution in the feet and hands. The etiology can include advancing age, diabetes, heavy metal poisoning, long-standing hypertension, and congenital defect. This condition can usually be diagnosed with EMG/nerve conduction studies. Both axonal loss and demyelination can occur to varying degrees.

Periradicular Sheath: The covering of the nerve root that is continous with the dura. See Nerve Root Sheath.

Permanent Impairment: This is defined by the AMA Guides to the Evaluation of Permanent Impairment as impairment which is not likely to change despite medical treatment. Permanent impairment is given in percentages. With respect to the spine, these percentages are in whole person units. See Impairment Rating.

peron. brevis: An abbreviation for *peroneus brevis.*

peron. long.: An abbreviation for *peroneus longus.*

PERRLA: Pupils Equal, Round, Reactive to Light and Accommodation.

Petit's Triangle: An anatomic triangle located just above the ilium. The borders are the latissimus dorsi, the external oblique, and the ilium. See Lumbar Triangle.

Petrissage: A type of massage which involves deep circular movements and is applied with the tips of the thumbs, the three middle fingers, or the knuckles.

Pettibon Technique: A chiropractic technique which uses complex formulas to ascertain various misalignment angles. Specific manual and instrument adjustments are used to correct these misalignments. This technique is used by only 6% of U.S. chiropractors.

Pg: An abbreviation for *pregnant.*

PGF Listing System: The most common way to list or record chiropractic vertebral malpositions. See Palmer-Gonstead-Firth Listing System.

PH: An abbreviation for *past history* or *personal history.*

Phenol: A caustic neurolytic agent used in some prolotherapy solutions. Phenol causes a long-lasting segmental demyelination when injected around peripheral nerves. See P2G, Prolotherapy.

Philadelphia Collar: A hard cervical orthosis which immobilizes the cervical spine by extending from the chin/occiput to the upper thoracic spine. This has intermediate effectiveness in controlling cervical range of motion, most specifically in flexion/extension and lateral bending. This provides better cervical immobilization than a soft cervical collar.

Phlebolith: Concretions of thrombi attached to the walls of veins which appear on x-ray as dense, round-to-oval, well-defined nodules often with a lucent center. They are most commonly seen on an AP pelvic view just superior to the pubis. By the fourth decade, at least one pelvic phlebolith will be seen in approximately one third of all x-rays. They commonly occur in the perirectal and perivesical venous plexuses.

Phonophoresis: The delivery of a medication (usually an anesthetic or anti-inflammatory steroid) using ultrasound to push medication into a specific area. This is most effective when treating superficial structures because penetration is less than 1 cm. This delivery system is less effective in overweight patients. This is thought to be less effective than iontophoresis. This is commonly used to treat inflammatory conditions such as tendonitis.

Physiatrist: An M.D. or D.O. who has completed residency training in physical medicine and rehabilitation. A specialist in rehabilitation and outpatient nonoperative orthopedics. Board certification is given by the American Academy of Physical Medicine and Rehabilitation.

Physical Capacity Evaluation: A test of physical strength and stamina used to determine working restrictions and work tolerance. See Functional Capacity Evaluation.

Physical Work Capacity Assessment: A test which measures physical fitness. The relationship between heart rate, work output, and oxygen consumption are used to evaluate the cardiovascular fitness of the individual relative to the cardiovascular demands of the job.

Physician's Desk Reference: A proprietary name for a comprehensive drug reference text.

Physioball: A large, brightly colored rubber ball used in many lumbar stabilization programs. See Swiss Ball.

Physiologic Barrier: The line at which active range of motion ends and passive range of motion begins. Each vertebral segment has an active range. This active range is as far as the musculature can move that particular segment. However, the vertebral segment can be pushed into the passive range using manual pressure.

Physiologic Movement: Normal movements such as flexion, extension, rotation, abduction, and adduction.

Physiologic Therapeutics: A chiropractic term which refers to passive modalities such as heat, cold, electricity, vibration, and massage. This can also refer to exercise.

PI: An abbreviation for *personal injury* and *present illness.*

Pia: A vascular membrane covering the spinal cord. See Pia Mater.

Pial Ligaments: A sheath-like connective tissue which provides additional mechanical support for the anterior spinal artery in the lower thoracic and lumbosacral regions. This system protects the radicular vasculature from repeated but temporary loss of blood flow due to traction with spinal movements. See Pial Sheath at the Anterior Spinal Artery.

Pial Sheath at the Anterior Spinal Artery: A sheath-like connective tissue which provides additional mechanical support for the anterior spinal artery in the lower thoracic and lumbosacral regions. See Pial Ligaments.

Pia Mater: A vascular membrane covering the spinal cord. Its inner layer contains a network of fine elastic fibers, and its outer layer is a loose meshwork of collagen fibers continuous with parts of the arachnoid membrane. In the cervical and thoracic regions, the pia mater thickens to form the dentate ligaments. See Pia.

PICR: The point about which a rigid body rotates at a given instance of time. This terminology is used by therapists who work on muscle imbalances. It is thought that a muscle imbalance can change the point of rotation of a joint or the fulcrum of a system like the scapulae.

Pierce-Stillwagon Technique: A chiropractic technique that is considered "full spine." This technique uses specific x-ray analysis and instrumentation and high-velocity, low-amplitude adjusting procedures developed by Pierce and Stillwagon. This technique is used by just under 20% of U.S. chiropractors.

PIEX: A chiropractic term which refers to an ASIS which is posterior, inferior, and externally rotated. This would be equivalent to an osteopathic outflare combined with an anteriorly rotated ilium.

PIEx: A chiropractic term which refers to an ASIS which is posterior, inferior, and externally rotated. See PIEX.

PIEx Ilium: A chiropractic term which refers to an ASIS which is posterior, inferior, and externally rotated. See PIEX.

Pigeon Breast: A prominent sternum produced by an anterior displacement of that bone. See Pectus Carinatum.

Pigeon-toed: A condition in which the feet point inward. See Intoeing.

PI Ilium: A chiropractic term which refers to an SI joint dysfunction. The ilium is found to be posterior and inferior relative to the sacrum. The most common landmark is the ASIS. It is thought that there is a short leg on the side of the dysfunction and the gluteal fold is lower on the side of the PI ilium. See Sacroiliac Flexion Fixation.

PIIN: A chiropractic term which denotes an ASIS which is posterior, inferior, and internally rotated. This would be equivalent to an osteopathic inflare combined with an anteriorly rotated ilium.

PIIn: A chiropractic term which denotes an ASIS which is posterior, inferior, and internally rotated. See PIIN.

PIIn Ilium: A chiropractic term which denotes an ASIS which is posterior, inferior, and internally rotated. See PIIN.

PI-L: A chiropractic notation for an SI joint dysfunction. The sacrum is found to be posterior and inferior on the left. This is similar to an osteopathic torsion combined with a left side bent sacrum.

Pilates: A rehabilitation technique first described by Joseph Pilates. This technique emphasizes balance and truncal stability with strengthening. Perfection in movement is stressed during exercise, and special equipment is used including sleds, benches, and beams.

Pilates Bench: One of the more common pieces of Pilates equipment. See Universal Reformer.

Pillar: Referring to the articular pillar. See Articular Pillar.

Pillar Fractures: A fracture of the articular pillars of the cervical spine. See Articular Pillar, Articular Pillar Fracture.

Pillar View: An AP x-ray view of the spine with rotation and a 20–30° caudal tilt. The articular pillars of the cervical spine are better visualized since these are not seen on standard x-ray views. The articular pillars are rhomboidal shaped structures that are often the site of occult fracture.

Pincer Rouler: A physical examination technique in which the thumb and index finger are used to grasp the paravertebral skin and "roll" this tissue from inferior to superior. See Skin Rolling.

Pinched Nerve: Dysfunction of a nerve root. See Radiculopathy, Radiculitis.

Pinwheel Examination: A sensory examination in which a Wartenburg wheel or pinwheel is used to determine if there is sensory loss.

PI-R: A chiropractic listing for an SI joint dysfunction in which the sacrum has moved posterior and inferior on the right. This is similar to an osteopathic sacral torsion combined with a right side bent sacrum.

Piriformis Muscle: An external rotator of the hip which originates from the anterior sacrum and inserts on the upper part of the greater trochanter, filling the greater sciatic foramen. It is innervated by S1 or S2. In a small percentage of the population, the peroneal portion of the sciatic nerve passes through the piriformis muscle. See Piriformis Syndrome.

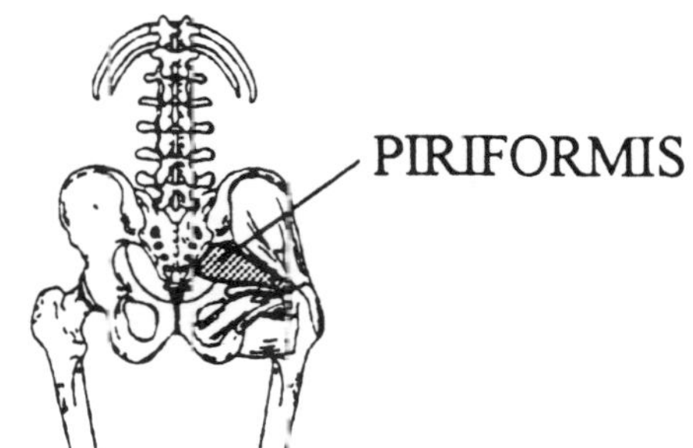

Piriformis Release: The surgical sectioning of the piriformis muscle performed to "free" an entrapped sciatic nerve. See Piriformis Syndrome.

Piriformis Stretch: A stretch for the piriformis muscle that may be helpful in treating SI joint syndrome. The patient starts in a long sit position. One leg is crossed over the other with the foot and ankle on the lateral side of the opposite knee. The elbow is placed on the outside of the bent knee and is pushed across the body to increase the stretch.

Piriformis Syndrome: A constellation of symptoms involving posterior hip pain localized in the piriformis muscle that may include radiating numbness or tingling down one leg. A small segment of the population has a sciatic nerve which pierces through the piriformis muscle, and this may get irritated when inflammation occurs within the muscle. The piriformis is an external rotator and abductor of the hip and can be symptomatic with these movements. Piriformis muscle spasm can be associated with a forward sacral torsion. SI joint pathology should be ruled out. Common treatments include piriformis stretches, strengthening of the internal rotators of the hip, correcting an SI joint syndrome, muscle energy techniques, Jones strain-counterstrain, and injection of anesthetic or corticosteroids into the piriformis muscle belly. Surgical release of the piriformis has been described but is uncommon.

Piroxicam: A nonsteroidal anti-inflammatory drug. See Feldene.

PIS: An abbreviation for *pre-injury status.*

Pixel: The tiny squares that make up a digital image. For instance, an MRI image is made up of many thousands of pixels.

PKB: An abbreviation for *prone knee bend*. The prone knee bend is an adverse neural tension test performed with the patient in the prone position while the knee is flexed passively. A positive response is pain in the quadriceps or tingling in the front of the thigh. Most patients can tolerate the ankle taken to the buttocks. However, caution must be used in interpreting this test because some patients will complain of pain in the anterior thigh due to a tight quadriceps or tight rectus femoris. This test can also be performed with the patient side lying and with a slump test added. See Prone Knee Bend, Femoral Nerve Stretch Test, Femoral Nerve Traction Test, Hyperextension Test, Passive Knee Flexion.

PL: A chiropractic listing which refers to a spinous process, transverse process, or mamillary process which is found to be posterior and left of center. See SP PL.

Platybasia: A congenital defect in the development of the sphenoid or occipital bones. There is a flattening of the skull base, and this can sometimes be confused with basilar impression. On a lateral x-ray of the skull, the angle formed by the plane of the clivus and the plane of the floor of the anterior fossa is unusually flat.

Platyspondyly: An extreme flattening of the lumbar vertebral bodies seen in Morquio's syndrome.

PLD: Percutaneous lumbar discectomy. See Percutaneous Discectomy.

Plexopathy: Dysfunction of usually the brachial or lumbar plexus. This can be due to direct nerve injury, compression, or systemic causes. Since many different nerve roots cross over and reorganize in both of these plexuses, the resulting clinical presentation is numbness or weakness that extends over multiple nerve root and peripheral nerve territories.

PLF: A surgical technique used for spinal fusion. See Posterior Lateral Fusion.

PLI: A chiropractic listing which refers to a spinous process which is found to be posterior, left of midline, and inferior. See SP PLI, Spinous PLI.

PLIF: A surgical technique used for spinal fusion which involves excising the disc through the spinal canal posteriorly and then inserting a bone graft into the intervertebral space. See Posterior Lumbar Interbody Fusion.

PLL: The ligament extending most of the length of the spine affixed to the posterior vertebral bodies. See Posterior Longitudinal Ligament.

PLS: A chiropractic listing which refers to a spinous process which is found to be posterior, left of midline, and superior. See SP PLS, Spinous PLS.

P-L-Sacrum: A chiropractic notation for a sacrum with the left lateral border posterior.

Plumb Line Analysis: A technique used to assess upright posture. A string with a weight is suspended in front of a clear grid, and the patient is asked to stand such that the string would be centered at the spine. Posture is then analyzed versus this line.

Plyometrics: Strength training that involves explosive movements such as jumping or trampoline work. This form of exercise can increase strength quickly in a physiologic manner, but there is a higher incidence of injuries.

pm: An abbreviation for *physical medicine*.

PMD: Percutaneous microdiscectomy. The removal of bulging disc material percutaneously through a large-bore needle inserted into the disc space. See Percutaneous Discectomy.

PN: The removal of disc material. See Percutaneous Nucleoectomy.

Pn: An abbreviation for *pain*.

PNF: A physical exam maneuver first described by Brudzinski as one of the clinical signs of meningitis. This is used today as an adverse neural tension sign for the dura. The patient lies supine with arms at sides and legs together. Passive neck flexion is applied. This test can be combined with others including SLR, DF, and PF. This is also a major test for sensitizing upper limb tension tests. See Passive Neck Flexion.

PNF: Patterns of movement. See Proprioceptive Neuromuscular Facilitation.

Poker Spine: A radiographic term associated with ankylosing spondylitis in which the spine on an AP view looks like a bamboo shaft. See Bamboo Spine.

Polymyalgia Rheumatica: A diffuse aching which is usually described as stiffness in the neck, hip girdle, or shoulder girdle. It is usually associated with an increased ESR and is promptly responsive to steroids.

Posimetric Relaxation: Treatment based on correcting joint position by effecting changes in neuromuscular reflexes. See Muscle Energy Technique.

Positional Diagnosis: An osteopathic or manual physical therapy term for naming a vertebral segment in the direction in which it is found. For instance, an ERSL would denote a vertebral segment which is extended, rotated, and side bent to the left. This would mean that, functionally, that segment has decreased range of motion in flexion, side bending, or rotation to the right. See Positional Dysfunction.

Positional Dysfunction: An osteopathic or manual physical therapy term for naming a dysfunction in the position it is found. For instance, if a segment was noted to be flexed, it would be named a flexion dysfunction. Or, if the ilium was noted to be anterior, it would be named an anterior ilium. This is in contrast to a movement dysfunction which is named for the direction in which motion does not occur. See Positional Diagnosis.

Positional Dyskinesia: A chiropractic term which refers to a vertebral segment that has moved into a position which is not within its normal physiologic range of motion.

Positional Fault: Loss of normal joint biomechanics. See Somatic Dysfunction.

Possibility: A legal term commonly used to imply a likelihood of less than 50%.

Postconcussive Syndrome: A mild brain injury which is self-limited (resolves on its own). Symptoms can include confusion, headaches, short-term memory loss, decreased visual and spatial abilities, and decreased comprehension. This syndrome can occur after a direct blow to the head but has also been noted in patients in rear-end MVAs of low-to-moderate impact.

Posterior: Of or pertaining to the back or dorsum of the body. See Dorsal.

Posterior Arch Fracture: A fracture of the posterior portion of the arch of the atlas. See Posterior Arch of C1 Fracture.

Posterior Arch of C1 Fracture: A fracture of the posterior portion of the arch of the atlas. See Fracture of the Posterior Arch of C1.

Posterior Atlantoaxial Membrane: This ligament courses from the posterior ring of C1 to the posterior ring of C2. See Posterior Atlanto-occipital Membrane.

Posterior Atlanto-occipital Ligament: An elastic ligament which attaches to the posterior ring of C1 and courses up to the posterior portion of the foramen magnum. See Posterior Atlanto-occipital Membrane.

Posterior Atlanto-occipital Membrane: An elastic ligament which attaches to the posterior ring of C1 and courses up to the posterior portion of the foramen magnum. This ligament is analogous to the yellow ligament/ligamentum flavum. It is well suited to allow rotation because a traditional yellow ligament would be too stiff and would not allow significant axial rotation to occur among C0, C1, and C2. The vertebrobasilar artery must pass through this ligament to gain access to the foramen magnum. See Posterior Atlanto-occipital Ligament.

Posterior Body Line: A radiographic sign used to detect abnormal vertebral alignment. See George's Line.

Posterior C1–C2 Subluxation: Posterior subluxation of the arch of C1 on C2. This is a rare complication of rheumatoid arthritis that can also be caused by defects in the arch of C1. It usually involves extensive erosion of the dens.

Posterior Cervical Line: A line drawn on lateral cervical x-rays along the spinolaminar junction. This is the place where the spinous process meets the lamina. A smooth curve is anticipated. If the curve is not continuous at any level, a true subluxation is suspected. Cervical flexion/extension views can be helpful. See Spinolaminar Junction Line.

Posterior Cervical Sympathetic Syndrome: A relatively uncommon syndrome characterized by dizziness, light-headedness, vertigo, vasomotor face disturbances, retro-orbital pain, disturbances of vision, and other symptoms. See Syndrome of Barre-Lieou.

Posterior Elements: Everything posterior to the pedicles. This includes the superior articular facet, the inferior articular facet, the transverse process, and the spinous process. The transverse processes are not usually regarded as part of the posterior elements due to their slightly different embryologic origin. The musculature of the lumbar spine attaches to the posterior elements, and the muscles that act on this area all pull downward. This muscular action is transmitted from the vertebral bodies to the pedicles.

Posterior Fusion: A surgical technique of spinal fusion which involves decorticating (removing the bony cortex) and bone grafting the neural arches and the facet joints. See Spinal Fusion.

Posterior Iliac Shear: An osteopathic or manual physical therapy term that denotes a condition where the ilium is posterior in relation to the sacrum. See Posterior Shear.

Posterior Ilial Rotation: A movement dysfunction of the pelvis in which the ilium moves too much in the direction of posterior rotation on the sacrum. See Posterior Ilium.

Posterior Iliosacral Rotation: A movement dysfunction of the pelvis in which the ilium moves too much in the direction of posterior rotation on the sacrum. See Posterior Ilium.

Posterior Ilium: A movement dysfunction of the pelvis in which the ilium rotates too far in a posterior direction on the sacrum. The ASIS on one side is noted to be superior, posterior, and lateral. The PSIS is noted to be inferior, posterior, and medial. In essence, posterior rotation of the ilium is increased while anterior rotation is decreased. Ilial rotations can be traumatic or compensatory for a number of conditions including a long leg or scoliotic deformities within the lumbar spine. See Backward Innominate, Posterior Innominate, Posterior Ilial Rotation, Posteriorly Rotated Ilium, Backward Ilium, Posterior Iliosacral Rotation.

Posterior Innominate: A movement dysfunction of the pelvis in which the ilium rotates too far posterior on the sacrum. See Posterior Ilium.

Posterior Innominate Shear: An osteopathic or manual physical therapy term that denotes a condition where the ilium is posterior in relation to the sacrum. See Posterior Shear.

Posteriority: A chiropractic term which refers to a part which is posterior (toward the back).

Posterior Joint: Posterior to the pedicles. See Facet Joint, Posterior Elements.

Posterior Lateral Fusion: A surgical technique used for spinal fusion in which the transverse processes are decorticated (outer layer of bone removed to promote bony growth) and bone graft is placed lateral to the posterior elements and between the spinous processes. This is usually combined with a posterior fusion. See Spinal Fusion, PLF.

Posterior Longitudinal Ligament: The ligament extending most of the length of the spine that is affixed to the posterior vertebral bodies. A disc herniation must pass through the posterior longitudinal ligament to qualify as extruded. This ligament is one of the constraints to forward flexion. In some ethnic groups, this ligament can become calcified. See PLL, OPLL.

Posterior Lumbar Interbody Fusion: A surgical technique used for spinal fusion which involves excising the disc through the spinal canal posteriorly and then inserting a bone graft into the intervertebral space. The bone graft is inserted through the same posterior approach. The disadvantages include scar formation around the exiting nerve roots (perineural fibrosis) causing persistent radicular pain. See Spinal Fusion, PLIF.

Posterior Nutation: Moving in a posterior or backward direction. See Counternutation.

Posterior Pubic Ligament: One of the supporting ligaments of the pubic symphysis.

Posterior Ramus Block: The injection of anesthetic and, usually, a steroid to block the medial branch of the sinuvertebral nerve (innervation of the facet joint). See Medial Branch Block.

Posterior Rim Fracture: A fracture of the posterior rim of the acetabulum which usually occurs after a blow to the knee with the knee in flexion and the hip abducted. This is often associated with posterior dislocation of the hip and is most commonly caused by the knee suddenly striking the dashboard in an MVA. This represents approximately one third of all acetabular fractures. See Dashboard Fracture.

Posterior Sacral Nutation: An osteopathic or manual physical therapy term which denotes a sacral base which is superior and posterior. See Bilateral Sacral Extension.

Posterior Sacrum: An osteopathic or manual physical therapy term which refers to a sacrum in which the sacral base has rotated backward and is bent to the side opposite the rotation. This is named for the side on which the rotation occurs. For example, a posterior sacrum left is when the sacrum is rotated left and side bent right. The sacrum moves more freely in rotation left and side bending right and is restricted in rotation right and side bending left. See Unilaterally Extended Sacrum.

Posterior Shear: An osteopathic or manual physical therapy term that denotes a condition where the ilium is posterior in relation to the sacrum. The pubic tubercle on that side is felt to be posterior when the pubic tubercles are palpated bilaterally. See Posterior Innominate Shear, Posterior Iliac Shear.

Posterior Spinal Fusion: A common fusion technique for the lumbar spine. Bone graft is added and packed into the area around the medial facets, lamina, and spinous processes. This technique is often combined with pedicle screw fixation. Nonunion rates (rate of bone not fusing together) are higher in smokers. See Pedicle Screws.

Posterior Subluxation: A chiropractic term which refers to a vertebral body which has moved posteriorly in relation to the one above and below. Due to the orientation of the facets, the segment has a tendency to move inferiorly. Therefore, the spinous process is noted to be more pronounced and inferior.

Posterior Superior Iliac Spine: The posterior superior bump felt on the ilium just lateral to the sacrum. See PSIS.

Posterior Torsion: An osteopathic or manual physical therapy term which describes a sacral torsion found in lumbar extension. See Backward Sacral Torsion.

Posterior Translated Sacrum: An osteopathic term which refers to a sacrum that has moved backward relative to the ilia. See Translated Sacrum—Posterior.

Posteriorly Rotated Ilium: A movement dysfunction of the pelvis in which the ilium has "moved" posterior on the sacrum. See Posterior Ilium.

Posteroanterior View: An x-ray which is taken with the patient's right side against the x-ray cartridge. The x-ray beam passes from posterior to anterior. See PA View, PA.

Posteroinferior Subluxation: A chiropractic term which refers to a vertebra which is "extended" relative to the adjacent vertebrae. See Extension Malposition.

Posterolateral Disc Herniation: The most common type of lumbar HNP (disc herniation). The nucleus pulposus (gel-like center of the disc) ruptures through the annulus (outer covering of the disc) posterolaterally.

In the lumbar spine, this portion of the disc is considered to be biomechanically weaker and more prone to disc herniation.

Posterosuperior Subluxation: A chiropractic term which refers to a segment which is noted to be statically "flexed" relative to the adjacent vertebrae. See Flexion Malposition.

Postfacilitation Stretch: Treatment based on correcting joint position by effecting changes in neuromuscular reflexes. See Muscle Energy Technique.

Postisometric Relaxation: Treatment based on correcting joint position by effecting changes in neuromuscular reflexes. See Muscle Energy Technique.

Postlaminectomy Instability: Segmental instability which occurs after a laminectomy due to removal of the medial portion of the facet joints. This has been postulated as one cause of worsened back pain after laminectomy. See Failed Back Syndrome, Instability—Postlaminectomy.

Postlaminectomy Syndrome: ICD-9 diagnosis for chronic and disabling pain thought secondary to a laminectomy or laminectomy and discectomy done for HNP or a disc bulge. See Failed Back Syndrome.

Postoperative Spondylolisthesis: The development or progression of spondylolisthesis after a surgical decompression. This occurs most commonly at L4–L5 after a decompressive procedure for spinal stenosis. See Spondylolisthesis.

Postsurgical Spondylolisthesis: A stress fracture of the pars interarticularis one level above or below a spinal fusion. This happens due to shunting of biomechanical forces to the pars above and/or below the fused segment. This problem occurs more commonly with an anterior interbody fusion than a posterior lateral fusion. This also occurs when too wide a laminectomy is performed causing weakness in the pars interarticularis. This term is often loosely interchanged with postoperative spondylolisthesis. See Iatrogenic Spondylolisthesis, Spondylolisthesis Acquisita.

Posttraumatic Dystrophy: A clinical syndrome characterized by the presence of pain out of proportion to the severity of the injury. See Reflex Sympathetic Dystrophy.

Posttraumatic Stress Disorder: An abnormal amount of psychological stress related to some traumatic event. This commonly occurs after MVAs. In this particular instance, the patient experiences anxiety with driving and especially in situations which might reproduce another MVA. Psychological intervention is usually not necessary because this is often self-limited. However, psychological intervention may be helpful if the syndrome does not subside on its own. The use of short-term benzodiazepines or nonbenzodiazepine antianxiety drugs may also be helpful. See PTSD.

Postural Alignment: The relationship of the spine to the rest of the body. This is the position of the spine and its ability to counteract the effects of gravity. See Posture.

Postural Balance: The idea that the normal posture of the body allows the spinal column to be balanced relative to gravity. This is supported by the concept that very little active muscle contraction is needed for normal standing. When this balance is thrown off by injury, overwork of the musculature, or joint misalignment, overloading of the supporting structures can develop.

Postural Decompensation: Posture which has given in to the effects of gravity. The usual presentation is a patient with a forward head, rounded shoulders, and a flattened lumbar lordosis (flat back). The cause is usually overload of the supporting musculature, fascial tightness that maintains this abnormal position, and, sometimes, joint restriction.

Postural Fault: A posture without structural limitations that deviates from normal alignment.

Postural Strain: A syndrome which occurs in patients with significant degenerative disc disease and excess biomechanical creep. The patient usually reports that one position held for any length of time will increase pain. This is especially noted in flexion postures. There may be a normal or almost normal low back examination. Range of motion may be essentially normal. Common treatments include McKenzie extension; manual medicine to correct specific segmental lesions; use of ergonomic devices while seated such as a lumbar roll or special chair; training in body mechanics; strength work to increase proper posture; and lumbar stabilization. See McKenzie Exercises, Postural Syndrome.

Postural Syndrome: A McKenzie physical therapy term in which the pain increases after being in one position for any significant length of time. The patient usually reports that activity decreases pain. It is thought that this syndrome occurs due to disc degeneration which causes more biomechanical "creep" (usually into flexion). See Degenerative Disc Disease, McKenzie Exercises.

Posture: The position of the body used to function. For instance, normal standing posture is used to combat gravity. See Postural Alignment.

Posture Analysis: A systematic approach to evaluating posture or the biomechanical relationships of one body part to another.

Posture Dysfunction: Shortening of the soft tissues and muscles in at attempt to adapt once muscle weakness has occurred. These adaptions can cause an inefficient posture and pain.

Posture Grid: A series of perpendicular and horizontal lines which are used as a reference when determing upright posture. The patient stands in front of or behind a structure with lines or wires used to represent postural ideals. For instance, there are usually horizontal lines that are leveled with normal shoulders and iliac crests.

POSTURE GRID

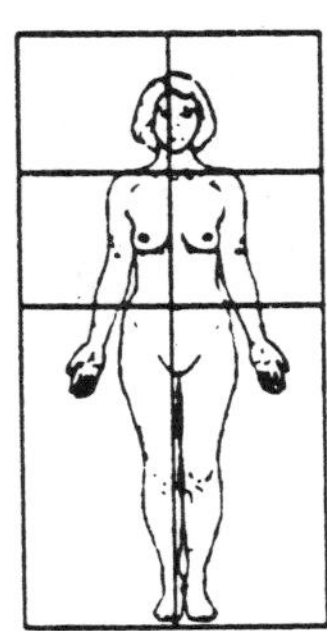

Pott's Disease: A tuberculosis infection involving the spine which can cause collapse of the vertebral bodies. This can be associated with a structural scoliosis. See Tuberculous Spondylitis.

Poupart's Ligament: An older name for the inguinal ligament.

Power Spectrum Analysis: A biofeedback term which refers to the computerized analysis of a wide range of muscle recruitment frequencies. It is thought that in sustained muscle contraction or fatigue, there is a shift to lower recruitment frequencies.

PPD: An abbreviation for *permanent partial disability.*

PPO: Preferred Provider Organization.

PPP: Points along the periosteal attachments of muscle to bone (entheses) which are noted to be tender with specific muscle overload or joint dysfunction. See Periosteal Pain Points.

PR: A chiropractic abbreviation which refers to a spinous process which is found to be posterior and right of center. See SP PR, Spinous PR.

PRAE: An abbreviation for *patient responding as expected.*

PRE: A technique for strength training that has been called heavy resistance exercise and progressive resistance exercise. See DeLorme Technique, Progressive Resistance Exercise.

Predental Interspace: The distance between the posterior margin of the anterior atlas and the anterior surface of the odontoid. See Atlanto-dental Interspace.

Predental Space: The distance between the posterior margin of the anterior atlas and the anterior surface of the odontoid. See ADI.

Prednisone: A synthetic glucocorticoid (steroid) which is a potent anti-inflammatory medication. See Steroid for drug interactions and precautions. With respect to the spine, prednisone and other synthetic glucocorticoids are often used for their anti-inflammatory effects in such conditions as radiculopathy and ankylosing spondylitis. See Deltasone.

preg: An abbreviation for *pregnant*.

Prespondylolisthesis: A defect in the pars interarticularis. See Spondylolysis.

Press-up: A McKenzie physical therapy exercise. The patient is in a prone position and presses up onto the elbows or wrists. The idea is that a disc bulge will be reduced in this position allowing pressure to be taken off the nerve root and thus centralization of the patient's pain. See McKenzie Exercises, Prone Press-up.

Pressure Algometry: The use of a pressure-reading device to estimate pain threshold from applied pressures. This is used most commonly to quantify myofascial trigger points.

Preventative: A medication used to treat headache which is taken before the pain starts to prevent the headache from starting. Examples would be calcium channel blockers or beta blockers.

Prevertebral: The area in front of the vertebral column.

Prevertebral Fascia: A fascial plane which lies anterior to the vertebral column.

Prevertebral Soft Tissues: The musculature, fascia, and neurovascular structures which occur anterior to the vertebral column in the cervical spine. This would include the esophagus. See Prevertebral Space, Retropharyngeal Interspace.

Prevertebral Space: The musculature, fascia, and neurovascular structures which occur anterior to the vertebral column in the cervical spine. See Prevertebral Soft Tissues.

PRI: A chiropractic listing which refers to a spinous process which is found to be posterior, right of midline, and inferior. See SP PRI, Spinous PRI.

Primary Basilar Impression: A basilar impression which is congenital in origin. This has been associated with numerous vertebral defects such as occipitalization of the atlas, spina bifida occulta of the atlas, Klippel-Feil syndrome, Chiari malformation, and various odontoid anomalies. See Basilar Impression.

Primary Curve: A scoliotic curve which is the earliest to occur. It is usually the longest curve in the scoliosis.

Primary Osteosarcoma: A malignant tumor of bone. Approximately 2% of all primary osteogenic sarcomas involve the spine. The five-year survival rate is very poor, and survival is perhaps more appropriately measured in months from the time of diagnosis. Radiographically, there are both lytic and sclerotic lesions with cortical destruction and soft tissue calcification. Advanced cases show collapse of these lesions and CT scan can show intraspinal and paraspinal soft tissue masses more clearly. In the spine, treatment usually consists of limited tumor excision and radiotherapy.

prn: An abbreviation for *as needed* (from the Latin *pro re nata*).

Probability: A legal term used to imply a likelihood of greater than 50%.

Procardia: A calcium channel blocker used primarily for angina but is also used for patients with migraine headaches and reflex sympathetic dystrophy. See Procardia XL, Adalat, Adalat CC.

Procardia XL: A calcium channel blocker used for angina. See Procardia, Adalat, Adalat CC.

Progressive Resistance Exercise: A technique for strength training that has been called heavy resistance exercise and progressive resistance exercise. See DeLorme Technique, PRE.

Prolapsed Disc: When the nucleus pulposus ruptures through most of the fibers of the annulus and is contained only by a few of the outermost fibers. The posterior longitudinal ligament is intact. This is synonymous with a large disc bulge. See Disc Protrusion, Disc Prolapse.

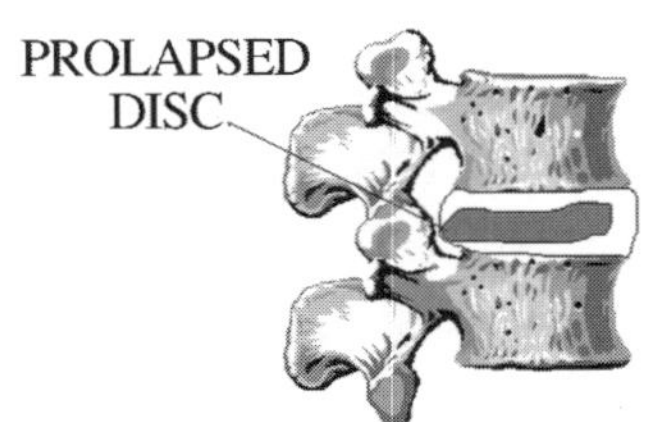

THE INNER GEL-LIKE MATERIAL (NUCLEUS PULPOSUS) HAS PUSHED THROUGH MOST OF THE ANNULUS (THE TOUGH FIBROUS TISSUE THAT HOLDS THE GEL INSIDE THE DISC). HOWEVER, THE GEL HAS NOT RUPTURED THROUGH THE ANNULUS.

Prolapse of the Intervertebral Disc: When the nucleus pulposus ruptures through most of the fibers of the annulus and is contained only by a few of the outermost fibers. See Prolapsed Disc.

Prolotherapy: The injection of specific solutions designed to cause scarring and the proliferation of new tissue (collagen) around joints. This has been used when joints are "hypermobile" to stabilize these areas. See P2G, Phenol, Sclerosant Injection.

PROM: In the spine, passive range of motion is measured in flexion, extension, side bending, or rotation. See Passive Range of Motion.

Promoatron: A brand name for an isometric dynamometer. This is a lift station which measures strength isometrically in several different lift positions including floor lifts, arm lifts, and above-shoulder lifts.

Pronated Foot: A foot that is turned in (sole of the foot points to the outside). There is eversion of the ankle. Excessive pronation of the foot can cause a functional short leg or functional leg length discrepancy. This can aggravate an SI joint dysfunction or spine pain. See Foot—Pronated.

Prone: The face-down position.

Prone Hip Extension: A lumbar stabilization exercise in which the patient lies prone on the stomach with knees straight and arms overhead (usually with a pillow under the stomach). The patient tightens the stomach and squeezes the buttocks as one leg is raised from the floor. This is repeated with the opposite leg. The spine must be stabilized during these maneuvers. This exercise can also be used to strengthen the gluteals in patients with an SI joint dysfunction. See Hip Extension—Prone.

Prone Knee Bend: An adverse neural tension test performed with the patient in the prone position while the knee is flexed passively. See PKB.

Prone Knee Flexion Test: The patient is in the prone position and the bilateral knees are flexed bringing the heels toward the buttocks. This causes some hyperextension within the lumbar spine and apparently intensifies an intervertebral disc protrusion into the spinal canal. A positive test is aggravation of the symptoms of radiculopathy. The patient can be held in that position for 45–60 seconds.

Prone on Elbows: A McKenzie physical therapy exercise in which the patient starts prone and props up on the elbows. See McKenzie Exercises.

Prone Opposite Arm and Leg Lift: A lumbar stabilization exercise in which the patient is in a prone position with knees extended and arms overhead (usually with a pillow under the stomach). The patient is asked to tighten the stomach and squeeze the buttocks as they simultaneously raise a straight leg and opposite arm from the floor. This is repeated on the opposite side. Spinal stability must be maintained during this exercise.

Prone Press-up: A McKenzie physical therapy exercise in which the patient presses up on the elbows while in the prone position. Sphinx Position: A manual physical therapy or osteopathic physical exam maneuver in which the patient is in the prone position and asked to perform a prone press-up such that the chin rests in the hands with the patient propped up on his or her elbows. The spine is then checked for rotational deformities level by level. This is a common position for testing the spinal segments for their position in extension. See Press-up.

Prone Reduction: A technique which attempts to "reduce" an acute disc injury. A patient that presents in a flexed position, is gradually placed in a prone position usually using a "high-low table." The prone position is then "reduced" by adding in further lumbar extension.

Pronex: An inflatable form of cervical traction. A plastic collar is placed around the patient's neck and secured with Velcro. The collar is then pumped up like a blood pressure cuff to increase traction.

Pron. quad.: An abbreviation for *pronator quadratus.*

Pron. ter.: An abbreviation for *pronator teres.*

Propoxyphene: A mild narcotic analgesic (pain reliever) which is used in the brand name drug Darvocet. Propoxyphene has approximately two-thirds the potency of codeine. There is a synergistic effect with aspirin and caffeine in that propoxyphene in combination with these drugs provides greater pain relief than what would be expected additively. See Darvocet-N 100.

Propranolol: A beta blocker drug normally used for hypertension but is also used for the prevention of migraine headache. See Inderal.

Proprioceptive Neuromuscular Facilitation: Patterns of movement involving large muscle groups and not individual muscles. These are functional patterns that are used in everyday activities. Many of the components of a lumbar stabilization program are borrowed from PNF. See PNF.

Prostrate Leg Raising Test: A physical exam maneuver. See Crossed Straight-Leg Raising Test.

Proteoglycan: The major chemical component of the nucleus pulposus. This is composed of chondroitin-6-sulfate, chondroitin-4-sulfate, and keratin sulfate. Some proteoglycans within the nucleus pulposus form large macromolecular aggregates with hyaluronic acid. These aggregating proteoglycans are in equilibrium between aggregating and nonaggregating states. As the normal intervertebral disc ages, the ability of the proteoglycans and the nucleus pulposus to hold onto water decreases thus leading to normal dehydration and degenerated discs. Also, as the disc ages, proteoglycan degradation takes over proteoglycan formation. This also likely increases "creep behavior" in the aging intervertebral disc.

Proton Density Film: An MRI sequence. See Spin Density Film.

Proton Density Image: An MRI imaging technique which is obtained in the early part of a T2 weighted sequence. This imaging sequence shows anatomic detail of the lumbar spine well without the noise problems usually seen with a T2 weighted image. This is a particularly good image sequence for showing the outermost annulus of the intervertebral disc. See Proton Spin Image.

Proton Spin Film: An MRI sequence. See Spin Density Film.

Proton Spin Image: An MRI imaging technique. See Proton Density Image.

Protruded Disc: When the nucleus of the disc ruptures through the inner annular fibers but does not rupture through a majority of those fibers. This is synonymous with a small disc bulge. See Disc Protrusion, Disc Bulge, Contained Herniation.

Provocative Maneuver: A physical exam test which reproduces pain through movement, mobilization, pressure over a structure, or other means. For instance, cervical compression would be a provocative maneuver for a cervical radiculopathy.

Prozac: An antidepressant which is chemically unrelated to tricyclic, tetracyclic, or other available antidepressant agents. It is in the selective serotonin reuptake inhibitor class and blocks the uptake of serotonin into human platelets, thus increasing serotonin levels in the central nervous system. It is used primarily in clinical depression and obsessive compulsive disorder. It is contraindicated for use in patients on MAO inhibitors. It is also contraindicated for use in patients with significant heart disease and may alter control of blood sugars in diabetics. When administered with other antidepressants, there has been a greater than twofold increase in plasma levels of the other antidepressant. It has drug interactions with lithium, diazepam, phenytoin, and drugs tightly bound to plasma proteins. The recommended initial dose is 20 mg administered in the morning. A dose increase may be considered after several weeks if no clinical improvement is seen. The maximum dose should not exceed 80 mg a day. The full antidepressant effect may be delayed until four weeks of treatment or longer. A lower or less frequent dose should be used in patients with renal or hepatic impairment. A lower or less frequent dose should also be used in the elderly or with patients on multiple medications. See Fluoxetine.

PRS: A chiropractic listing which refers to a spinous process which is found to be posterior, right of midline, and superior. See SP PRS, Spinous PRS.

P-R-Sacrum: A chiropractic notation for a sacrum with the right lateral border posterior.

Pseudarthrosis: In the spine, pseudarthrosis refers to a failure to obtain a solid fusion after surgically attempting fusion. There may be excessive gross motion within the affected vertebral segment, but commonly the pseudarthrosis is "stiff," with micro-motion that cannot be demonstrated on flexion/extension radiographs.

Pseudobasilar Invagination: Progressive destruction and remodeling of the bony architecture of the OA joint which allows a vertical translocation of the dens. This can be a fatal complication of rheumatoid arthritis. See Chamberlain's Line, Basilar Invagination, Rheumatoid Arthritis.

Pseudogout: An arthritic condition. See Calcium Pyrophosphate Deposition Disease.

Pseudohypertrophy of the Ligamentum Flavum: A stiffening of the ligamentum flavum which causes it to fold or bend into the spinal canal. See Ligamentum Flavum.

Pseudo-Intermittent Claudication: Abnormal pressure on the bottom-most portion of the spinal cord. See Cauda Equina Syndrome.

Pseudoradicular Pain: Pain derived from the mesodermal tissues. See Mesodermal Pain, Sclerotomal Pain.

Pseudospondylolisthesis: A spondylolisthesis caused by severe degeneration of the facet joints. See Type III Spondylolisthesis.

PSIS : The posterior superior bump felt on the ilium just lateral to the sacrum. This is a helpful landmark in SI joint diagnosis. This protuberance is easily palpated on the posterior ilium, just supeior and lateral to the SI joint. See Posterior Superior Iliac Spine.

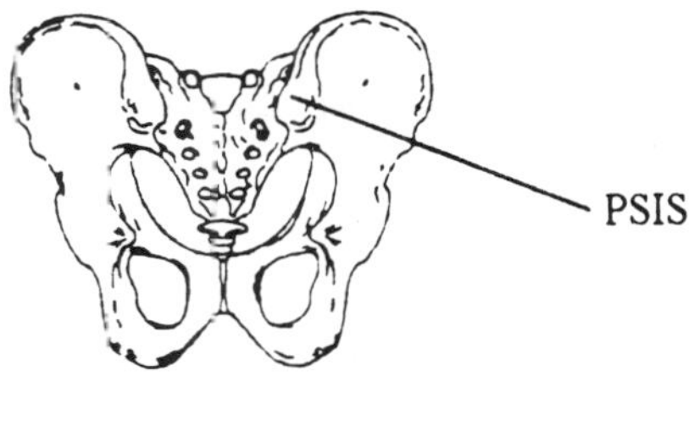

Psoas Abscess: A retroperitoneal mass which is a well-localized infection surrounded by fibrous tissue. This can be found in association with non-Hodgkin's lymphoma.

Psoriatic Arthritis: A seronegative spondyloarthropathy which occurs in about 60% of patients with psoriasis. Skin changes are generally seen first and can precede the symptoms of arthritis by as much as 20 years. Nail involvement predicts joint disease (80%). Spine involvement develops in about 20% of patients and involves the bilateral SI joints, lumbar spine, and upper cervical spine. Peripherally, this arthritis is most severe in the fingers and toes and is more intermittent and less disabling than RA. RF is negative. In a minority of patients, hands and feet can develop severe deformity (arthritis deformans). Radiographic signs include nonmarginal syndesmophytes, atlantoaxial subluxation, SI joint erosions, a hazy SI joint line, and SI sclerosis. See Psoriatic Arthropathy.

Psoriatic Arthropathy: A seronegative spondyloarthropathy. See Psoriatic Arthritis.

Psychologic Factors Affecting Physical Recovery: A statement often made to describe a patient with symptom magnification.

Psychometrics: A psychological testing instrument. See MMPI.

PT: Physical therapist.

PTA: Physical therapy aide.

PTD: An abbreviation for *permanent total disability*.

PTPW: An abbreviation for *patient tolerated procedure well.*

PTR: The reflex contraction of the quadriceps muscle with tapping of the patellar tendon. See Patellar Tendon Reflex.

PTSD: Posttraumatic stress disorder.

Pube: Slang for *pubic symphysis*.

Pubic Diastasis: A shearing separation of the pubic symphysis. If the separation exceeds 3 cm, it may be associated with an injury to the SI joint.

Pubic Spine: A bony protuberance. See Pubic Tubercle.

Pubic Symphysis: The place in the anterior pelvis where the two halves of the pelvis articulate. This area contains a disc similar in composition to the intervertebral disc. This is one axis of rotation for pelvic movement. The pubic symphysis can be tender in patients with SI joint pain or dysfunction. Osteopathic physicians and physical therapists often check to see if the pubic tubercles are level, inferior or superior, and anterior or posterior. See Symphysis Pubis.

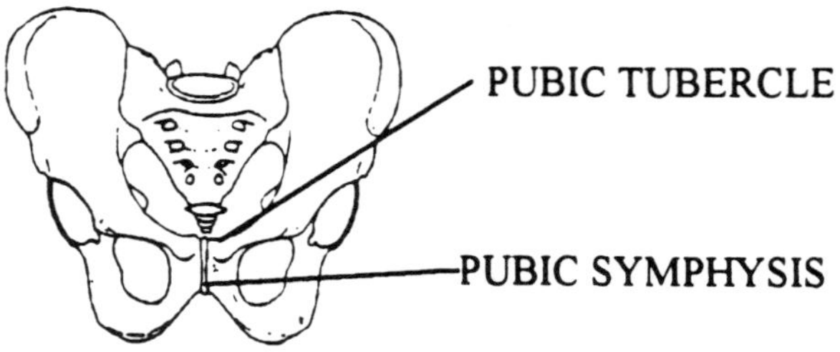

PUBIC TUBERCLE

PUBIC SYMPHYSIS

Pubic Tubercle: A bony protuberance on the upper border of the body of the pubic bone which is used as a landmark in manual medicine to determine if the "pubes" are uneven. The inguinal ligament is attached to this tubercle.

Pubis: One of three bones which are fused to form the innominate bone. The pubic bones come together anteriorly to form the pubic symphysis.

Pumice: One of the sclerosing agents used in prolotherapy. This is thought to be one of the more potent injectable substances for this purpose.

Pump Handle Restriction: An abnormality in the normal movement of the upper rib cage. An inhalation restriction is defined as the inability of the rib to elevate fully with inhalation. An exhalation restriction is considered to be the inability of the rib to depress fully with exhalation. See Inhalation Restriction, Exhalation Rib, Inhalation Rib, Pump Handle Rib Motion.

Pump Handle Rib Motion: The movement of the upper rib cage during respiration. With inhalation, the anterior aspect of the rib elevates, and with exhalation the anterior aspect of the rib depresses. See Pump Handle Restriction.

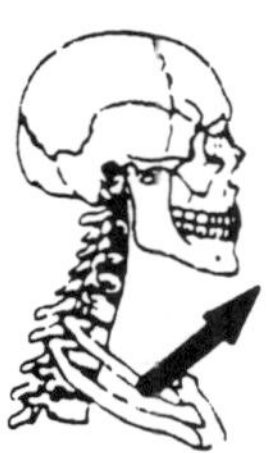

PUMP HANDLE RIB MOTION

Purdue Pegboard: An upper extremity dexterity test which measures gross movement and finger dexterity. This is sometimes performed during an upper extremity functional capacity evaluation.

Push/Pull Dynamometer: A testing device used to measure the force exerted with pushing or pulling. This can be measured either isometrically or dynamically. See Chatillion Gauge.

Px: An abbreviation for *plan.*

Pyramidal Tract: Nerve fibers. See Corticospinal Tract.

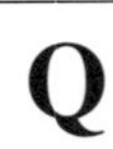

q4 hours: An abbreviation for *every four hours.*

q6 hours: An abbreviation for *every six hours.*

q8 hours: An abbreviation for *every eight hours.*

q12 hours: An abbreviation for *every twelve hours.*

QCT: A method for quantifying osteoporosis. See Quantitative Computerized Tomography.

q.d.: An abbreviation for *once a day.*

q.i.d.: An abbreviation for *four times a day.*

q.o.d.: An abbreviation for *every other day.*

Quadrant Test: A physical exam maneuver used to detect facet pain. The patient is asked to extend and side bend or extend and rotate to one side. This puts maximal pressure on the facet joint on that side. When overpressure is applied in this position, there is narrowing of the intervertebral foramen. Therefore, this can also be considered a test for foraminal stenosis.

Quadruped: Implies "on all fours." For instance, a dog is quadruped. This position is used in the transition from prone activities in a lumbar stabilization program. The patient performs exercises "on all fours" while keeping the spine stable. The next transition after quadruped would be to biped, or standing, activities.

Quadruped Arm Extension: A lumbar stabilization exercise in which the patient starts in a quadruped position and is asked to tighten the stomach and squeeze the buttocks as the straight arm is raised parallel to the floor. The pelvis is kept parallel to the floor and stabilized. This is repeated on the opposite side. See Arm Extension—Quadruped.

Quadruped Leg Extension: A lumbar stabilization exercise. The patient starts in the quadruped position and is asked to tighten the stomach and squeeze the buttocks as one straight leg is raised parallel to the floor. The pelvis is kept stabilized. This is then repeated on the opposite side. This exercise can also be an effective way to strengthen the gluteals. See Leg Extension—Quadruped.

Quadruped Opposite Arm and Leg Extension: A lumbar stabilization exercise. The patient starts in a quadruped position and is asked to tighten the stomach and squeeze the buttocks while simultaneously raising a straight leg and the opposite straight arm. Pelvic stability is maintained. This exercise is then repeated on the opposite side. See All Fours Opposite Arm and Leg Extension.

Quantitative Computerized Tomography: A method for quantifying osteoporosis which provides an accurate measure of the trabecular bone of a vertebral body as well as a measurement of true density. This method can provide a three-dimensional localization of density throughout the vertebral body. See QCT.

R

R: An abbreviation used in the PGF listing system which denotes a spinous process which is off to the right when the patient is in the prone position.

R: An abbreviation for *right.*

R+: A notation made during discography indicating that the patient reported a 2 or more decrease in usual pain on a visual analog pain scale (1–10) with instillation of anesthetic. See Discogram.

R+/− : A notation made during discography which describes that the patient had only a vague, uncertain response to instillation of anesthetic (no significant pain relief of the usual symptom complex) after the provocative portion of the test. See Discogram.

R++: A notation made during discography which describes that the patient reported complete ablation of usual symptoms with instillation of anesthetic. See Discogram.

R0: A notation made during discography which describes that the patient had no response to the instillation of anesthetic following the provocative portion of the test. See Discogram.

R1 Response: A notation made during a provocative procedure, such as a discogram. Local anesthetic is injected into the disc. If this does not significantly decrease the patient's familiar pain response, it is known as an R1 response. It is then assumed that the disc is not the pain generator. See R2 Response, P1 Response, P2 Response.

R2 Response: A notation made during a provocative procedure such as a discogram. Local anesthetic is injected into the patient's disc. If this significantly decreases the familiar pain response, this is known as an R2 response. It is then assumed that the disc is the pain generator. See R1 Response, P1 Response, P2 Response, Objective Discography.

RA: Rheumatoid arthritis.

Rachiometer: A device for measuring spinal curvature.

Rachischisis: A congenital defect of the spinal column in which the neural arch fails to fuse, resulting in a hole in the back of the vertebra that leaves the spinal cord and/or nerves exposed. See Spina Bifida.

rad: An abbreviation for *radiating*.

Radial Reflex: A physical exam maneuver that tests the integrity of the C6 nerve root. See Brachioradialis Reflex.

Radial Tear of the Annulus: A fissure that extends perpendicular to the fibers of the annulus. If the tear is complete, a herniated disc can ensue. This can be an important sign of early disc degeneration or acute disc trauma. See Annular Rent, Annular Tear, Internal Disc Disruption.

Radiate Ligament: The ligament which attaches the head of the rib to the vertebra and the intervertebral disc. The fibers of this ligament "radiate" out from the center of the attachment.

Radiculalgia: Pain due to disease or dysfunction of the spinal nerve roots. See Radiculitis, Radiculopathy.

Radicular: Of or pertaining to a root. With respect to the spine, this refers to a nerve root.

Radicular Canal: A portion of the vertebral canal recognized by surgeons because of its relationship to the nerve root. This is a curved channel that runs around the medial portion of each pedicle and follows a course (with the nerve root) into the intervertebral foramina. There are three segments: the upper-most or retrodiscal, the parapedicular segment, and the upper part of the intervertebral foramen. The nerve root can be compromised by bony hypertrophy of one of the structures that forms the boundaries of the canal. See Lateral Recess.

Radicular Pain: Pain caused by a radiculopathy or radiculitis. This pain refers in a dermatomal distribution that corresponds to a specific nerve root. See Dermatome, Nerve Root.

Radicular Symptoms: Symptoms such as pain radiating down an extremity that follows a dermatomal pattern. For instance, in a patient with an L5 radiculopathy, radicular symptoms would be numbness or tingling sensations in the big toe on the side of the lesion. See Radiculopathy.

Radiculitis: Inflammation of a nerve root which causes irritation. The symptoms can include numbness, tingling, pain, or weakness in the distribution of that root. This is usually considered a neuropraxic lesion that does not involve true axonal loss. This is considered to be less severe than radiculopathy. See Radiculopathy, Pinched Nerve.

Radiculoneuritis: Dysfunction of a nerve root. See Radiculopathy, Radiculitis.

Radiculoneuropathy: Dysfunction of a nerve root. See Radiculopathy.

Radiculopathy: Dysfunction of a nerve root that can cause (1) radiating pain, numbness, or tingling in a specific pattern corresponding to that nerve root or (2) muscle weakness in the muscles supplied by that nerve root. This can be caused by a herniated disc causing inflammation or pressure on the nerve, bony pressure through spondylosis (bone spurs), enlarged facet joints, or other causes. This is usually treated nonoperatively with injection of epidural steroids or selective nerve root block combined with a rehabilitation program. If caused by bony impingement, radiculopathy may be less responsive to conservative therapy. Surgical treatment includes a variety of treatments along a spectrum of invasiveness. Least invasive would be a microdiscectomy, most invasive would be a decompressive laminectomy with fusion. See Acute Sciatica, Cervical Radiculopathy, Lumbosacral Neuropathy and Radiculopathy, Nerve Root and Plexus Disorders, Nerve Root Compression, Nerve Root Compromise, Radiculitis, Pinched Nerve, Radicular Symptoms, Root Pain, Root Signs.

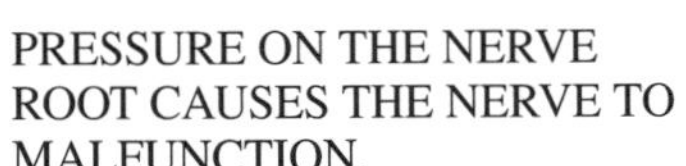

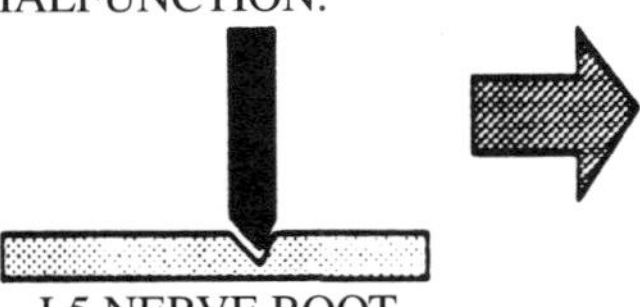

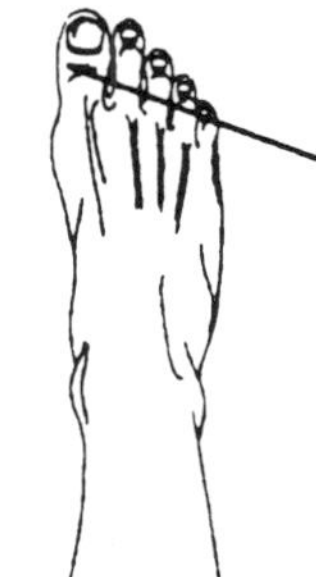

Radiculopathy—Cervical: Dysfunction of a cervical nerve root. See Cervical Radiculopathy, Radiculopathy.

Radiographic Instability: Abnormal translation in flexion or extension due to severe degenerative disc disease due to increased creep or ligamentous trauma. This concept is often used by surgeons to define clinical instability and to determine which candidates would be best for lumbar fusion.

Radiolucency: A darker appearing image on standard x-ray that represents an area of decreased density. For instance, osteoporotic bones (those with less calcium) are often said to be radiolucent. See Osteoporosis.

Radionuclide Bone Scanning: See Bone Scan.

RA Factor: See Rheumatoid Factor.

Rami Communicantes: Postganglionic fibers that emerge from the sympathetic ganglia and connect to corresponding spinal nerves or to other fibers in the sympathetic chain. See Gray Rami Communicantes.

Ramrod Spine: A marked restriction of movement of the spine in all directions.

RAO: An x-ray term. See Right Anterior Oblique.

Rating of Perceived Capacity: A quantification of the patient's perception of his ability to perform physical tasks as measured by a West tool sort. The patient is shown various pictures of tools and told to sort them into categories based on his/her ability to use the tool. This rating is then compared with standardized percentiles for sex and age. See RPC.

Ratio Method: A measurement of the size of the cervical spinal canal. See Canal–Body Ratio.

Razorback Deformity: A severe, unilateral rib hump deformity seen in severe scoliosis. This rib deformity becomes more prominent in forward flexion of the spine.

RC: An abbreviation for *rotator cuff.*

Reactivation: Getting an inactive patient more physically active.

Reactive Arthropathy: An aseptic arthritis that develops during or after an infection in another location. There are many extra-articular features including conjunctivitis, iritis, urethritis, and uveitis.

Reciprocal Inhibition: The inhibition (decrease in muscle tone) of the agonist muscles by firing the antagonist muscles.

Reclination: Another word for extension at the atlanto-occipital joint.

Recoil Adjustment: A chiropractic manipulative technique which is a variation of the elbow extension method. This is accomplished by immediately jerking the hands away from the contact after the thrust has been given. See Toggle Recoil.

Reconditioning: A supervised exercise program designed to promote physical conditioning through strength, flexibility, and increasing aerobic capacity.

Recruitment: The extent to which a muscle can be activated. In normal movement, only a small portion of the many available motor units of a muscle are used. Increasing the recruitment of a muscle increases the number of motor units within the muscle that are activated during a contraction. See Recruitment Pattern.

Recruitment Pattern: The extent to which a muscle can be activated. See Recruitment.

Recumbent Exercise Bicycle: An exercise bike in which the patient is in a seated position with back support. Instead of riding on top of the peddling mechanism, the patient sits with the lower extremities out in front and extended. This can be helpful in the rehabilitation of low back patients since this provides back support while exercising. It also can be helpful in rehabilitating patients with SI joint dysfunctions because the pelvis is stabilized during this exercise.

Recurrent Disc Herniation: A disc extrusion (herniation) which occurs more than once. See Recurrent HNP.

Recurrent Herniated Disc: A disc extrusion (herniation) which occurs more than once. See Recurrent HNP.

Recurrent HNP: A disc extrusion (herniation) which occurs more than once. The natural course of HNP is that the body naturally resorbs the disc material. However, it has been noted for decades that reherniations are common. See Recurrent Herniated Disc, Recurrent Disc Herniation, Recurrent Ruptured Disc, HNP.

Recurrent Meningeal Nerve: The sinuvertebral nerve that emerges from the dorsal root just distal to the dorsal root ganglion. See Sinuvertebral Nerve.

Recurrent Ruptured Disc: A disc extrusion (herniation) which occurs more than once. See Recurrent HNP.

ref: An abbreviation for *refer* or *referred.*

Referred Autonomic Phenomenon: Autonomic changes which are referred to another area of the body by a trigger point. This can include vasoconstriction, coldness, sweating, ptosis, or a pilomotor response. These changes usually occur in the same area of referred pain associated with that trigger point.

Referred Pain: Pain that originates in one tissue but is perceived in another part of the body. The referred pain phenomenon is thought to occur because different areas of the body share the same portions of the brain. When pain sensation arrives from one area, the body cannot differentiate between that area and other areas of the body that are perceived at that point in the cortex. There are many different types of referred pain. The classic example is a dermatome. It is also well documented that mesodermal pain exists. This is a referred pain phenomenon from the soft tissues. However, these maps of referred pain tend to be less reliable than dermatomal maps.

Reflex Arc: A term which refers to the simplest reflex which loops through the spinal cord. A sensory impulse is detected; this travels through an afferent neuron through the spinal cord, synapses with an efferent neuron, and then a motor response is provided.

Reflex Dystrophy: A clinical syndrome characterized by the presence of pain out of proportion to the severity of the injury. See Reflex Sympathetic Dystrophy.

Reflex Muscle Guarding: Spasm seen in the musculature which occurs in response to a painful stimulus. In the spine, that stimulus can be a facet joint, a herniated disc, or something from another part of the body (i.e., hip), or it can occur with abnormal positions of the vertebral segments. See Reflex Muscle Spasm.

Reflex Muscle Spasm: Spasm seen in the musculature that occurs in response to a painful stimulus. See Reflex Muscle Guarding.

Reflexology: A traditional Chinese therapy which connects various regions in the sole of the foot with different body parts. The theory is that life energy, or *chi,* is channeled through these zones, and stimulating any zone in the foot by applying pressure with the fingers affects that zone in the body. These areas are stimulated to bring about a state of balance.

Reflex Sympathetic Dystrophy: A clinical syndrome characterized by the presence of pain out of proportion to the severity of the injury. Burning, skin atrophy, and decreased range of motion are common. The etiology is usually trauma, including surgery. It is thought that there is an "autonomic overdrive" which causes burning pain and hypersensitivity. Abnormal pilomotor response (sweating) is also common. In the late stages, skin atrophy, muscle atrophy, and decreased joint range of motion may ensue. On x-ray, diffuse osteoporosis and characteristic areas of "spotty rarification" can be seen in late-stage RSD. Bone scan and stress thermography are reported to be sensitive indicators. See RSD, Sympathetic Dystrophy, Reflex Dystrophy, Sudeck's Atrophy, Causalgia, Posttraumatic Dystrophy, Shoulder-Hand Syndrome, Posttraumatic Dystrophy.

Reformatted CT: A CT scan which produces a computer-generated image in a sagittal plane. See Sagittal Reformatted CT, Sagittal Reconstruction.

Reformer: One of the more common pieces of Pilates equipment. See Universal Reformer.

Regional Enteritis: Another name for Crohn's disease. See Enteropathic Arthritis.

Reinforcement Maneuver: A physical exam maneuver designed to increase the amplitude of a deep tendon reflex. See Jendrassik's Maneuver.

Reiter's Syndrome: A triad of arthritis, urethritis, and uveitis. The male–female ratio is 50:1. There are two types: venereal and enteric. Asymmetric SI joint inflammation occurs in approximately one-third of patients with this syndrome. Spine involvement is usually limited to the thoracolumbar region. There is less involvement of the facet and costovertebral joints than in ankylosing spondylitis (AS) and enteric arthritis. Syndesmophyte formation is less prominent and more randomly distributed in Reiter's syndrome than in AS and inflammatory bowel disease (IBD). Also, patients with Reiter's syndrome who have spine involvement tend to have better functional outcomes than patients with AS or IBD. This syndrome is thought to be caused by *Shigella*, *Salmonella*, *Yersinia*, *Campylobacter*, and venereal-acquired *Chlamydia*.

rel: An abbreviation for *relief* or *relieved.*

Relafen: A nonsteroidal anti-inflammatory drug (NSAID) that exhibits anti-inflammatory, analgesic, and antipyretic properties. As with other NSAIDs, the probable mode of action is its ability to inhibit prostaglandin synthesis. There is a risk of GI side effects, including ulceration and renal and hepatic side effects. There are drug interactions with anticoagulant and thrombolytic agents. Recommended starting dose is 1,000 mg taken at a single dose with or without food. Common maintenance doses are between 1,000 and 2,000 mg per day given either as a single or twice-a-day dose. The maximum dose is 2,000 mg a day. The lowest effective dose should be used for maintenance therapy. See Nabumetone.

Relative Stenosis: A type of central canal stenosis in which there is a congenitally small canal with stenosis superimposed on abnormal anatomy. The congenitally small canal (usually due to short pedicles) allows for less room in the central canal. The elements that can cause stenosis including herniated disc, facet hypertrophy, pseudohypertrophy of the ligamentum flavum (when this ligament buckles into the canal), or spondylosis are likely to cause symptoms due to the smaller space available.

Release Phenomenon: Painful paresthesias which are experienced after pressure is removed from a nerve. When pressure is supplied to a nerve, a faint tingling and numbness can be experienced followed by lack of sensation. When pressure is released, the lack of sensation is followed by painful paresthesias.

Rep EIL: A McKenzie physical therapy test maneuver. See EIL, Repetitive Extension in Lying.

Rep EIS: A McKenzie physical therapy maneuver involving repetitive backward bending to determine if this reproduces the patient's characteristic pain. See Repetitive Extension in Standing, EIS.

Repetition Maximum: The greatest amount of weight that a muscle can move through a range of motion a specified number of times in an exercise routine. See RM.

Repetitive Extension in Lying: A McKenzie physical therapy test maneuver. See EIL, Rep EIL.

Repetitive Extension in Standing: A McKenzie physical therapy test maneuver. See EIS, Rep EIS.

Repetitive Flexion in Lying: A McKenzie physical therapy test maneuver. See FIL, Rep FIL.

Repetitive Flexion in Standing: A McKenzie physical therapy test maneuver. See FIS, Rep FIS.

Repetitive Side Glide in Standing: A McKenzie physical therapy test maneuver which involves repetitive side glide in standing. See SGIS, Rep SGIS.

Rep FIL: A McKenzie physical therapy test maneuver where the only difference is that repetitive flexion in lying maneuvers are performed. See FIL, Repetitive Flexion in Lying.

Rep FIS: A McKenzie physical therapy test maneuver involving repetitive forward bending to determine if this reproduces the patient's pain. See FIS, Repetitive Flexion in Standing.

Rep SGIS: A McKenzie physical therapy test maneuver involving repetitive side glide in standing maneuvers. See SGIS, Repetitive Side Glide in Standing.

resp: An abbreviation for *respiration*.

Restriction: A chiropractic term denoting limitation of movement. This is used to describe dysfunctional joints and can be restricted in flexion, extension, lateral flexion (right or left), or rotation (right or left).

Restriction of Activities: Limiting the patient's physical movements, positions, and lifting after an injury for the purposes of healing. See Activity Restriction.

Reticulum Cell Sarcoma: This is an older term for an isolated bony tumor which is classified as a lymphoma. See Lymphoma.

Retrocollis: An abnormal extension posture of the cervical spine often associated with cervical dystonia.

Retroflexion: Extension of the spine.

Retrograde Transport: The transport of materials along a nerve axon from the periphery to the cell body. This is a system designed to carry recycled transmitter vesicles and extracellular materials from the nerve terminal. It is also thought that "trophic messages" about the status of the axon are carried back to the cell body. If this retrograde flow is altered from ischemia or compression, there are changes in the cell body. Viruses such as herpes can be transported via retrograde transport.

Retroligamentous Herniation: A disc extrusion or sequestration that migrates posterior to the posterior longitudinal ligament.

Retrolisthesis: A chiropractic term which refers to a vertebral body which has moved posterior relative to the vertebral body above and below. Also, due to the orientation of the facets, the vertebral segment tends to move inferiorly.

Retrolisthesis Positional Dyskinesia: A chiropractic term which denotes a segment which has moved back in relation to the segment below it. It is thought that this occurs because of the increased creep of a degenerated disc combined with the normal lumbar lordosis. There is a shift in weight bearing from the anterior portion of the intervertebral disc to the facets. This position may narrow the spinal canal.

Retrolisthetic Deformity: A spondylolisthesis where one vertebra has fallen back relative to the vertebral body below. This occurs more often in the upper lumbar spine. See Retrolisthesis.

Retropharyngeal Hemorrhage: Bleeding into the area behind the pharynx and in front of the cervical spine due to significant cervical spine trauma. See Retropharyngeal Interspace.

Retropharyngeal Interspace: The soft tissue in front of the cervical vertebral bodies and behind the air shadow of the pharynx. An increase in the prevertebral soft tissue may indicate a significant posttraumatic hematoma due to fracture or significant ligamentous damage, retropharyngeal abscess, or neoplasm. In neutral, the following measurements are considered normal: C1—10 mm, C2—5 mm, C3—7 mm, C4—7 mm, C5—20 mm, C6—20 mm, and C7—20 mm. See RPI, Retrotracheal Space, Prevertebral Soft Tissues, Retropharyngeal Hemorrhage.

Retropulsed: Fragments of a vertebral body fracture which are pushed posteriorly into the spinal canal. This can cause spinal cord compression and may be a true surgical emergency requiring decompressive and stabilization procedures.

Retropulsion: Fragments of a burst fracture which have been pushed backward into the spinal canal.

Retrotracheal Space: The soft tissue in front of the cervical vertebral bodies and behind the air shadow of the pharynx. See Retropharyngeal Interspace.

Retroversion: A decreased angle between the neck and shaft of the hip in the transverse plane. In simpler terms, this amounts to a hip joint which is facing too far backward. There can be an increased internal tibial torsion and excess supination at the foot and ankle. The internal rotators will be shortened and weak and there will be an out-toeing gait. This can be associated with low back pain and SI joint dysfunctions. Treatment includes strengthening the internal rotators, stretching tight external rotators, mobilizations into internal rotation, correcting the SI joint dysfunction, orthotics to correct the foot and ankle supination, or correcting the leg length discrepancy.

Retroverted: Tilted backward. This is commonly used to describe hips with an acetabulum facing backward or more posterior than usual.

Reversal: A radiographic term which describes a curve which has been reversed to the opposite direction, e.g., the straightening of a lordotic curve. This phenomenon can occur with muscle spasm in the anterior cervical spine after a whiplash injury.

Reverse Double Crush: A syndrome characterized by a more distal nerve entrapment which leads to nerve dysfunction more proximally. For example, ulnar nerve entrapment at Guyon's canal causes ulnar nerve entrapment at the cubital tunnel.

Reversible Conduction Block: See Conduction Block. Less pressure is applied per unit area for less time. When the pressure is released, nerve conduction returns.

Revision: A surgical term referring to a second operation done to "revise" the original operation because of continued symptoms.

Revision Decompression: A surgical term used to denote a second decompressive laminectomy after inadequate decompression of the spinal cord or nerve roots.

RF: An abbreviation for *rheumatoid factor.*

Rheumatoid Arthritis: A common type of symmetrical, inflammatory arthritis thought to be an autoimmune process which selectively targets the synovial tissue of the hands and feet as well as the cervical spine. The onset occurs between the ages of 20 and 60 years. There is a predilection for women (3:1 between 20 and 40 years and 1:1 over 40 years). An inflammatory response is initiated, which starts an inflammatory cascade. An intense inflammatory process ensues, and, after it subsides, repair takes place. Scar tissue is laid down and some element of joint destruction over the long term takes place. This process occurs in the cervical spine, distal upper extremities, knee, hip, ankle, and shoulder. SI joint involvement is possible but uncommon. Rheumatoid factor is positive in 70% of patients. Anemia, elevated or normal leukocyte count, elevated ESR and CRP are typical. Upper cervical subluxation is possible in late-stage rheumatoid arthritis. See Pseudobasilar Invagination, Atlantoaxial Instability.

Rheumatoid Discitis: A combination of decreased disc height and end plate erosion seen in rheumatoid arthritis.

Rheumatoid Factor: A laboratory blood test for rheumatoid arthritis. As a screening test in patients with low back pain, many more false-positive results will be obtained than true-positive results. There is a less than 1-in-5 chance that routine screening with a positive rheumatoid factor will detect true rheumatoid arthritis.

Rheumatoid Nodules: Nontender, firm nodules which are seen in patients with rheumatoid arthritis. They frequently occur over the extensor surfaces and synovial tissues.

Rheumatoid Spondylitis: An inflammatory disease of the spine that greatly restricts spinal movement and is often associated with morning pain. It occurs primarily in young adults. See Ankylosing Spondylitis, AS, Von Bechterew Disease, Marie-Strumpell Disease, Pelvospondylitis Ossificans.

Rheumatoid Spondylodiscitis: The extensive erosion of adjacent vertebral end plates in the absence of osteophytes associated with severe rheumatoid arthritis. See Spondylodiscitis.

RI: A chiropractic term which refers to a vertebra which is displaced laterally to the right and inferior. See Right Inferior Subluxation.

Rib Cage: The 12 ribs connected to the thoracic vertebra and sternum. This forms a protective "cage" around the lungs and heart. The expansion of the lungs is due in part to expansion of the rib cage. The upper rib cage expands in an anterior/posterior direction while the lower rib cage expands in a lateral direction. See Bucket Handle Rib Motion, Pump Handle Rib Motion.

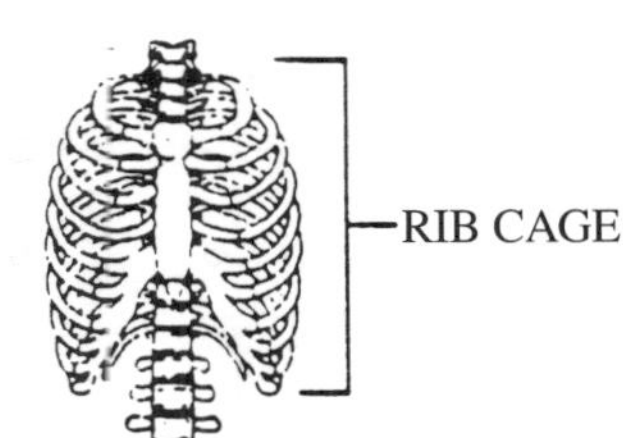

Rib Facet: The area where the rib attaches to the transverse process of the thoracic vertebra. This is the costovertebral joint and is a common point of palpation to access manual lesions of the ribs.

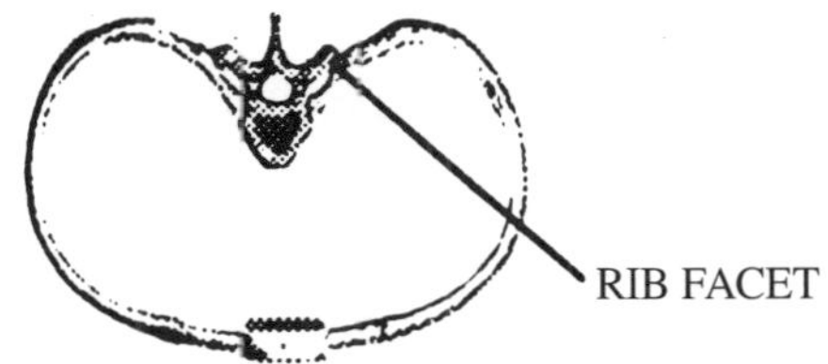

Rib Hump: A prominent hump seen posteriorly in the ribs on the convexity of a scoliotic curvature. This is caused by the vertebral rotation that occurs due to the scoliosis. This is easiest to detect clinically with the spine in a flexed position.

Rib Motion Test: A test for symmetrical movement of the costovertebral joints. The patient is supine, and the examiner's hands are placed over the chest. The anterior/posterior movement of the ribs is monitored as the patient inhales and exhales. Any restriction or side-to-side difference is noted. A rib which is restricted during exhalation is considered an elevated rib. One that is restricted in inhalation is considered a depressed rib. Depressed ribs are usually seen in the upper rib cage while elevated ribs are more commonly seen in the lower rib cage. This testing is not dissimilar to the osteopathic equivalent of looking for pump handle and bucket handle restrictions in the rib cage.

Rib Resection: A surgical technique used to remove the first rib in thoracic outlet syndrome. This is usually reserved for severe cases that are either neurogenic or vascular. This can be done through an anterior approach and combined with a scalenectomy or done through a separate transaxillary approach.

Rib Synostosis: The congenital fusion of two adjacent ribs that can cause a thoracic or thoracolumbar scoliosis.

Rib Vertebral Angle Difference: The angle between the rib and the vertebra in the thoracic spine used to predict the progression of infantile scoliosis. See Mehta Angle.

Rider's Bone: Avulsion of the apophysis of the ischial tuberosity as a result of a large contraction of the hamstrings. See Avulsion Fracture of the Ischial Tuberosity.

Right Angle Test Line: A radiographic line for determining if there is anterolisthesis of L5 on S1 (spondylolisthesis). See Ullmann's Line.

Right Anterior Innominate: One of the many dysfunctions of the SI joint. See Anteriorly Rotated Ilium, Anterior Ilial Rotation.

Right Anterior Oblique: An x-ray term in which the patient faces the x-ray cartridge with the right shoulder touching the cartridge and left shoulder positioned posteriorly and away from the cartridge. The x-ray beam then passes through the left posterior portion first and the right anterior portion last. See RAO.

Right Anterior Sacrum: An osteopathic or manual physical therapy term which refers to a sacrum in which the right sacral base is restricted in flexion. See Unilateral Sacral Extension—Right.

Right Backward Sacral Torsion: A right-on-left sacral torsion in which a right-facing sacrum is on a left oblique axis. L5 is unable to extend on the sacrum. The left sacral base is anterior, and the right inferior lateral angle is posterior and inferior. On lumbar extension the left sacral base is noted to be anterior. Right-on-Left Sacral Torsion, Right Posterior Sacral Torsion.

Right-Facing Sacrum: An osteopathic or manual physical therapy term. See Forward Sacral Torsion, Backward Sacral Torsion, Right-on-Left Sacral Torsion, Right-on-Right Sacral Torsion.

Right Forward Sacral Torsion: Also known as a right-on-right sacral torsion. A right-facing sacrum is on a right oblique axis. The left piriformis is thought to be tight, causing the dysfunction. The left sacral base is anterior in neutral and corrects on lumbar extension. Flexion causes the base to be more anterior on one side.

Right Inferior Subluxation: A chiropractic term which refers to a laterally "flexed" vertebra to the right. There is also some rotation to the right due to the plane of the facets. See Lateral Flexion Malposition, RI.

Right Lateral: A radiographic term in which the patient's right side is against the x-ray cartridge and left side is toward the x-ray beam. The beam then passes from left to right.

Right Lateral Subluxation: A chiropractic term which denotes a vertebral segment which has moved laterally to the right in relation to the vertebral segment above and below. See Lateralisthesis.

Right-on-Left Sacral Torsion: A right-on-left sacral torsion in which a right-facing sacrum is on a left oblique axis. See Right Backward Sacral Torsion.

Right-on-Right Sacral Torsion: An osteopathic or manual physical therapy term which describes a sacral torsion along an oblique sacral axis (from one sacral base to the opposite ILA). See Forward Sacral Torsion.

Right Posterior Oblique: An x-ray term in which the patient is facing away from the x-ray cartridge. The right shoulder is touching the x-ray cartridge, and the patient is positioned obliquely so that the left shoulder is forward. The x-ray beam passes through the left side first and then the right side.

Right Posterior Sacral Torsion: A right-on-left sacral torsion in which there is a right-facing sacrum on a left oblique axis. L5 is unable to extend on the sacrum. See Right Backward Sacral Torsion.

Right Posterior Subluxation: A chiropractic term that refers to a vertebra which is rotated to the right (right-facing or the right side of the vertebra has rotated posteriorly). Due to the orientation of the facets, the side that is posterior is also inferior. See Rotation Malposition, RP.

Right Superior Sacral Shear: An osteopathic or manual physical therapy term which refers to a sacrum in which the right sacral base is restricted in flexion. See Unilateral Sacral Extension—Right, Unilateral Sacral Flexion—Right.

Right Unilateral Sacral Extension: An osteopathic or manual physical therapy term which refers to a sacrum in which the right sacral base is restricted in flexion. See Unilateral Sacral Extension—Right.

Right Unilateral Sacral Flexion: An osteopathic or manual physical therapy term which refers to a sacrum in which the right sacral base is found in flexion. See Unilateral Sacral Flexion—Right.

Rigid Orthotic: An orthotic which is fabricated of inflexible materials. This is to provide more precise foot control and support. See Orthotic.

Rim Lesion: An injury to the intervertebral disc in which the outer portion of the rim of the disc is separated from the vertebral body. This is usually caused by a flexion/extension injury or a distraction injury.

Ring Apophysis: The narrow rim of bone which surrounds the superior and inferior surfaces of each vertebral body. This is the secondary ossification center of the vertebral body. See Vertebral Ring Apophysis.

Risser-Ferguson Method: One technique for measuring a scoliotic curve on AP radiography. The end vertebra is the same as in the Cobb method. This is a vertebra that is at the far extreme of the scoliotic curve on either end. An apical vertebra is also chosen which is the most laterally displaced segment. The center of these three vertebral bodies is determined by drawing intersecting diagonal lines connecting the opposing points. See Ferguson Method.

Risser Jacket: An orthosis used for conservatively correcting a scoliotic curve. See Risser Localizer Cast.

Risser Localizer Cast: An orthosis used for conservatively correcting a scoliotic curve. Localized pressure is placed laterally over the rib cage at the apex of the curve, while traction is exerted on the head and pelvis. This is often used presurgically. See Risser Jacket.

Risser Sign: A radiographic sign used to determine when vertebral growth is complete. This occurs when the iliac epiphysis (growth plate) has fused and is no longer visible on AP radiographs. See Apophysis Sign.

Risser Turnbuckle: A casting technique used to correct spinal scoliosis.

RLI: The soft tissue in front of the vertebral bodies and behind the air shadow of the pharynx. See Retropharyngeal Interspace.

RM: The greatest amount of weight that a muscle can move through a range of motion for a specified number of times in an exercise routine. See Repetition Maximum.

RN: Registered nurse.

Robaxin: A muscle relaxant which decreases muscle tone by causing sedation. It does not act directly on skeletal muscle. This drug should not be used with alcohol. It is available in 500-mg and 750-mg tablets. Initial dosage is one to two tablets three to four times a day. See Methocarbamol.

Robinson-Smith Procedure: A technique for cervical fusion which involves anterior disc excision followed by insertion of a (cortical/cancellous) horseshoe-shaped bone graft into the disc space. This is similar to the Bailey-Badgley procedure, but no attempt is made to remove posterior or posterolateral osteophytes.

Roentgenometrics: A chiropractic x-ray technique which involves biomechanical analysis by using markers on static spinal views or acetate overlays on bending views.

Rolfing: A body work system created by Ida Rolf used to correct posture and integrate structure. The technique involves manual soft tissue manipulation to balance "the body" in the gravitational field. It is thought that there are adhesions or restrictions in the fascial layers of the body which need to be corrected through very deep tissue massage and mobilization. Rolfing is a standardized approach that is not symptom-specific. The technique involves ten 1-hour sessions, each emphasizing a different aspect of posture. These ten sessions include respiration, lower extremity balance, front-to-back balance, left and right balance, rectus abdominis–psoas balance, sacrum, occiput–atlas relationship, upper and lower half of the body relationship (two sessions), and balance throughout the system. See Structural Integration.

Roman Bench: A stationary piece of exercise equipment on which the patient lies face down with the legs hooked under a bar. The patient then flexes at the hips and re-extends to strengthen the erector spinae. This piece of equipment is used in the Oldfeldt protocol. It should be noted that this type of erector spinae strengthening is very difficult.

Romanus Lesion: An x-ray sign in ankylosing spondylitis. This is an erosion of the anterior vertebral body margin which occurs just prior to the formation of syndesmophytes. These erosions occur at the anterior–superior and anterior–inferior corners of the vertebral bodies and can be seen in conjunction with a "shiny corner" sign. See Shiny Corner Sign, Ankylosing Spondylitis.

Roos Test: A test for thoracic outlet syndrome (TOS) in which the shoulder is abducted to 90° and the glenohumeral joint is externally rotated. The fingers are then rapidly flexed and extended. If this test elicits arm pain, vascular thoracic outlet syndrome may be implicated. The pulse is also monitored. This is thought to be more sensitive for vascular TOS and pulse changes than the classic Adson's test or costoclavicular maneuvers. See Abduction External Rotation Test.

Root Pain: The sensory portion of a radiculopathy with pain in a specific dermatomal distribution corresponding to the affected nerve root. See Radiculopathy.

Root Signs: Weakness or numbness in a specific nerve root distribution due to a radiculopathy. See Radiculopathy.

Root Sleeve Fibrosis: Scarring around nerve roots which can occur after a surgical procedure. See Perineural Fibrosis.

Rosary Bead Appearance: A radiographic sign in ankylosing spondylitis. There is an undulating appearance of the SI joint margins due to erosions.

Rosen Body Work: A type of body work which is less invasive and structured than most and is often performed in conjunction with psychotherapy.

Rose's Gluteal Reflex: A physical exam maneuver used to indicate the presence of sciatica. The gluteus maximus is percussed at or near its attachment to the sacrum. A positive test is an exaggerated contraction which is localized and indicates the presence of sciatica. A negative test would be a generalized contraction of the muscle.

Rot: An abbreviation for *rotation*.

Rotary: A chiropractic term which refers to manipulation which induces rotation.

Rotatory Subluxation of C1 on C2: A traumatic subluxation of the atlantoaxial articulation. See Atlantoaxial Rotatory Subluxation.

Rotated: An osteopathic, chiropractic, or manual physical therapy slang term that refers to a vertebral segment which has abnormal biomechanics. For instance, if a vertebral segment is said to be rotated right, the vertebral segment is noted to be facing toward the right in either flexion, extension, or neutral. This is a nonspecific term.

Rotated Dysfunction of the Sacrum: An osteopathic term. See Rotated Sacrum.

Rotated Sacrum: An osteopathic term which refers to a sacrum that has rotated about the y-axis. Movement is freer in the direction that rotation has occured and is restricted in the opposite direction. See Rotated Dysfunction of the Sacrum.

Rotational Subluxation: An orthopedic spine term. An asymmetric erosion of the lateral masses of C1 or C2 that results in a rotation of C1 with respect to C2. The principal symptom is pain. A nonreducible rotational head tilt due to lateral mass collapse is seen in up to 10% of patients with advanced rheumatoid arthritis. On radiographs, the sizes of the lateral masses of C1 and C2 are asymmetrical.

Rotation at _______ [vertebral level]: A manual physical therapy, osteopathic, or chiropractic term which refers to a vertebral segment which has abnormal motion and is facing right or left in flexion, extension, or neutral.

Rotation Malposition: A chiropractic term which refers to a vertebra which is noted to be rotated either to the right or to the left on static testing. This is in relation to the adjacent vertebrae. See Left Posterior Subluxation, Right Posterior Subluxation.

Rotator Cuff Impingement: Compression of the supraspinatus and subacromial bursa underneath the coracoacromial arch. See Impingement Syndrome.

Rotator Cuff Tendinitis: Compression of the supraspinatus and subacromial bursa underneath the coracoacromial arch. See Impingement Syndrome.

Rotodextro Scoliosis: A lateral curvature of the spine which also has a rotatory component. The convexity is toward the right.

Rotolevo Scoliosis: A lateral curvature of the spine which has a rotatory component. The convexity is toward the left.

Rotoscoliosis: A lateral curvature of the spine which has a rotatory component. This is usually considered to be either structural or functional. A structural rotoscoliosis is caused by bony changes in the spine. A functional rotoscoliosis is usually adaptive in nature and caused by biomechanical changes elsewhere in the spine or in the lower extremities.

Round Back Posture: A posture characterized by an increased thoracic curve, protracted scapulae, and a forward head. See Kyphotic Posture.

Roy-Camille Plates: One type of pedicle screw fixation which uses a posterior plate and screw system. The system is adjustable, and pedicle screws are used. However, there is a significant screw breakage rate, and slippage has been noted. See Pedicle Screw Fixation.

RP: A chiropractic term which refers to a vertebra which has rotated toward the right. See Right Posterior Subluxation.

RPC: A quantification of the patient's perception of his/her ability to perform physical tasks. See Rating of Perceived Capacity.

RPI: The soft tissue in front of the vertebral bodies and behind the air shadow of the pharynx. See Retropharyngeal Interspace.

RPO: An x-ray term in which the patient is facing away from the x-ray cartridge. See Right Posterior Oblique.

RPT: Registered Physical Therapist.

RSD: A clinical syndrome characterized by the presence of pain out of proportion to the severity of the injury. See Reflex Sympathetic Dystrophy.

RT: Recreational therapist.

RTI: The soft tissue in front of the vertebral bodies and behind the air shadow of the pharynx. See Retropharyngeal Interspace.

RTW: An abbreviation for *return to work.*

Ruffini End Organs: Mechanoreceptors which are found within the joint capsule and around the joint. Each is responsible for an angle of approximately 15° with some degree of overlap with the adjacent Ruffini end organ. They are not easily fatigued, and they are progressively recruited as the joint moves. The prime function of these end organs is to maintain prolonged postures and to provide information to the CNS about the direction of movement. See Type 1 Mechanoreceptors.

Ruptured Disc: A "slipped" disc. See Herniated Disc, HNP.

Ruptured Intervertebral Disc: A "slipped" disc. See Herniated Disc, HNP.

Rupture of the Transverse Ligament: An isolated traumatic disruption of the transverse ligament is not common. Since the ligament is strong, the dens will probably fracture before the ligament is completely ruptured. Rupture of the ligament does occur in association with a Jefferson fracture, inflammatory arthritis, and, not uncommonly, in Down syndrome. There is an abnormal atlanto-dental interspace (greater than 3 mm in adults and 5 mm in children). Since the spinal cord at the atlas takes up approximately one third of the space and the dens one third, there can be considerable anterior displacement of the atlas (up to 1 cm) before significant cord damage occurs. See ADI, Transverse Ligament Rupture.

Rust's Sign: A physical exam sign which is positive in a patient with a markedly splinted cervical spine who needs to support the weight of the head with both hands. Removal of the support cannot be tolerated, and this suggests instability of the upper cervical spine due to fracture or severe cervicothoracic sprain or strain.

R Vision: The brand name for a videotape composer that tapes from videodisc. Exercises are chosen from a videodisc and then copied onto a videotape so that the patient has a home program on videotape.

Rx: An abbreviation for *drug* or *prescription.*

S

S: An abbreviation for *sharp pain.*

S&C: An abbreviation for *strength and conditioning.*

S-1: Referring to the first sacral nerve root or first sacral vertebra.

S1 Nerve Root: The first sacral nerve root that exits between L5 and S1. It supplies numerous muscles including the gastrocnemius, gluteus maximus, and semimembranosus. It supplies sensation to the lateral foot. See S1 Root, Nerve Root—S1.

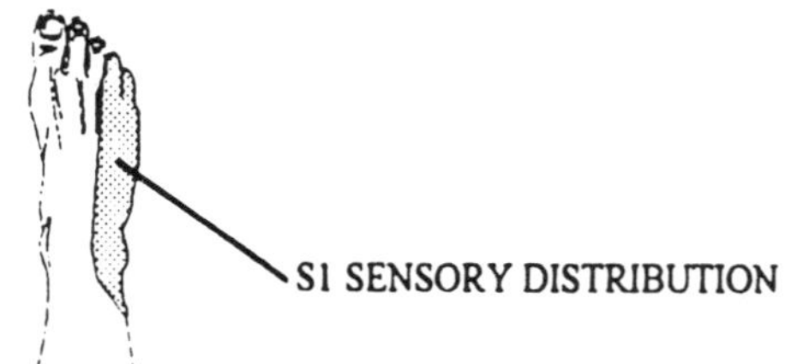

S1 Root: The first sacral nerve root that exits between L5 and S1. See S1 Nerve Root.

SABA: A Norwegian brand of exercise equipment which is common in medical exercise therapy programs. An inclined sled is used in conjunction with pulleys. See MET, Medical Exercise Therapy.

sac: An abbreviation for *sacrum.*

Sacral Agenesis: A congenital malformation in which all or part of the sacrum is absent. This rare condition, which is detected at birth, is characterized by scoliosis, pelvic instability, hip dislocation, deficient lower extremity musculature, and lower extremity contracture at the knee and hip.

Sacral Ala: The large lateral mass of the first sacral vertebral body. See Ala of the Sacrum.

Sacral Apex: The most inferior portion of the sacrum that articulates with the coccyx. See Apex of the Sacrum.

Sacral Backward Bending: When the base of the sacrum (top of the sacrum) moves posteriorly in relation to the ilia. See Sacral Counternutation.

Sacral Base: The superior most portion of the sacrum that is the inferior portion of the L5–S1 disc space. This also refers to the end plate of the first sacral vertebra. It is flanked by the alae of the sacrum. This is a landmark used in manual medicine tests. See Base of the Sacrum.

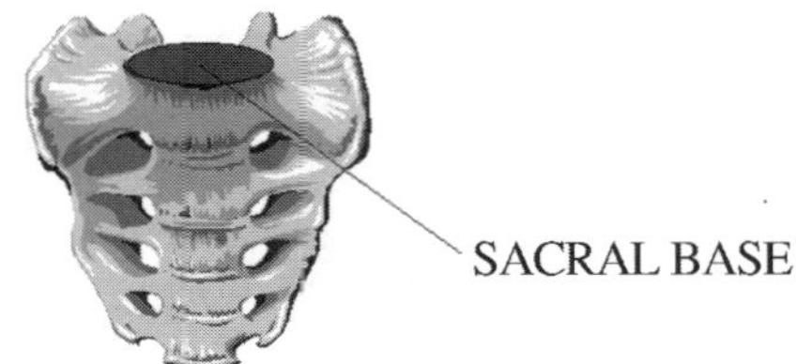

Sacral Base Anterior: An osteopathic or manual physical therapy term used to denote a sacral position such that the sacral base is anterior and inferior and the apex is posterior and superior. See Bilaterally Extended Sacrum.

Sacral Base Posterior: An osteopathic or manual physical therapy term used to denote a sacral position such that the sacral base is extended or posterior and the apex is anterior. See Bilaterally Flexed Sacrum.

Sacral Canal: The continuation of the lumbar spinal canal which extends through the sacrum ending in the sacral hiatus at the inferior-most portion of the sacrum. The sacral canal contains the cauda equina.

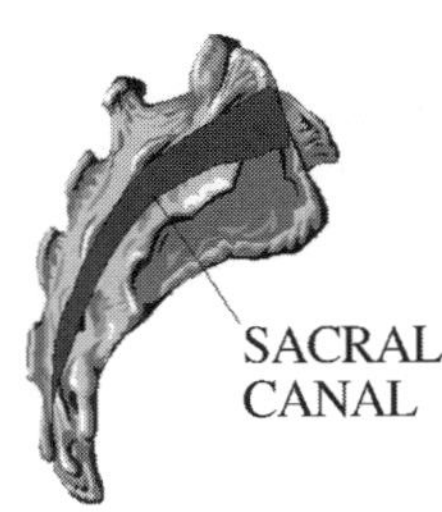

Sacral Coccygeal Pubic Line: The line passing from the sacrococcygeal joint to the inferior point of the pubic bone on a lateral radiograph. See Scipp Line, Sacrococcygeal Pubic Line.

Sacral Cornua: Rudimentary inferior facets which lie on either side of the sacral hiatus and articulate with the cornua of the coccyx.

Sacral Counternutation: When the base of the sacrum (top of the sacrum) moves posteriorly in relation to the ilia. See Sacral Extension, Extension—Sacral, Sacral Backward Bending.

Sacral Extension: When the base of the sacrum (top of the sacrum) moves posteriorly in relation to the ilia. See Sacral Counternutation, Extension—Sacral, Sacral Backward Bending.

Sacral Femoral Angle: A radiographic measurement of the amount of pelvic rotation–derotation present in stance. Lateral standing x-rays are taken of the lumbar spine, pelvis, and hip. One line is drawn along the superior aspect of the sacrum, the other along the femoral shaft. If this angle is less than 35°, a significant hip flexion deformity is present. The normal angle is 50–65°. See Fick Method.

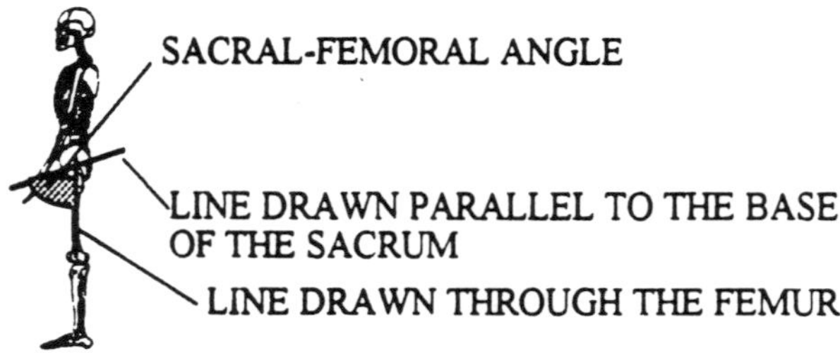

Sacral Flexion: When the base of the sacrum (top of the sacrum) moves anteriorly in relation to the ilia. See Sacral Nutation, Sacral Forward Bending, Flexion—Sacral.

Sacral Flexion—Bilateral: An osteopathic or manual physical therapy term used to denote a sacral position such that the base is anterior and inferior and the apex posterior and superior. See Bilateral Flexed Sacrum.

Sacral Flexion–Extension Test: A test for sacral mobility. The patient is seated on a stool with feet supported. The examiner kneels behind the patient and places the thumb pads on the inferior lateral angles of the sacrum. The examiner monitors ILA movement with nutation and counternutation of the sacrum as the patient backward bends and forward bends. This movement should be bilaterally symmetrical. Presence of one posterior ILA suggests a torsion on that same side. If the posterior ILA is found during nutation (backward bending) this suggests a backward torsion. If the posterior ILA is found in counternutation (forward bending) and becomes symmetric in nutation (backward bending) a forward torsion is suspected. If the asymmetric ILA does not become symmetric in either nutation or counternutation, then a seated flexion test should be performed. If this test is positive, then a unilateral sacral flexion or extension is suggested as the diagnosis.

Sacral Foramina: Foramina or openings which occur bilaterally and segmentally on the anterior sacrum through which pass the anterior branches of the sacral nerve roots. See Anterior Sacral Foramina.

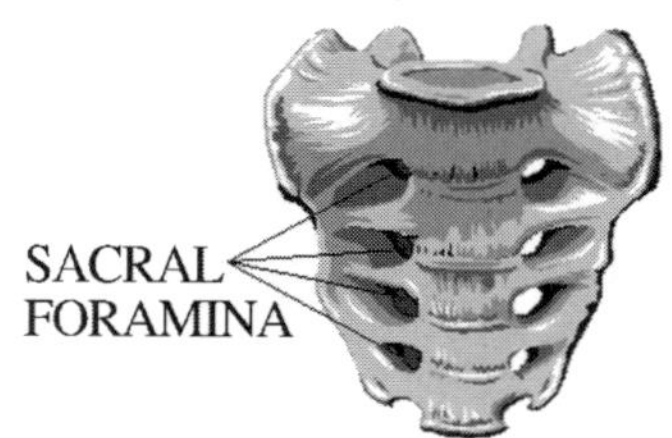

Sacral Forward Bending: When the base of the sacrum (top of the sacrum) moves anteriorly in relation to the ilia. See Sacral Flexion, Sacral Nutation, Flexion—Sacral.

Sacral Fracture—Vertical: A fracture of the sacrum which usually occurs due to indirect trauma to the pelvis. See Vertical Fracture of the Sacrum, Fracture Sacral—Vertical, Vertical Sacral Fracture.

Sacral Hiatus: A hiatus or opening on the posterior surface of the sacrum located at the inferior tip. This is formed by the unfused lamina of the last sacral segment. The sacral hiatus is a common delivery site for sacral epidural steroids.

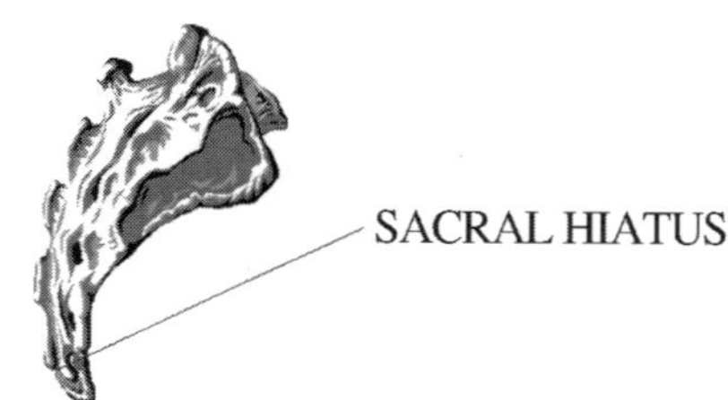

Sacral Horizontal Plane Line: A chiropractic x-ray analysis technique. See SHPL.

Sacral Inclination: A radiographic sign used in the assessment of sacral position and pelvic tilt. A lateral lumbar spine–sacral view is used. A line is drawn on the posterior surface of the sacrum. A vertical intersecting line is then drawn. The average sacral inclination is 46° with the range between 30 and 72°.

Sacralization: A congenital defect which is a normal variation of lumbar spine anatomy. The L5 vertebral body is fused to the sacrum making L4–L5 the first mobile segment rather than the usual L5–S1. This is a normal variant in 3–6% of the population.

Sacral Line: A line drawn through the vertical axis of the sacrum on AP radiographs and drawn perpendicularly to the level of the iliac crest. This is used to detect pelvic obliquities.

Sacral Mob: A mobilization of the sacroiliac joint by mobilizing the sacrum.

Sacral Nerves: The S1 through S5 nerves.

Sacral Nutation: When the base of the sacrum (top of the sacrum) moves anteriorly in relation to the ilia. See Sacral Flexion, Sacral Forward Bending, Flexion—Sacral.

Sacral Occipital Technique: A chiropractic technique that incorporates wedge-shaped blocks in conjunction with a pumping motion to make sacral corrections. See SOT.

Sacral Plexus: A complicated plexus of nerves which receives contributions from L4 through S5. The sacral plexus consists of the L4 root, the lumbosacral trunk, the superior gluteal nerve, the inferior gluteal nerve, the sciatic nerve, the nerve to quadratus femoris and inferior gemellus, the nerve to obturator internus and superior gemellus, posterior cutaneous femoral nerve, penetrating cutaneous nerve, the pudendal nerve, and the S5 root. See Lumbosacral Plexus.

Sacral Promontory: A prominent anterior enlargement of the upper portion of the body of the sacrum.

Sacral Respiratory Motion: The normal movement of the sacrum with inspiration and expiration. With inspiration, the base of the sacrum moves posteriorly, or seems to lift upward in the prone position. With expiration, the base moves anteriorly, or seems to fall in the prone position. It is thought that a backward sacral torsion inhibits sacral respiratory motion due to the involvement at L5–S1. See Sacral Respiratory Rhythm.

Sacral Respiratory Rhythm: The normal movement of the sacrum with inspiration and expiration. See Sacral Respiratory Motion.

Sacral Sciatic Notch: A notch formed between the sacrum and the ilium. See Sciatic Notch.

Sacral Screw Fixation: The placement of screws into the sacrum for the purpose of stabilizing a disruption of the posterior pelvic ring, or a screw placed into the sacrum to provide fixation for lumbosacral fusions with instrumentation.

Sacral Shear: An osteopathic abnormality of sacral motion. See Unilateral Sacral Flexion.

Sacral Torsion: An osteopathic or manual physical therapy term used to describe a sacrum which is facing right or left along an oblique (diagonal) axis through the sacrum. Forward sacral torsions normally occur during the gait cycle. However, when used in the context of an SI joint dysfunction, they refer to a joint which is not moving properly and is displaced along an oblique axis. Sacral torsions are usually treated with muscle energy technique correction, stretching, and other manual (mobilization or manipulative) treatments. These dysfunctions can be described as forward or backward and left- or right-facing. The terms *left-on-left*, *left-on-right*, *right-on-right*, and *right-on-left* are used to describe sacral torsions. The first position given is the direction the sacrum is facing and the second is the axis of displacement.

Sacral Tuberosity: The upper two tubercles that present laterally to the sacral foramina on the posterior portion of the sacrum. This is the attachment site of the posterior sacroiliac ligament.

Sacral Vertebrae: The vertebrae that are usually fused to form the sacrum. The five sacral vertebrae are denoted S1 to S5.

Sacral Vertebral Angle: The angle measured between two radiographic lines, one drawn parallel to the sacral base and one drawn parallel to the inferior end plate of L5.

Sacrococcygeal Pubic Line: A line passing from the sacrococcygeal joint to the inferior point of the pubic bone on a lateral radiograph. See Sacral Cococcygeal Pubic Line, Scipp Line.

Sacrofemoral Angle: A radiographic measurement of the amount of pelvic rotation–derotation present in stance. See Sacral Femoral Angle, Fick Method.

Sacroiliac Arthrodesis: A surgical procedure. See SI Joint Fusion, SI Arthrodesis, Fusion—SI Joint, Sacroiliac Fusion.

Sacroiliac Extension Fixation: A chiropractic term denoting an SI joint in which the PSIS has moved anteriorly and superiorly with the ilium fixed in extension in relation to the sacrum. The axis of rotation has thus shifted inferior and the superior portion of the joint remains mobile. See AS.

Sacroiliac Fixation: A chiropractic term describing abnormal motion at the SI joint found by motion palpation. The axis of rotation of the joint has shifted either superiorly or inferiorly and has caused locking within the joint. See Sacroiliac Joint Locking.

Sacroiliac Flexion Fixation: A chiropractic term denoting an SI joint in which the PSIS is inferior and posterior. The ilium is noted to be flexed in relation to the sacrum. The axis of rotation has shifted superiorly, and the inferior portion of the joint remains mobile. See PI Ilium.

Sacroiliac Fusion: A surgical procedure. See SI Arthrodesis, SI Joint Fusion, Sacroiliac Arthrodesis, Fusion—SI Joint.

Sacroiliac Joint: Referring to the area where the sacrum and the iliac bones form a joint. These areas are on either side of the spine in the lower back region. The muscles and ligaments in the region are exceptionally prone to injury. See Lumbosacral Joint.

Sacroiliac Joint Disease: Degenerative changes seen in the SI joint.

Sacroiliac Joint Locking: A chiropractic term describing abnormal motion at the SI joint found by motion palpation. See Sacroiliac Fixation.

Sacroiliac Joint Provocation Tests: One of many physical exam maneuvers designed to produce pain within the SI joint and to determine if the SI joint is a pain generator. The most common of these are Patrick's maneuver, FABER maneuver, open book test, and squish test.

Sacroiliac Somatic Dysfunction: A biomechanical abnormality which is intrinsic to the SI joint(s) and alters normal movement (or viscoelasticity) within the SI joint(s). See SI Dysfunction.

Sacroiliac Sprain: Pain emanating from the sacroiliac joint(s). See SI Joint Syndrome.

Sacroiliitis: Inflammation within the SI joint. This is also used in place of the terms *SI joint syndrome* or *SI joint dysfunction*. It is implied that pain is emanating from the SI joint.

Sacrolisthesis: A sacral fracture which occurs more often in patients after the second decade of life. There is an anterior dislocation of the proximal part of the sacrum, and there may be injury of the cauda equina with perianal anesthesia and paralysis of the sphincter.

Sacropubic Diameter: A measurement of the diameter of the pelvic inlet, usually measured on lateral radiographs. This is the distance between the lower margin of the symphysis pubis and the tip of the sacrum. See Anterior Posterior Diameter of the Pelvis, AP Diameter of the Pelvis.

Sacrospinous Ligament: An important stabilizing ligament of the SI joint which extends from the ILA of the sacrum to the spine of the ischium. There are slips to the coccyx, and the coccygeus muscle forms the anterior surface of this ligament. The sacrospinous ligament has a pain referral pattern which can mimic an S1 radiculopathy.

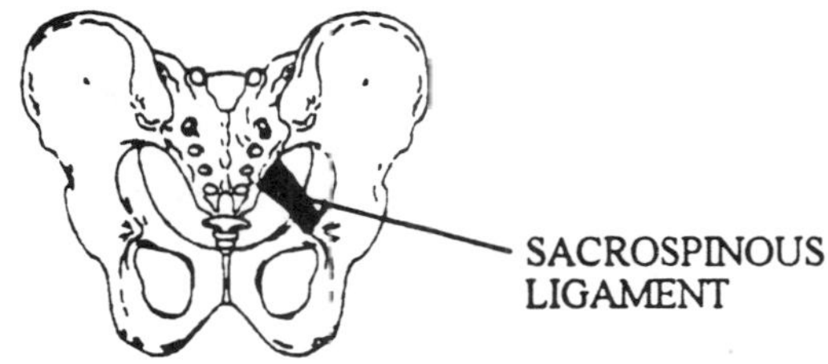

Sacrotuberous Ligament: An important stabilizing ligament of the SI joint. This connects the sacrum to the ischial tuberosity and has slips that travel into the coccyx. It inserts near the inferior lateral angle of the sacrum. It is pierced by the S2 and S3 sensory nerves, which supply the medial and inferior buttock. The referral pattern of this ligament is down the back of the leg. Movement of the sacrum independent of the pelvis will cause changes in the tension of the sacrotuberous ligament. Decreased tension in one sacrotuberous ligament may indicate an up-slip of the pubis. In some patients, there is thought to be a partial connection of the biceps femoris and gluteus maximus with the sacrotuberous ligament.

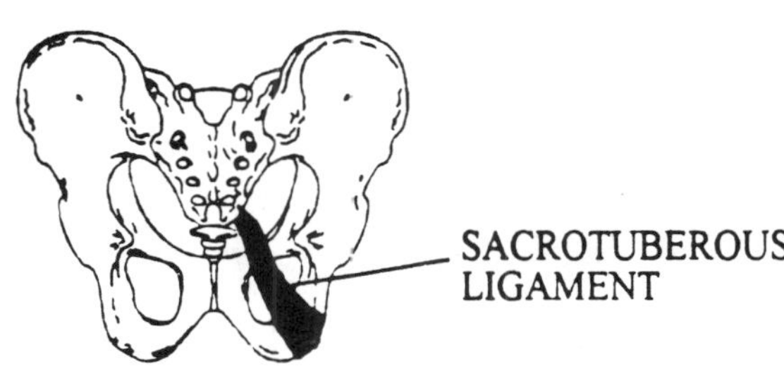

Sacrotuberous Ligament Test: A physical exam test used to determine the tension in the sacrotuberous ligament. The sacrotuberous ligament extends from the sacrum to the ischial tuberosity. Movement of the sacrum independent of the hemipelvis, or vice versa, will cause changes in the tension in the sacrotuberous ligament. The ischial tuberosities are identified and then the thumb pads are moved medially and posteriorly to lie over the sacrotuberous ligament. The tension in this area is noted. The sacrotuberous ligament has a pain referral pattern which travels down the back of the leg, and this pain referral pattern may be noted. Decreased tension in one sacrotuberous ligament may indicate an up-slip of the pubis. This needs to be correlated with other tests.

Sacrum: The base of support for the spine. This bone is made up of the S1 through S5 vertebrae, which are fused to form a triangular bone. The sacrum articulates with the L5 vertebra through the L5–S1 intervertebral disc superiorly. Inferiorly, it articulates with the coccyx. Laterally, it articulates with the ilium on either side. See Ala of the Sacrum.

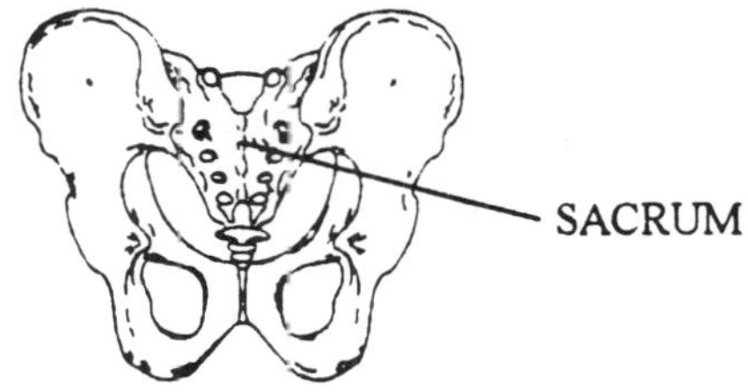

Sacrum Fracture—Horizontal: The most common type of sacral fracture usually seen at the level of the third and fourth sacral segments near the lower end of the SI joint. See Horizontal Fracture of the Sacrum.

Sacrum Fracture—Transverse: The most common type of sacral fracture usually seen at the level of the third and fourth sacral segments near the lower end of the SI joint. See Horizontal Fracture of the Sacrum.

SAD: This is the diameter across the spinal canal from the tip of a posterior osteophyte to the opposing lamina. The general concept is that an osteophyte on the vertebral body will narrow the diameter of the central canal and reduce the space for the spinal cord possibly causing spinal stenosis. A smaller DAD or developmental anteroposterior distance would predispose more clinical significance for spinal stenosis. See DAD, Developmental Anteroposterior Diameter, Spondylitic Anteroposterior Diameter.

Sagittal Curve: One of the three normal curves present in the adult spine. These are the cervical lordosis, lumbar lordosis, and thoracic kyphosis. Since this occurs in the sagittal plane (front/back plane), this is called the sagittal curve. This is the view seen on a lateral x-ray.

Sagittal Diameter: A common measurement in cervical stenosis. This is the anterior/posterior diameter of the cervical spinal canal. This is usually measured on lateral radiographs, CT scan, or MRI.

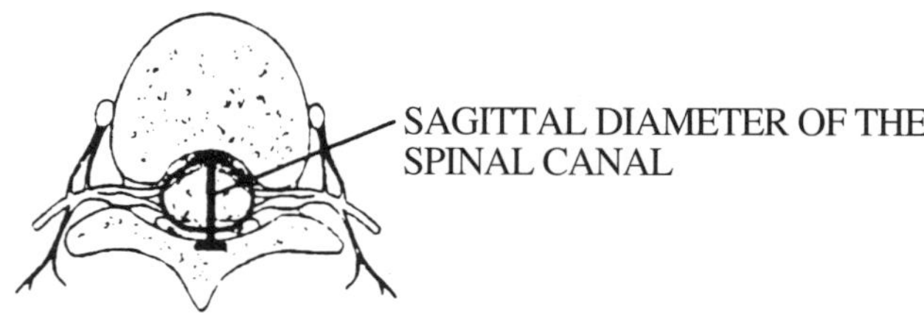

Sagittal Dimension of the Cervical Spinal Canal: The anterior/posterior diameter of the cervical spinal canal measured on lateral radiographs. This measurement is from the posterior surface of the mid-vertebral body to the spinolaminar junction line. The measurement varies at each level with the maximum measurement at C1 being 31 mm and the minimum measurement at C7 being 12 mm. Central canal stenosis is said to be present when the measurement is less than 12 mm. If degenerative osteophytes are present, the measurement is taken from the tip of the osteophyte to the opposing side.

Sagittal Mobility: The overall flexibility or range of motion in the sagittal plane. With respect to the spine, this is flexion/extension.

Sagittal Plane Rotation: The movement of the vertebral bodies as they rotate around a fixed point in the anterior annulus or the anterior longitudinal ligament. This measurement is used as part of a checklist for clinical instability proposed by White and Panjabi.

Sagittal Plane Translation: The movement of one vertebral body on another in flexion or extension with the end plates remaining roughly parallel. This distance can be used as a measure of clinical instability.

Sagittal Reconstruction: A CT scan with a computer-generated image in a sagittal plane (rather than the standard axial). See Sagittal Reformatted CT, Reformatted CT.

Sagittal Reformatted CT: A CT scan with a computer-generated image in a sagittal plane (rather than the standard axial). Information is obtained from axial images and reconstructed through a computer to yield a sagittal image. This type of image can be used to view the foramina for surgical planning. See Reformatted CT.

Salsalate: A nonsteroidal anti-inflammatory drug of the salicylic acid group. See Disalcid.

Saphenous Nerve: The terminal branch of the femoral nerve which is purely sensory. It supplies sensation to the medial border of the foot and ankle as well as the medial side of the proximal tibia.

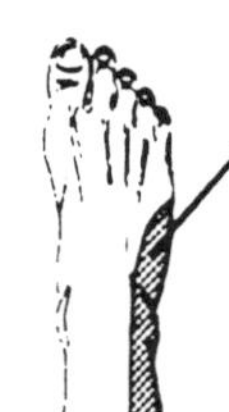

Satellite Trigger Point: A trigger point located in the zone of referral of another trigger point. A satellite trigger point becomes active because it is located in the zone of reference or referral of the primary trigger point.

Sayre Jacket: A plaster orthosis used to immobilize the vertebral column. The patient is suspended by the head and axilla during the application of a cast to allow for full spinal elongation before immobilization.

SC: An abbreviation for *splenius capitis*.

SCAAPF: An abbreviation for *simultaneously combined anterior and posterior fusions*. An anterior lumbar fusion where the excised disc is replaced with bone graft while distraction is applied to the intervertebral space. Under the same anesthetic, the corresponding posterior spinal segments are exposed and fused with instrumentation. The lateral gutters are prepared and packed with large volumes of bone graft material. See Simultaneously Combined Anterior and Posterior Fusions.

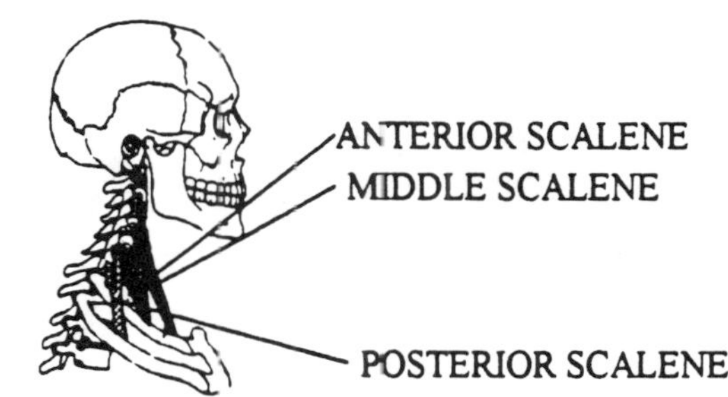

Scalene: One of a group of three anterior neck muscles (anterior, middle, and posterior) which originate from the C1–C6 anterior tubercles of the transverse processes and insert on the first and second ribs. The brachial plexus and subclavian artery pass between the anterior and middle scalene muscles. It is because of this that these muscles are implicated in thoracic outlet syndrome. They have multiple actions depending on whether the origin or insertion is fixed. With the rib cage fixed, they side bend the neck and rotate it slightly to the opposite side. With the neck fixed, they are accessory muscles of respiration, fixing the first two ribs in quiet respiration or raising them in forced inspiration. Innervation is through the ventral rami that correspond to their origin.

Scalene Anticus Syndrome: Compression of the neurovascular bundle as it passes between the anterior and middle scalenes in the thoracic outlet. Irritation of the neurovascular bundle is thought to occur because of taut bands or tightness within the anterior scalene. The roof of the thoracic outlet is the clavicle and the floor is the first rib. Symptoms include numbness and tingling in the arm, hand, or fingers; weakness of finger movements and grip; and a deep, dull, aching pain in the arm and hand. These symptoms occur most frequently at night, but also can and do occur during the day. An Adson's test which is also known as a scalene anticus test, can be performed. This consists of turning the head to the same side as the symptoms, extending the head, abducting the arm, and having the patient take a deep breath. Rotation of the head toward the same side will decrease the space in the thoracic outlet by causing the scalenes on that side to become taut. Symptoms are usually seen with this maneuver. There may be trigger points located within the scalene musculature. EMG/NCS is notoriously nonsensitive for the majority of patients with TOS. This test is usually performed to rule out true neurogenic TOS (rare) or peripheral nerve entrapment that might be masquerading as TOS. Common treatments include spray and stretch of the scalenes, ischemic compression of trigger points in the scalenes, deep tissue mobilization of the scalenes, first rib mobilizations, clavicular mobilizations, correction of sternoclavicular restrictions, passive modalities, scalene stretches, injection and stretch, postural exercises, muscle energy techniques, Jones strain–counterstrain, and other treatments. Scalenectomy and first rib resection have also been performed. See Anterior Scalene Syndrome, Thoracic Outlet Syndrome, Scalenius Anticus Syndrome.

Scalenectomy: A relatively controversial surgical technique, which involves removal of the scalenes, is usually combined with a first rib resection. This is done to decompress the thoracic outlet in patients with neurogenic or vascular thoracic outlet syndrome. Scar tissue is not uncommon after this surgical procedure and can lead to recurrence of symptoms.

Scalenius Anticus Syndrome: Compression of the neurovascular bundle as it passes between the anterior and middle scalenes in the thoracic outlet. See Anterior Scalene Syndrome, Thoracic Outlet Syndrome, Scalene Anticus Syndrome.

Scalloped Vertebra: An abnormal exaggeration of the concavity of the posterior vertebral body surface.

Scapulocostal Syndrome: Pain at the insertion of the levator scapulae muscle caused by a rounded-shoulders posture. Symptoms can include referral of pain to the posterolateral neck and along the border of the scapula as well as to the posterior shoulder. There can be decreased range of motion of the cervical spine secondary to the pain in the levator scapulae. There is usually local pain as well as trigger point activity within the levator scapulae. Common treatments include postural exercises, a figure-of-8 harness, posture corrector, anti-inflammatory medication, injection and stretch, spray and stretch, ischemic compression, correction of thoracic dysfunctions, and correction of rib restrictions.

Scapulohumeral Periarthritis: A marked decrease in range of motion usually in one shoulder. Etiology is usually unknown. See Adhesive Capsulitis, Frozen Shoulder.

Scapulohumeral Reflex: A deep tendon reflex where the tip of the spine of the scapula or acromion is tapped with a reflex hammer. This is thought to be mediated through the upper cervical spine, testing the cervical spine above C3. Abnormal response is elevation of the scapula or abduction of the humerus, and, if these are present, the reflex is considered hyperactive. Hypoactivity cannot be distinguished from normal activity. See SHR.

Scapulothoracic Fibrositis: A rheumatology term which usually refers to myofascial pain of the scapular stabilizers. This is due to tissue overload as a consequence of other postural abnormalities, including a protracted shoulder or thoracic spine problems. This is somewhat of a catchall term.

Scarpa's Triangle: An anatomic triangle bounded by the inguinal ligament, the sartorius muscle, and the medial border of the adductor longus muscle. See Femoral Triangle.

Schepelmann's Sign: A physical exam maneuver during which the patient is seated comfortably and then fully abducts the shoulders bringing the hands overhead. The patient is then asked to laterally bend at the thoracic spine. Pain on the side of the lateral bend indicates intercostal neuritis while pain on the convex side indicates intercostal myofascial pain. The test is then performed bilaterally and the sides are compared.

Scheuermann's Disease: A disorder of growing vertebral bodies (onset 10–13 yrs) that affects about 8–10% of the population. Inflammation of the bone and cartilage occurs in the vertebral end plates. The condition can lead to increased thoracic kyphosis and Schmorl's nodes. In more severe conditions, the vertebral bodies can show anterior wedging. The radiographic criteria for diagnosis are kyphosis due to at least three contiguous segments, wedging of 5° or more (each vertebral body), irregular end plates, loss of disc height, and increased thoracic kyphosis.

Schmorl's Node: A break in the vertebral end plate which causes a portion of the disc to protrude into the vertebral body. It may be traumatic in origin or degenerative in nature. It can be associated with Scheuermann's disease. See Vertebral End Plate Fracture.

Schober's Test: A method to measure true lumbar flexion. With the patient standing, a mark is made on the skin at the lumbosacral junction. Another mark is made 10 cm above this point. The patient then bends forward to touch his or her toes. The distance between the two points is measured. Normally, the measurement is greater than 15 cm.

SCI: An abbreviation for *spinal cord injury.*

Sciatica: A general term which is more accurately and specifically described by the term radiculopathy (pinched nerve in the spine). This is a clinical syndrome associated with an HNP (herniated disc) causing nerve root irritation and neurologic findings such as motor weakness or decreased sensation in a dermatomal distribution. (Numbness or tingling in specific areas of the skin that correspond to nerve roots. For instance, if the big toe is numb, this is usually associated with the L5 nerve root.)

Sciatic Foramen: One of two foramina formed by the sacrotuberous and sacrospinous ligaments in the sciatic notch. There is a greater and lesser sciatic foramen.

Sciatic Nerve: The major nerve supplying motor and sensory functions to the lower extremity. This is the largest peripheral nerve in the body. This later divides to form the tibial and peroneal nerve. It arises from the L4, L5, and S1–S3 nerve roots. It emerges from the lumbar spine and sacrum into the gluteal region through the sciatic notch.

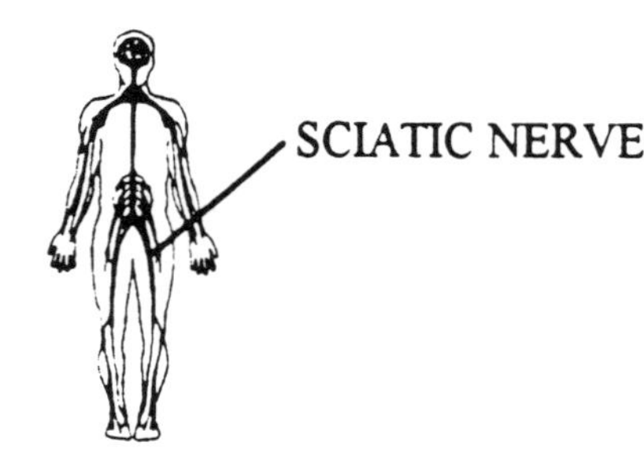

Sciatic NMEPs: A type of neurogenic motor evoked potential in which the sciatic nerve is stimulated.

Sciatic Notch: A notch between the sacrum and the ilium. The sciatic nerve travels through this notch. This is a common point of palpation on physical exam for sciatic irritation. See Sacral Sciatic Notch.

Sciatic Phenomenon: A physical exam maneuver. See Crossed Straight-Leg Raising Test.

Sciatic Stress Test: Any one of a number of physical exam tests designed to stretch the sciatic nerve. All of these tests are graded as positive if radiating pain or numbness in a nerve distribution occurs. The most common of these would be a straight-leg raising maneuver. All of these tests would be positive in a radiculopathy or HNP.

Scipp Line: The line passing from the sacrococcygeal joint to the inferior point of the pubic bone on a lateral radiograph. See Sacral Cococcygeal Pubic Line, Sacrococcygeal Pubic Line.

SCJ: The joint between the upper lateral portion of the sternum and the clavicle (breast bone and collar bone). See Sternoclavicular Joint.

SC Joint: The joint between the upper lateral portion of the sternum and the clavicle (breast bone and collar bone). See Sternoclavicular Joint.

Scleromate: A mixture of the sodium salts of cod liver oil used for prolotherapy or sclerotherapy. This drug has been demonstrated to increase collagen deposition, and it is approved for use by the FDA for the obliteration of varicose veins. Caution should be used when injecting this agent, because it is possible to induce thrombosis if a vein is encountered. It is contraindicated in patients with uncontrolled diabetes mellitus, thyrotoxicosis, tuberculosis, asthma, sepsis, or blood dyscrasias and in bedridden patients. The drug is supplied in 30-ml multiple-use vials. See Morrhuate Sodium Injection.

Sclerosant Injection: This term was used by Cyriax. See Prolotherapy, Sclerotherapy.

Sclerosis: An increase in the density of bone usually due to an increase in mechanical loading. See Eburnation.

Sclerosis—Vertebral Body: Increased density within the vertebral body adjacent to the site of disc narrowing. This can be confused with neoplasm. See Vertebral Body Sclerosis.

Sclerotomal Pain: Bony pain that refers to other sites in a specific distribution. See Splanchnic Pain.

SCM: An anterior neck muscle which originates from the sternum and clavicle (two heads) and inserts on the mastoid process of the skull. See Sternocleidomastoid Muscle.

Scoliometer: An inclinometer used to measure trunk asymmetry or axial trunk rotation in forward bending. This is used for the screening and assessing the progression of scoliosis.

Scoliometry: A technique for measuring the degree of scoliosis or lateral curvature of the spine. This quantifies the deformity of the rib cage associated with axial rotation of the vertebrae. The differences from side to side are measured in millimeters or in degrees of deformity. Usually, a large bubble goniometer, which is known as a scoliometer, is used. This measures the degree of scoliosis based on the amount of posterior rib hump.

Scoliosis: An abnormal curvature and/or rotation of the spine. Most of the scoliosis seen clinically is idiopathic. Scoliosis can also be caused by neuromuscular diseases such as muscular dystrophy. Since this is a common finding in the thoracic spine, the shape of the rib cage is also altered, decreasing pulmonary function in severe cases. A Cobb angle is commonly used to measure scoliosis on x-rays. Muscle fatigue and ligamentous strain can develop on the convex side of the curve, while nerve root irritation can develop on the side of the concavity. There are usually tight structures on the concave side of the curve and weak structures on the convex side of the curve. See Scoliosis—Congenital, Scoliosis—Decompensated, Scoliosis—Functional, Scoliosis—S-curve, Scoliosis—Structural, Lordoscoliosis, Structural Curve.

Scoliosis—Congenital: A structural scoliosis caused by an anomalous or malformed vertebra. See Congenital Scoliosis.

Scoliosis—Decompensated: When the angle of the compensatory scoliotic curve does not equal the angle of the major curve the scoliosis is termed decompensated. See Decompensated Scoliosis.

Scoliosis—Functional: A reversible scoliosis of the spine which is not caused by bony changes. See Functional Scoliosis.

Scoliosis—S-curve: A type of scoliosis which involves a major curve and a compensatory curve. See S-curve Scoliosis.

Scoliosis—Structural: An irreversible curvature of the spine with bony changes and a fixed rotation of the vertebrae. See Structural Scoliosis.

Scoliotic Index: A complex multifaceted measurement of scoliosis with multiple points taken along the scoliotic curve. A scoliotic index of 0 is normal while numbers greater than 0 are present in scoliosis.

Scopolamine Patch: A transdermal patch delivery system which is designed for continuous release of scopolamine. See Transderm Scōp.

Scottie Dog Sign: A radiographic sign of spondylolysis or spondylolisthesis. On oblique x-rays of the spine, the posterior elements take the outline of a Scottish terrier. The nose of the dog is the transverse process, the ear is the superior articular process, the neck is the pars interarticularis, the leg is the inferior articular facet, the eye is the pedicle seen end on, and the body is the lamina. In spondylolysis, the Scottie dog appears as if wearing a collar. In spondylolisthesis, the Scottie dog appears to be decapitated. This is due to defects in the pars interarticularis, which is seen as the Scottie dog's neck. See Pars Interarticularis Defect, Collar Sign, Obliques.

Screen: A quick physical exam. See Screening Exam.

Screening Exam: A quick physical exam to look for easily identifiable pathology or to guide a more detailed exam. See Screen.

SCS: An electrical device implanted near the spinal cord with leads that stimulate the dura to block intractable chronic pain. See Epidural Stimulator, Spinal Cord Stimulation.

S-curve Scoliosis: A type of scoliosis which involves a major curve and a compensatory curve. This is the most common form of idiopathic scoliosis. It is usually a right thoracic curve and a left lumbar curve and involves structural changes in the vertebrae of the major curve. See Scoliosis—S-curve, Scoliosis.

Seat Belt Fracture: A fracture of the thoracolumbar spine which is caused by a flexion-distraction force. The fracture can result from an MVA in which the patient was wearing an old style lap belt. See Chance Fracture, Lap Seat Belt Fracture, Lap Belt Injury.

Seated Flexion Test: A physical maneuver for SI hypomobility. See Seated Forward Flexion Test.

Seated Forward Flexion Test: A physical maneuver for SI hypomobility. The patient is seated on a stool with feet supported. The examiner places the thumb pads beneath the PSISs bilaterally. The upper excursion of the PSIS is monitored as the patient bends forward with hands between knees. The side that presents with the greatest upper excursion or that moves first is positive for hypomobility. It should be noted that a forward sacral torsion will show a positive finding on the opposite side. Backward sacral torsions will show a positive finding on the same side as the direction of the torsion. See Sitting Flexion Test.

Seated Hamstring Stretch: A physical therapy stretch. The patient is seated, and the leg to be stretched is straight while the opposite knee is flexed with the foot tucked into the groin. The patient reaches down toward the straight leg until a stretch is felt in the hamstring area. Another variation of this excercise is with the patient sitting over the edge of a table and extending the knee of the leg to be stretched while maintaining the lumbar spine in a neutral or extended position.

Seated Low Back Stretch: A physical therapy stretch. The patient is seated, and the knees are spread apart while the patient bends toward the floor. A comfortable stretch can be felt in the lumbar and gluteal area. This excercise is also used to stretch the gluteus maximus.

Seated Straight-Leg Raising Test: A physical examination maneuver. See Lasegue Sitting Test.

Secondary Basilar Impression: An acquired basilar impression. This is associated with diseases which cause softening of the bone such as Paget's disease, osteomalacia, and fibrous dysplasia. See Basilar Impression.

Secondary Gain: An external gain which arises from an illness and perpetuates an illness. The illness can secure monetary gain or attention for the patient.

Secondary Osteosarcoma: A malignant tumor of the spine which usually occurs secondarily in Paget's disease or previously irradiated bone. Patients usually present with sarcoma in their 40s or 50s while those with Paget's sarcoma are usually in their 60s. This group consists of approximately one-third of the osteosarcomas. These tumors are rapidly progressive, producing extensive bony destruction and metastasizing early. In Paget's disease, long-term survival is less than 5%. The tumors that occur usually occur in patients who have received more than 5,000 rads, and a majority of these patients were originally radiated for nonosseous disease such as Hodgkin's lymphoma or breast cancer. Survival in postradiation tumors is slightly better than Paget's disease, with a 5-year survival of approximately 17%. There can sometimes be a long latency period of years between irradiation and presentation of the tumor.

Secondary Trigger Point: A trigger point that occurs due to muscle overload. As the synergist becomes weak, the muscle containing the secondary trigger point compensates and becomes overloaded.

Sedentary Work: A NIOSH work category with lifts up to 10 pounds. Most of the job is spent sitting, but there are aspects which involve occasional walking and standing.

Sed Rate: A laboratory blood test that measures the approximate amount of inflammation in the body. See ESR.

Segmental Dysfunction: A term used by chiropractors, osteopathic physicians, or manual physical therapists to describe a spinal segment which is not positioned or moving correctly.

Segmental Instability: Motion of a spinal segment which exceeds normal physiologic range of motion for that segment. This may occur secondary to degenerative disc disease, spondylosis, or trauma. This usually refers to degenerative disease but can also be used to describe gross instability after trauma. Lumbar fusions are often performed to stabilize the unstable spinal segments. It is believed that segmental instability can lead to hypertrophied facet joints and spondylosis, which can cause foraminal stenosis and central canal stenosis. See Degenerative Disc Disease, Spinal Instability.

Segmental Spinal Instrumentation: Any of a number of spinal implants, such as cables, wires, steel rods, rods and hooks, and pedicle instrumentation, that have points of fixation at multiple spinal segments. See SSI.

Segmental Wiring: A wiring system used to add further stability to a hook-rod construct which spans many motion segments. This may be used in the management of scoliosis, trauma, or tumors. There is a small risk of dural or cord injury since these wires encircle the lamina. See Harrington Rods.

Selective Nerve Root Block: Injection of corticosteroid (anti-inflammatories) and local anesthetic onto the nerve root sleeve surrounding a nerve root. This is usually done as a treatment for radiculopathy of that specific nerve root or as a diagnostic procedure to determine if that nerve root is causing symptoms. In a recent series, approximately 20% of patients had long-term (greater than 3 months) pain relief. Since the injection is into to the epidural space, other areas are also bathed in the solution injected as it migrates through this space.

Self-mobilization: A technique by which the patient is taught to perform joint mobilizations on restricted joints using gliding techniques. The patient performs these mobilizations on him- or herself through the use of positioning or special equipment.

Semicircular Canals: Three circular structures that are part of the labyrinth of the inner ear. They are oriented in three different planes (x-, y-, and z-axes). They are important in maintaining balance and equilibrium. It is thought that this system is integrated with the proprioceptive ability of the head and neck complex.

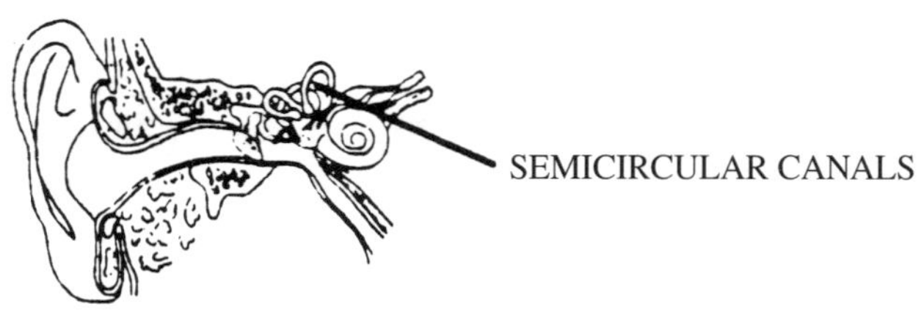

Senile Ankylosis: A joint which has been completely fused due to natural aging. In the spine, a common example would be the SI joint.

Senile Kyphosis: A degenerative disease of the spine which is usually equated with the normal aging process. See Spondylosis.

Sensorcaine: An amino amide anesthetic. See Bupivacaine.

Sensory Deficit: A decrease in sensation noted on physical exam. This can be associated with a radiculopathy (pinched nerve in spine) or other disorders such as thoracic outlet syndrome.

SEP: A diagnostic technique used to detect a sensory radiculopathy or significant myelopathy. See Somatosensory Evoked Potentials.

Sequestered Disc: Material from the nucleus pulposus which is outside of the disc and separated from the disc. This is synonymous with a free fragment or free nuclear material. Sequestered discs can often be missed on imaging studies. See Disc Sequestration, Free Fragment.

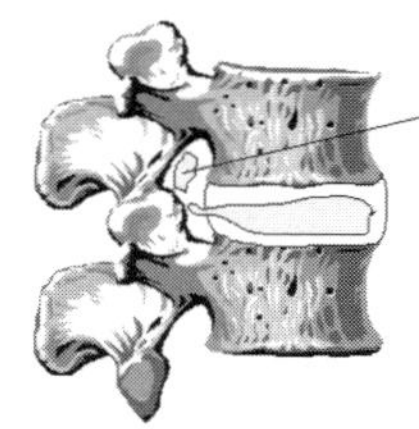

Ser. ant.: An abbreviation for *serratus anterior.*

Serapin: A volatile sodium salt of pitcher plant extract that is sometimes used in trigger point injections. It is thought that this is a longer-acting agent than anesthetic alone.

Seronegative Arthropathy: An arthritic condition with a negative rheumatoid factor. Examples would include psoriatic arthritis, Reiter's syndrome, ankylosing spondylitis, Behçet's syndrome, and enteropathic arthritis.

Seronegative Spondyloarthropathies: A varied group of arthritic conditions with a predilection for spinal and SI joint involvement which are associated with a negative rheumatoid factor. This includes ankylosing spondylitis, psoriatic arthritis, and Reiter's syndrome.

Sertraline Hydrochloride: An antidepressant in the SSRI (selective serotonin reuptake inhibitor) class. See Zoloft.

sev: An abbreviation for *severe.*

SF: An abbreviation for *spinal fluid.*

SGIS: An abbreviation for *side glide in standing.* A physical therapy test maneuver attributed to McKenzie which is used to reproduce the combined movements of lateral bending and rotation to one side. One hand is placed on the patient's shoulders while the other hand is placed on the opposite iliac crest. The patient is pushed by the shoulder into a side glide to one direction and then the other. The patient's characteristic pain is observed during these maneuvers for centralization or peripheralization. This maneuver can also be used by the patient for treatment. See Side Glide in Standing.

Sharpey's Fibers: The portion of the outer annulus that attaches to the vertebral body.

Sharp-Pursor Test: A physical exam test for the integrity of the transverse ligament and for the evaluation of atlantoaxial instability. The patient is seated, and the examiner places the palm of one hand on the patient's forehead and the thumb of the other hand on the atlas (space between the occiput and C2). As the patient slowly flexes the neck, the examiner presses backward on the forehead and checks for a backward sliding motion of the head. A positive test is an abrupt shift forward and can be associated with a palpable clunk. Cord signs or nausea also denote a positive test. See Atlantoaxial Subluxation.

Sharp Wave: An EMG finding which corresponds to partial or complete loss of nerve supply to a given muscle. This finding found across several muscles can then be traced to a single nerve root in a radiculopathy. Sharp waves can also be associated with primary muscular pathology. See EMG/NCS.

Shear: An osteopathic or manual physical therapy term that refers to movement of the ilium in relation to the sacrum. The displacement of the ilium is in one of the following planes: anterior, posterior, superior, and inferior. For instance, an inferior innominate shear describes an innominate which moves more freely in an inferior direction than in the superior direction. In some circles, the term is used to describe abnormalities in the pubic bones and anterior/posterior ilium movement.

Shiatsu: A style of acupressure that stimulates points along meridians and focuses on balancing *chi.* See Acupuncture, Acupressure, Ischemic Compression.

Shiny Corner Sign: An x-ray sign in ankylosing spondylitis. A dense reactive sclerosis at the vertebral body margins occurs just prior to syndesmophyte formation. This disappears once interbody fusion occurs. This appears as a "shiny corner" of the vertebral body. See Romanus Lesion.

Shiny Odontoid Sign: An x-ray sign which implies upper cervical involvement in ankylosing spondylitis. There is increased density of the odontoid, often with erosions. Transverse ligament laxity should be ruled out by measuring the atlanto-dental interspace on flexion films. See Atlanto-dental Interspace.

Shoe Lift: An orthotic to correct a short leg, which can sometimes cause back pain. These can be custom-molded out of several different soft or hard materials. Temporary shoe lifts are also used in clinic. See Functional Leg Length Discrepancy, Structural Leg Length Discrepancy, Heel Lift, In-shoe Lift.

Short Leg Syndrome: A difference in length between the lower extremities. See Leg Length Discrepancy.

Short Lever Thrust: A chiropractic treatment technique which involves a direct thrust of the spinal segment to restore normal anatomic motion. This is a direct technique.

Short Tau Inversion Recovery: An MR imaging technique. See STIR Image.

Shotgun SI Treatment: A nonspecific treatment for SI joint dysfunction. See Symphysis Pubis Shotgun Method.

Shotgun Treatment: A nonspecific treatment for SI joint dysfunction. See Symphysis Pubis Shotgun Method.

Shoulder Abduction Test: A physical exam test for a nerve root syndrome. The patient is asked to abduct and externally rotate the ipsilateral shoulder by moving the hand toward the head then placing the hand on top of the head. If this position relieves radicular pain, it is considered a positive sign for a nerve root syndrome. See Bakody Sign.

Shoulder Bursitis: Compression of the supraspinatus and subacromial bursa beneath the coracoacromial arch. See Impingement Syndrome.

Shoulder Depression Test: A physical exam maneuver used to detect radiculitis. The patient is seated with the head and neck in neutral position. One hand is placed on the parietal region of the skull, and the other hand is placed over the ipsilateral shoulder. The examiner depresses the shoulder while flexing the head. The head then is slowly moved toward the opposite shoulder. Reproduction of radicular or dural complaints is a positive test.

Shoulder Drop: A chiropractic adjusting technique. See Shoulder Drop Adjustment.

Shoulder Drop Adjustment: A chiropractic adjusting technique in which the upper part of the body drops from the knees. The arms are held straight and locked at the elbows. The upper trunk is dropped. See Shoulder Drop Method, Shoulder Drop.

Shoulder Drop Method: A chiropractic adjusting technique. See Shoulder Drop Adjustment.

Shoulder-Hand Syndrome: A clinical syndrome characterized by the presence of pain out of proportion to the severity of the injury. See Reflex Sympathetic Dystrophy.

Shoulder to Overhead: A type of lift tested during a functional capacity evaluation. The patient is asked to lift above the shoulder.

SHPL: A chiropractic x-ray analysis technique. Two dots are placed at the superior portion of the sacrum at the junction of the sacral facet and the alae. A line is then drawn to connect these two dots. This is reported to illustrate whether the sacral base is level or misaligned. See Sacral Horizontal Plane Line.

SHR: A deep tendon reflex. See Scapulohumeral Reflex.

SHx: An abbreviation for *social history*.

SI Arthrodesis: A surgical procedure. See SI Joint Fusion, Sacroiliac Arthrodesis, Fusion—SI Joint, Sacroiliac Fusion.

SI Belt: A pelvic belt used in SI joint syndrome where hypermobility is suspected. The belt is used to "lock-in" the SI joints. There are many different types of SI belts. The belt usually encircles the pelvis at the level of the iliac wings putting additional pressure over the sacrum with the use of a sacral pad. See Lumbopelvic Support, Pelvic Belt.

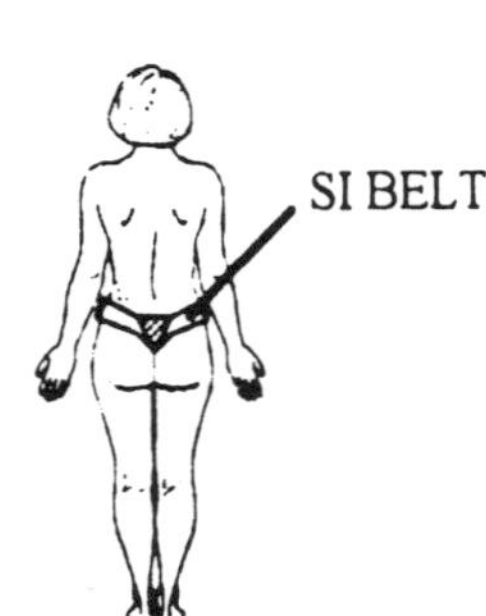

Sicard Sign: A physical exam test for sciatica. The patient is supine and asked to raise the extended leg to the point just short of producing pain or radiating symptoms. In a positive test, dorsiflexion of the big toe elicits sciatic pain.

Sick Headache: A migraine headache without the prodrome (symptoms which occur prior to migraine). See Common Migraine, Migraine without Aura.

Side Bending: Bending to the right or left. This is movement in the coronal plane. In the spine, side bending is coupled with rotation (when the spine bends to one side, it also rotates). See Lateral Flexion, Lateroflexion, Flexion Right, Flexion Left.

Side Bent: Referring to a segment in which side bending has occurred. For instance, in a vertebral segment which is side bent right, the right superior corner is lateral and the right inferior corner is medial.

Side Bent Sacrum: An osteopathic or manual physical therapy term which refers to a sacrum in which the base is pointing to the left or to the right. This is synonymous with a unilateral sacral flexion or a unilateral sacral extension.

Side Flexion: Bending to the right or left. See Lateral Bending.

Side Glide: A lateral translation of the spine. The spine is pushed laterally and not allowed into side bending. This stimulates the combined movements of lateral bending and rotation to one side. See Translatory Gliding Motion.

Side Glide in Standing: A physical therapy test maneuver. See SGIS.

Side Posture Push Adjustment: A common type of chiropractic manipulation to correct an SI dysfunction.

Sidely Slump: A physical exam maneuver. See PKB, Slump Test.

SI Dysfunction: A biomechanical abnormality which is intrinsic to the SI joint(s) and alters normal movement (or viscoelasticity) within the SI joint(s). This can be differentiated from an SI joint syndrome by the fact that pain does not need to be present with an SI dysfunction. This change in joint mechanics can cause overload of other structures. For instance, after a traumatic rotational injury, the joint can be slightly unstable in the anterior direction (ilium moves too far anteriorly). That leg would be slightly longer, and the ankle would have to pronate to shorten the leg. It is conceivable that once the SI joint heals, the ankle could be the only symptomatic part. See SI Joint Syndrome, Sacroiliac Somatic Dysfunction, Strained Sacroiliac Joint.

SI Joint: The joint between the sacrum and ilium (base of the spine and the back of the hip). There is a variable nerve supply which is not consistent from individual to individual. It is thought that the wide range of segmental innervation of the joint accounts for some of the variability and referred pain patterns seen in SI joint syndrome. This is a synovial joint which gives with movement. See SI Joint Syndrome.

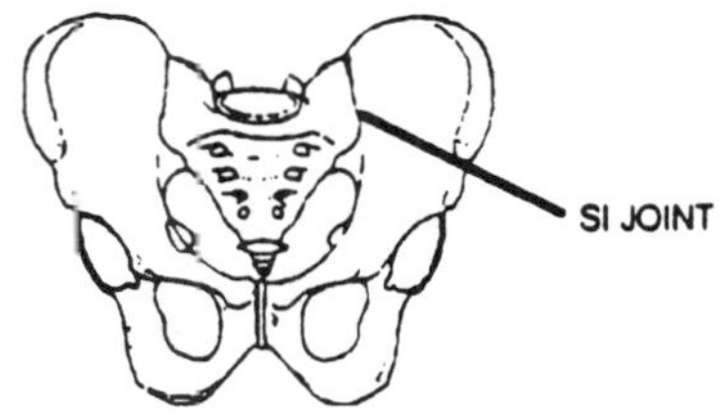

SI Joint Block: See SI Joint Injection.

SI Joint Fusion: A surgical procedure in which the SI joint is fused, usually through the use of instrumentation (screws) and bone grafting. This is considered for severe primary SI joint pain or traumatic SI hypermobility that does not respond to conservative management. This is a surgery of last resort. The SI joint is identified as a pain generator through blocks once all aggressive conservative therapy has failed. There is some controversy as to the long-term effects of this operation because the SI joint is generally considered to have a shock-absorbing role. It is thought that this procedure removes the shock-absorbing ability of the joint. The patient is usually kept non–weight bearing for 2–3 months depending on the progression of the fusion. See SI Arthrodesis, Sacroiliac Arthrodesis, Fusion—SI Joint, Sacroiliac Fusion.

SI Joint Injection: The injection of steroid and anesthetic into the SI joint to reduce pain and inflammation. This is also commonly performed as a diagnostic test to determine if the SI joint is causing pain. Fluoroscopy or CT guidance are used to ensure the accuracy of the injection technique.

SI Joint Syndrome: Pain emanating from the sacroiliac joint(s). There are many symptoms associated with this diagnosis including the possibility of referred pain to the anterior thigh, pain in the SI joint, cracking or popping in the SI joint, and pain or dysfunction in muscles that cross the SI joint and pelvis. Common treatments include lumbar stabilization, muscle energy techniques, Jones strain-counterstrain, joint mobilization (mobs), strengthening, chiropractic manipulation, piriformis injections, SI joint injections, movement retraining, and myofascial release. An SI joint can be either hyper- or hypomobile. Some controversy exists within the medical community as to how much the SI joint actually moves. However, the SI joint is a viscoelastic structure that gives. See SI Dysfunction, Strained Sacroiliac Joint.

SI Ligaments: The ligaments which hold the SI joint together. These include the interosseous, dorsal, sacrotuberous, and sacrospinous ligaments. See Dorsal Sacroiliac Ligament.

Simmon's Procedure: A technique for anterior cervical discectomy and fusion. This differs from Cloward's technique in that a keystone square or rectangular trough is created into which similarly shaped bone graft is inserted. See Gore Procedure.

Simultaneously Combined Anterior and Posterior Fusion: An anterior lumbar fusion with replacement of the excised disc with bone graft while distraction is applied to the intervertebral space. See SCAAPF.

Sinequan: A tricyclic antidepressant often used for chronic pain. This is a sedating antidepressant and is usually given at night to aid sleep. See Doxepin.

Single-coiled Vessel AVM: A type of arteriovenous malformation. See Type 1 AVM.

Single Leg Bridging: A lumbar stabilization exercise. The patient first contracts the abs to stabilize then performs a bridging maneuver by squeezing the buttocks and then straightening one knee. This is more difficult than a routine bridging maneuver and is useful with gluteal strengthening. The exercise is repeated on the opposite side. See Bridging—Single Leg.

Single Photon Absorptiometry: A reliable method for quantifying osteoporosis. See SPA.

Sinuvertebral Block: An injection technique described by Cyriax which is used as a local anesthetic block of the sinuvertebral nerve. Cyriax considered this injection helpful in patients who had failed epidural injection, postlaminectomy patients, patients requiring spinal arthrodesis, or before arthrodesis for planning.

Sinuvertebral Nerve: One of the major nerves of the spine. It emerges from the dorsal root just distal to the dorsal root ganglion. It then merges with the gray rami communicantes or a sympathetic ganglion and pursues a course back into the intervertebral foramen following the blood vessels. The sinuvertebral nerve supplies sensation to the dura, posterior longitudinal ligament, periosteum, blood vessels, and parts of the annulus. In innervating the dura, it forms a mesh-like network. See Recurrent Meningeal Nerve, Von Luschka's Nerve.

SI Shotgun: A nonspecific treatment for SI joint dysfunction. See Symphysis Pubis Shotgun Method.

SI Stabilization Belt: A pelvic belt used in SI joint syndrome where hypermobility is suspected. See SI Belt.

Sitting Flexion Test: A physical exam maneuver for SI hypomobility. See Seated Forward Flexion Test.

Skin Drag: An osteopathic term which refers to a sense of resistance in the skin with light traction. This is thought to be related to the hydration and sympathetic activity in that region.

Skin Rolling: A physical examination technique in which the thumb and index finger are used to grasp the paravertebral skin and roll this tissue from inferior to superior. The ease of displacement of both skin and subcutaneous tissue is evaluated, as are the thickness of the skin and pain manifestations. It is thought that areas of thickness or decreased displacement might indicate an osteopathic lesion at that level. See Kibler-Fold, Pincer Rouler.

Skin Rolling at the Angle of the Mandible: A physical exam maneuver in which a skin fold between the thumb and index finger is formed at the angle of the mandible. Increase in tenderness and/or turgor in this area is thought to be related to problems in the C2–C3 motor unit.

Skull Tongs: A technique for providing traction in which a large tong is inserted into the bones of the skull in order to pull traction on the cervical spine.

sl: An abbreviation for *slight.*

Sleeping Posture: The position of the spine while sleeping. The use of special cervical pillows or rolls has been advocated to keep the cervical spine in a neutral position. Also, some practitioners advocate that patients sleep with a pillow between the legs and with hips and knees in a flexed position. Body rolls are also used. The sleeping posture recommended depends on the presenting condition.

Slice Fracture: A "three-column" fracture in the lumbar spine produced by a flexion-rotation injury. The fracture line is through the upper border of the vertebral body, which extends into the articular process of the vertebra above. This is an unstable fracture.

Slip Angle: A radiographic method for quantifying spondylolisthesis. An angle is formed by lines drawn parallel to the inferior aspect of the L5 vertebral body and parallel to the sacral base. Obviously, a higher angle indicates more severe spondylolisthesis.

Slip Angle Percentage: This is similar to the grading method for spondylolisthesis used by Taillard. Rather than grade 1 through 4, the percentage of slip (0–100%) is used. This is determined by comparing the distance the vertebra is displaced relative to the adjacent vertebral body.

Slipped Disc: A herniated or extruded disc. The term "slipped disc" is actually not correct because there is nothing to slip out of place. Instead, the disc is like a gel-filled, tough, fibrous sack that gets a hole in it, causing the toothpaste-like gel to squirt out, or herniate. This can cause pressure on the exiting nerve root and/or cause a significant inflammatory reaction that can lead to radiculopathy (dysfunction of the nerve root that can cause weakness, numbness, and/or tingling in one extremity). See HNP, Herniated Disc.

SLP: An abbreviation for *short leg, prone.*

SLR: A physical exam maneuver which tests for nerve irritation and for radiculopathy. A positive test is when the patient's lower extremity becomes numb or tingles in a specific root distribution when the extended leg is raised in the supine position. A similar maneuver is often used by physical therapists to check for hamstring length and not radiculopathy. This test can also be used in conjunction with other dural tension signs. See Straight-Leg Raising, Straight-Leg Raise, Lasegue Test.

SLS: An abbreviation for *short leg, supine.*

Slump LS: A slump test where the tension in the nervous system from the legs and lower trunk is taken up first. See Slump Test, Slump Test in Long Sitting.

Slump Test: A physical exam maneuver to test for dural irritation or tension. The patient sits on the edge of a table and slumps forward. The examiner then places pressure on the patient's shoulders and pushes the head forward. Overpressure is applied to the head and cervical spine. The examiner then extends the patient's knee and dorsiflexes the foot. In a positive test the patient extends the head or experiences symptoms. This test is graded in many ways by different practitioners. Some would say that an increase in patient symptoms indicates increased dural irritation. Others would grade this test positive for dural tension if there is an opposite relationship between neck flexion and knee extension. For instance, if the knee is extended and the patient must extend the neck to decrease symptoms, the test would be positive. See Braggard's Sign, Deyerle Sciatic Tension Test, Femoral Nerve Traction Test.

Slump Test in Long Sitting: A slump test where the tension in the nervous system from the legs and lower trunk is taken up first. See Slump LS.

Small Sensory Nerve Evoked Potentials: A diagnostic technique. See SSEP.

SMT: An abbreviation for *spinal manipulative therapy.*

Snapping Hip: A condition that produces an audible click or a palpable snap with hip flexion and extension (primarily with walking). This may be painful and is more frequent in females. A chronic bursitis either of the trochanteric bursa or of the iliopsoas bursa can cause thickening of the bursal walls. This can also be caused by tightness in the iliotibial band or spasm in the tensor fasciae latae. This can be confused with an SI joint syndrome. Common treatments include stretching of the ITB, muscle balancing, ice, anti-inflammatory medications, injections of corticosteroids, iontophoresis, or surgical release.

Snapping Palpation: An examination technique which involves suddenly rolling the taut band of a trigger point underneath the fingers at right angles to the muscle fiber. The motion is said to be similar to plucking guitar strings. This is done to elicit a local twitch response.

Snook Percentiles: Tables which contain normal lifting and grip strength measurements and percentile ratings. See Snook Tables.

Snook Tables: Tables which contain normal lifting and grip strength measurements and percentile ratings. For example, a patient who can lift 70 pounds in a floor to knuckle lift can be compared with a table of normal values for that amount of weight in that style. The percentage of the population that can lift that amount has been determined so that the patient's ability can be compared. See Snook Percentiles.

SO: An abbreviation for *suboccipital.*

SOAP: An abbreviation for a method of patient assessment: *s*ubjective, *o*bjective, *a*ssessment, *p*lan.

SOB: An abbreviation for *short of breath.*

Soft Cervical Collar: A soft cervical orthosis made of foam rubber covered with fabric which provides little immobilization. This brace is often given to patients with acute whiplash injuries in the emergency room. There likely is some proprioceptive benefit, in that the patient gets pressure feedback with neck motion. Also, some collars may unload some of the weight of the head. See Soft Collar, Soft Neck Brace.

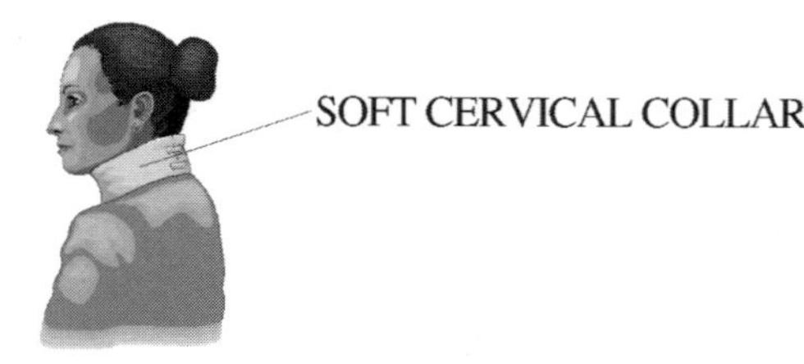

Soft Collar: A soft cervical orthosis. See Soft Cervical Collar.

Soft Disc: A herniated disc without a bone spur. This is in contrast to a hard disc. See Hard Disc, HNP.

Soft Neck Brace: A soft cervical orthosis. See Soft Cervical Collar.

Soft Tissue Approximation: A type of end feel described by Cyriax in which a joint cannot be pushed further because of contact with another part of the body. An example is elbow flexion being limited by contact with the muscle belly of the biceps brachii.

Soft Tissue Injury: A traumatic injury to the muscles, ligaments, or tendons.

Soft Tissue Mobilization: This term encompasses many different types of hands-on soft tissue techniques. See Myofascial Release.

Soft Tissue Window: CT scan image which shows soft tissues more clearly than bony structures.

Soft Tissue Work: A general term for any one of a number of hands-on therapy techniques that are performed to decrese muscle spasm or lengthen tissues. Massage therapy, myofascial release, ischemic compression, myotherapy, spray and stretch, and stretching can all be forms of soft tissue work.

sol.: An abbreviation for *soleus*.

Soleus Stretch: A physical therapy stretch designed to lengthen the soleus. The patient places one leg back and one leg forward and presses against a wall. Both knees are kept bent. The heel to be stretched is on the floor and turned slightly outward. The patient then leans into the wall until a stretch is felt in the gastrocsoleus area.

Solid Fusion: An orthopedic term which refers to a fusion that has healed and is radiographically or clinically stable, providing excellent rigidity to the levels fused.

Solitary Plasmacytoma: One of a continuum of B cell lymphoproliferative diseases which can occur in the spine. This is a rare disease process making up only 3% of all plasma cell neoplasms. Unlike malignant multiple myeloma, which is rapidly progressive and lethal, patients with this disease process may have prolonged survival despite slow eventual progression. This is usually seen as an isolated lesion, and treatment may provide long-term disease-free survival or even cure. There is up to a 60% five-year survival rate. Patients with survival of up to 20 years or more are not uncommon. Treatment of choice is radiation.

Soma: A muscle relaxant which has sedative properties (causes drowsiness). This does not directly relax tense skeletal muscles in humans; instead, most of its muscle relaxant effects are linked to the fact that it is a CNS depressant. The use of this medication is contraindicated in patients with acute intermittent porphyria. The usual adult dosage is 350 mg three times a day and at bedtime. It should be noted that there is a significant CNS depressant effect and that this may be quite severe in some patients. See Carisoprodol.

SOMA: A proprietary name for a gravity-unloading system. The actual name is the Zuni incremental weight-bearing system. See Medical Exercise Therapy, Zuni, Gravity Unloading.

Soma Compound: A muscle relaxant which has sedative properties (causes drowsiness) and contains 200 mg of carisoprodol plus 325 mg of aspirin. Please note that because this contains aspirin, GI side effects are possible. The use of this drug is contraindicated in patients with acute intermittent porphyria or bleeding disorders. There are drug interactions with oral anticoagulants, methotrexate, probenecid and sulfinpyrazone, oral hypoglycemic agents, antacids, ammonium chloride, alcohol, and corticosteroids. The usual adult dosage is one to two tablets four times a day. See Carisoprodol–Aspirin Tablets.

Soma Compound with Codeine: A muscle relaxant with a narcotic additive which has sedative properties (causes drowsiness). This compound contains 200 mg of carisoprodol, 325 mg of aspirin, and 16 mg of codeine phosphate. The usual adult dosage is one to two tablets four times daily. See Soma Compound.

Somasensory Evoked Potentials: An electrical test used to determine the integrity of the sensory pathways in the spinal cord or cauda equina. A sensory signal is applied to a specific area in the lower extremity; this is then recorded from electrodes placed over the cranium. This test can sometimes be helpful when used to identify a spinal stenosis that does not involve the motor pathways or a sensory radiculopathy. See SEP.

Somatic Dysfunction: An osteopathic or manual physical therapy term which is defined as an alteration in the normal kinetic function of a joint or other component of the musculoskeletal system. This is the loss of normal joint biomechanics. Dysfunctions usually occur as a result of forces that exceed the limit of joint tissues. This leads to an alteration in the quality and quantity of movement. Joints can be either hypomobile (not moving enough) or hypermobile (moving too much). They can also move too much in certain directions and not enough in others. See Osteopathic Lesion, Articular Dysfunction, Vertebral Subluxation Complex, Abnormal Spinal Segmental Motion, Joint Blockage, Loss of Joint Play, Positional Fault.

Somatic Lumbar Nerve Block: A local anesthetic block of the lumbar nerve roots as they exit from the foramen outside the epidural space. See Lumbar Nerve Block.

Somatization Disorder: A psychological condition characterized by multiple physical complaints without a clear physical cause which leads to multiple interactions with the medical system over a number of years. Common complaints can include back pain, palpitations, dizziness, pseudoneurologic symptoms, dysmenorrhea, and GI symptoms.

Somatoform Disorder: An older term which represents a number of different psychological problems and disorders which are characterized by the presence of pain or symptoms which have no physical cause. See Symptom Magnification Syndrome, Chronic Pain Syndrome, Somatoform Pain Disorder.

Somatoform Pain Disorder: An older term which represents a number of different psychological problems and disorders which are characterized by the presence of pain or symptoms which have no physical cause. This is different from malingering in that this is an unconscious deception. See Symptom Magnification Syndrome, Chronic Pain Syndrome, Somatoform Disorder.

Somatosensory Evoked Potentials: A diagnostic technique used commonly to detect a sensory radiculopathy or significant myelopathy. See SSEP, Large Mixed Nerve SEP.

SOMI Collar: A type of hard cervical/thoracic orthosis commonly used for rigid cervical immobilization. See Sternal Occipital Mandibular Immobilizer.

SOT: A chiropractic technique that incorporates wedge-shaped blocks in conjunction with a pumping motion to make sacral corrections. The idea behind this technique is to restore normal cerebral spinal fluid flow and to improve "spinal integrity." Sustained manual traction is also used. This technique is used by approximately 40% of the chiropractors in the U.S. See Sacral Occipital Technique, Nonforce Technique.

Soto Hall Test: A physical exam test in which the chin is brought to the chest to screen for dural irritation. Pain or numbness created in the spine is considered to be a positive test and may mean there is dural irritation at that level. See Adverse Neural Tension, Dejerine's Triad, Lindner's Sign.

SP: An abbreviation for *spine* or *spinous*.

sp: An abbreviation for *spinous process*.

SPA: A reliable method for quantifying osteoporosis. See Single Photon Absorptiometry.

Spasm: Increased local muscle tone due to irritation. An involuntary, sustained contraction of a muscle. See Localized Hypertonus, Muscle Spasm.

Spasmodic Torticollis: An abnormal neck posture due to the repetitive, clonic (spasmodic), and tonic (sustained) head movement. See Cervical Dystonia.

SPECT: An abbreviation for *single photon emission computed tomography*.

Sphincter Reflex: A physical exam maneuver which tests the integrity of the cauda equina. See Anal Wink.

Sphinx Position: An osteopathic manual medicine term which refers to a patient in the prone position with the elbows bent and the chin resting in the hands. This is used to look for type 2 FRS lesions in the spine.

Spin: Intrinsic joint movements around an axis perpendicular to the joint surface.

Spina Bifida: A congenital defect of the spinal column in which the neural arch fails to fuse resulting in a hole in the back of the vertebra that leaves the spinal cord and/or nerves exposed. This is usually associated with developmental defects of the spinal cord or meninges, which can cause disabling paralysis and/or bowel and bladder dysfunction. These patients are at a high risk of developing scoliosis. Protrusion of the neural elements through the defect is also possible. See Spina Bifida Occulta, Meningocele, Myelomeningocele, Rachischisis, Spinal Dysraphism, Spina Bifida Vera, Spina Bifida Manifesta.

Spina Bifida Manifesta: A congenital defect of the spinal column in which the neural arch fails to fuse. See Spina Bifida, Spina Bifida Occulta.

Spina Bifida Occulta: A very common congenital defect which involves a failure of the laminae to fuse leaving a defect in the neural arch without protrusion of the neural elements and without an external pouch or cyst. Unlike other forms of spina bifida, there is usually no damage or problem with the nervous system. Also, the spinal cord and/or nerves do not push out into a cyst. This is usually asymptomatic but is picked up on AP radiographs. There is no association with low back pain. Occasionally, there is a skin dimple, meningioma, or tuft of hair overlying this defect. This defect is much more common in males and occurs most commonly at L5 and S1. See Spina Bifida Vera, Spina Bifida Manifesta, Spina Bifida.

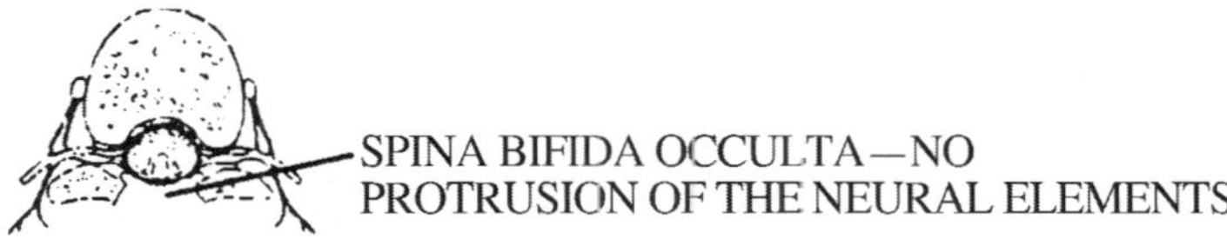

Spina Bifida Vera: A congenital defect of the spinal column in which the neural arch fails to fuse. See Spina Bifida.

Spinal: Medical slang for an epidural injection. See Epidural Steroid Injection.

Spinal Accessory Nerve: The eleventh cranial nerve.

Spinal Anesthesia: An injection of anesthetic or steroid into the epidural space. See Epidural Steroid Injection.

Spinal Arthrodesis: A surgical procedure. See Fusion.

Spinal Canal: The bony tunnel that houses the spinal cord and its coverings.

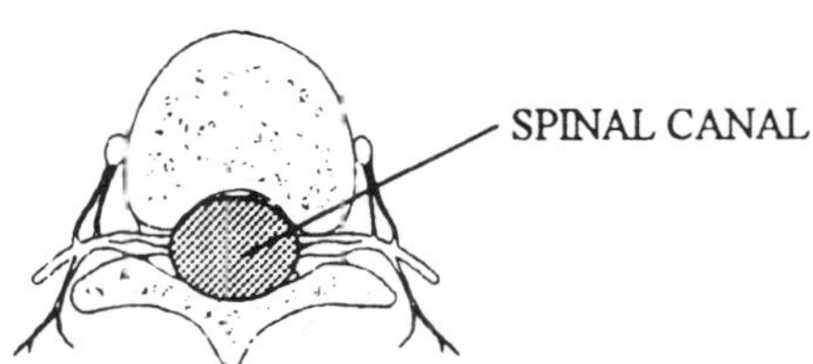

Spinal Claudication: A clinical symptom complex associated with lumbar central canal stenosis. See Neurogenic Claudication.

Spinal Column: Another name for the vertebral column.

Spinal Cord: The extension of the central nervous system which extends from the brain stem to the cauda equina and is surrounded by the spinal canal. This acts as a conduit for information to and from the brain. Significant spinal cord trauma usually produces paralysis and numbness below the level of the injury. There is a core of gray matter surrounded by white matter. The spinal cord usually ends at L2 and then extends in a horse's-tail configuration known as the cauda equina. The cervical and lumbar segments are larger than the thoracic segments. This corresponds to the increased nerve supply of the upper and lower limbs. There are 8 cervical nerves, 12 thoracic, 5 lumbar, 5 sacral, and 1 coccygeal nerve which exit in pairs. The spinal cord is surrounded by the dura, the arachnoid, and the pia mater.

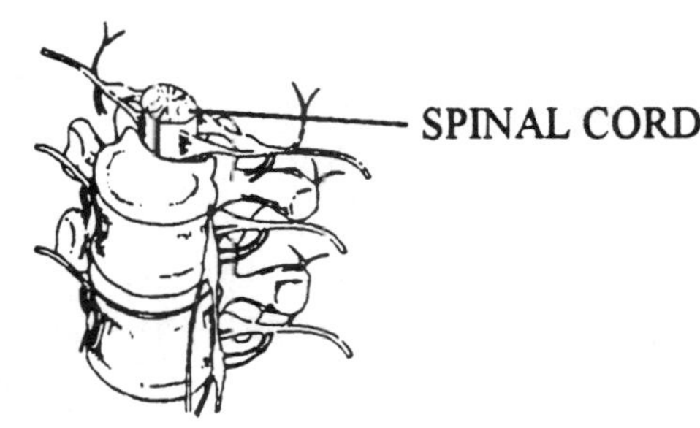

Spinal Cord Stimulation: An electrical device implanted near the spinal cord with leads that stimulate the dura to block intractable chronic pain. See Epidural Stimulator, SCS.

Spinal Cord Syndrome: A clinical syndrome that results from an incomplete spinal cord lesion. See

Brown-Sequard Syndrome, Anterior Cervical Cord Syndrome, Posterior Cervical Cord Syndrome, Central Spinal Cord Syndrome.

Spinal Dysraphism: A group of disorders which includes meningocele, myelomeningocele, and rachischisis. See Myelodysplasia, Spina Bifida.

Spinal Function Sort: A type of West tool sort. Physical tasks that use the spine are sorted by the patient into categories. See West Tool Sort.

Spinal Fusion: A surgical procedure performed to eliminate movement over painful or unstable spinal segments. Spinal fusion is often used to treat degenerative disc disease but is also used to treat scoliosis, kyphosis, fractures, and tumors. A bone graft is placed across a spinal segment (anterior, posterior, or posterolateral). The graft then grows together with the patient's bone, thus immobilizing that segment. The graft can be an autograft (bone taken from the patient) or an allograft (cadaver bone). The bony graft placed for fusion sometimes does not fuse. Many devices have been designed to aid fusion rates including magnetic stimulators and rigid instrumentation (to hold a section of spine in place to allow it to fuse). Also, posterior fusion rates seem to be lower in smokers. See Fusion, Posterior Fusion.

Spinal Fusion Implant: An electrical stimulator which is implanted at the time of surgery for enhancing the spinal fusion rate (bone growth) after fusion surgery.

Spinal Index: A method for assessing the diameter of the spinal canal on plain x-rays. The distance from the middle portion of the back of the vertebral body to the base of the opposing spinous process is measured on a lateral radiograph. Also, the distance between the pedicles is measured on an AP radiograph. These two values are multiplied together, and this product is compared as a ratio with the product of the anterior–posterior and transverse diameters of the adjacent vertebral body. See Canal–Body Index.

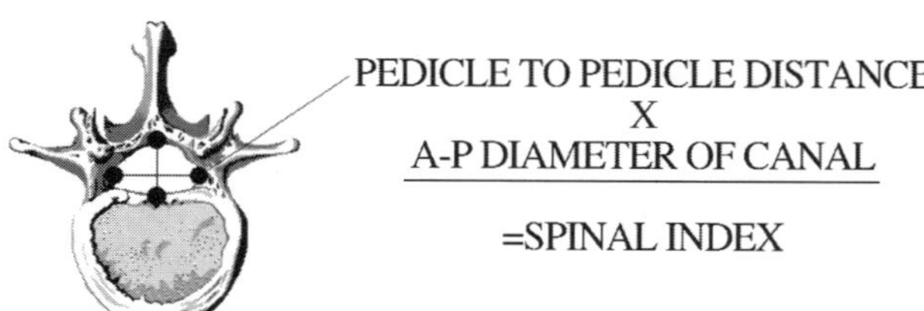

Spinal Instability: Abnormal excess motion in a spinal segment. See Spinal Instability Measurement, Segmental Instability, Van Adderveeken's Measurement of Lumbar Instability.

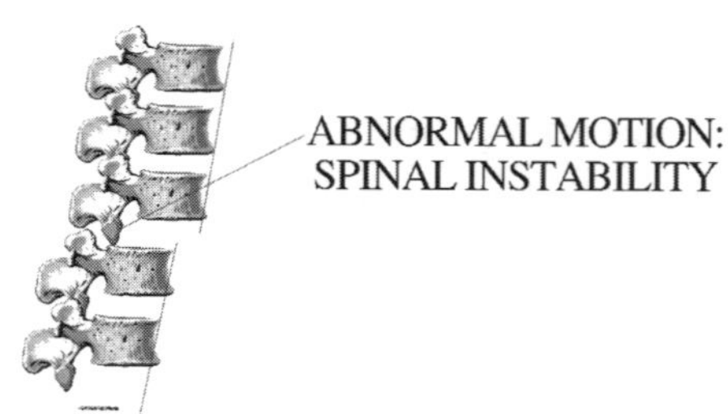

Spinal Instability Measurement: A radiographic method for detecting degenerative or traumatic instability (excess motion beyond normal movement) of the spine. A lateral lumbar view is obtained with flexion and extension views. There are many different measurements described. There is a gross assessment where the alignment of the posterior lumbar bodies is observed at the opposing posterior body corners. A more accurate measurement is horizontal displacement. The degree of "slippage" is measured by drawing lines along the posterior vertebral body margins. To avoid error due to magnification effects, the vertebral body width is also measured at the unstable vertebral body. The distance of the displacement is then divided by this width and multiplied by 100 to get a horizontal displacement percentage. Angular displacement can also be used. A line is drawn along the opposing end plates and the line is allowed to intersect posteriorly or anteriorly. This angle is then measured. See Clinical Instability, Degenerative Instability, Horizontal Displacement.

Spinal Motion Segment: Those structures that compose a functional unit of the spine. This includes two adjacent vertebrae, the intervertebral disc, the facet joints, all the interconnecting ligaments, two intervertebral foramens, and the spinal canal. A given spinal motion segment has specific movements that are allowed. For instance, much more flexion can occur at L5–S1 than can occur at L1–L2. A spinal motion segment is usually named by the vertebra on top followed by the vertebra on the bottom.

Spinal Nerve: One of the 31 pairs of nerves that exit the intervertebral foramina of the spine. The spinal nerves are composed of the dorsal and ventral root.

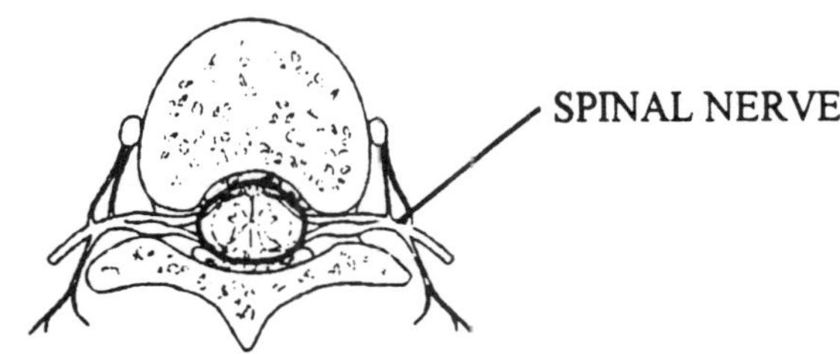

Spinal Nerve Root: A collection of nerve fibers that exits the spinal cord. See Nerve Root.

Spinal Percussion Test: A physical exam maneuver that tests for back sprains. The patient is seated and flexes the cervical spine forward. The examiner then percusses the spinous process of each vertebra either manually or with a reflex hammer. Localized pain is reported to be evidence of a sprain.

Spinal Puncture: The placement of a needle in the subarachnoid space.

Spinal Reflex: Any reflex mediated through the spinal cord without direct participation of the brain or brain stem. For example, a knee jerk, an ankle jerk, or a biceps reflex. See Deep Tendon Reflex.

Spinal Rotatory Manipulation: A side posture manipulation which involves a manipulative thrust into rotation. This is also known as a "million dollar roll." This is a nonspecific long-lever manipulation. See Million Dollar Roll.

Spinal Shock: A clinical syndrome of flaccid paralysis which immediately follows spinal cord trauma. All reflex activity is supressed.

Spinal Stenosis: Narrowing of the canal that contains the spinal cord and cauda equina. See Central Canal Stenosis.

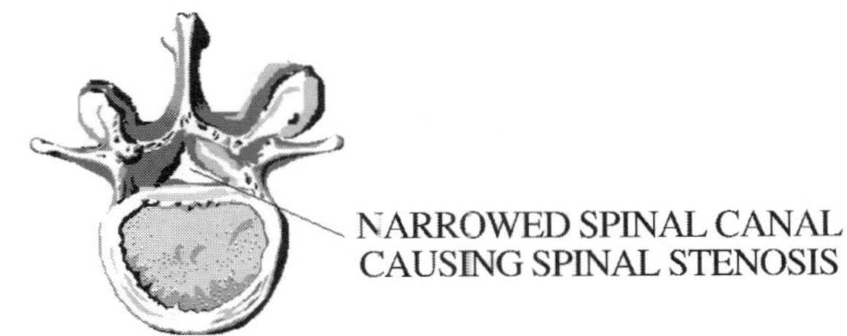

Spinal Stim: A brand name of electromagnetic spinal stimulator.

Spinal Stressology: A chiropractic term which refers to the study of stress in the spinal column and how it affects the function of the body.

Spinal Subluxation: A vertebral segment that does not move freely in all directions. See Fixation.

Spinal Tap: The introduction of a needle into the subarachnoid space for the purpose of sampling CSF for diagnosis, measuring CSF pressure, injecting medications such as anesthetics or steroids, or injecting contrast material such as in a myelogram. See Lumbar Puncture.

Spin Density Film: An MR image which depends on the density of hydrogen nuclei for signal strength. This is an excellent sequence for viewing anatomy. See Proton Density Film, Proton Spin Film.

Spine: The backbone. A bony structure composed of 25 bones which supports the axial skeleton. There are 4 main regions: cervical (neck), thoracic (upper back), lumbar (lower back), and sacral (pelvis and sacrum).

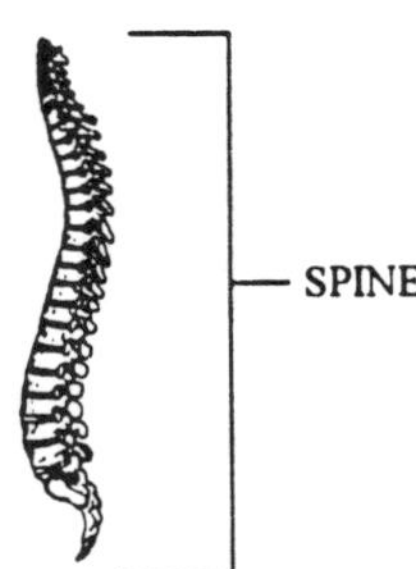

Spine of the Ischium: A protuberance on the posterior border of the body of the ischium that forms the lower border of the sciatic notch. See Ischial Spine.

Spinography: X-ray films which are taken in various positions for the purpose of accessing spinal motion.

Spinolaminar Junction Line: A line drawn on lateral cervical x-rays along the spinolaminar junction. See Posterior Cervical Line.

Spinothalamic Tract: A tract of neurons located anterolaterally in the spinal cord which travel to the VPL area of the thalamus and carry information concerning pain and temperature.

Spinous: A chiropractic term which refers to the spinous process. The position of the "spinous" is often referred to in Gonstead listings.

Spinous PL: A chiropractic listing which refers to a spinous process that is found to be posterior and left of center.

Spinous PLI: A chiropractic listing which refers to a spinous process that is found to be posterior, left of midline, and inferior. See SP PLI, PLI.

Spinous PLS: A chiropractic listing which refers to a spinous process that is found to be posterior, left of midline, and superior. See SP PLS, PLS.

Spinous PR: A chiropractic listing which refers to a spinous process that is found to be posterior and right of center. See SP PR, PR.

Spinous PRI: A chiropractic listing which refers to a spinous process that is found to be posterior, right of midline, and inferior. See SP PRI, PRI.

Spinous Process: A projection of bone which extends from the junction of the two laminae posteriorly (looks like a fin projecting off the back of the vertebra). The spinous processes in the lumbar spine project more posteriorly while in the thoracic spine they project more posteriorly and inferiorly. The spinous processes of the cervical spine can be difficult to palpate. The spinous processes of C2, C7, and T1 are easier to palpate.

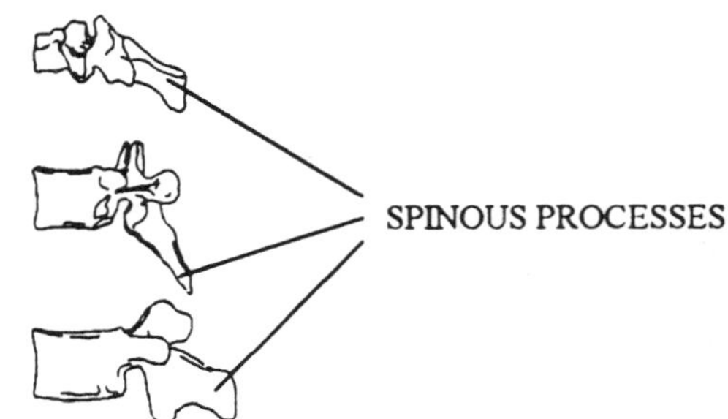

Spinous PRS: A chiropractic listing which refers to a spinous process that is found to be posterior, right of midline, and superior. See SP PRS, PRS.

Spin–Spin Relaxation Time: The same as a T2 relaxation time.

Splanchnic Pain: Visceral pain that is radiating. See Mesodermal Pain, Sclerotomal Pain.

Splinting: A generalized increased muscular tone or spasm that is a protective response to pain.

spondy: An abbreviation for *spondylolisthesis.*

Spondylitic Anteroposterior Diameter: The diameter across the spinal canal from the tip of a posterior osteophyte to the opposing lamina. See SAD, DAD.

Spondylitis: An inflammatory condition of the spine.

Spondylo-: A Latin prefix which means "spine."

Spondyloarthritis: An arthritic condition of the spine.

Spondyloarthropathy: Literally, arthritis of the spine. This is a group of related disorders characterized by a peripheral inflammatory arthritis, inflammation of the sacroiliac joints, diffuse spinal involvement, and sometimes extra-articular features such as uveitis or conjunctivitis. Rheumatoid factor is usually negative. There are also pathologic changes at the attachments of ligaments into bone (entheses). Spondyloarthropathies include ankylosing spondylitis, psoriatic arthropathy, the enteropathic arthropathies, and Reiter's syndrome. Ankylosing spondylitis is the most common of the spondyloarthropathies.

Spondyloarthrosis: Arthrosis of the synovial joints of the spine.

Spondylodiscitis: The extensive erosion of adjacent vertebral end plates in the absence of osteophytes associated with severe rheumatoid arthritis. There is loss of the disc space. This is a painful condition that often causes neurologic deficits and is difficult to distinguish from discitis due to infection. On radiographs, disc space narrowing and vertebral end plate sclerosis are seen without significant osteophytes or evidence of spondylosis. See Rheumatoid Spondylodiscitis.

Spondyloepiphyseal Dysplasia: A bone dysplasia which results from a defect in epiphyseal growth. The vertebra may be malformed. This includes spondyloepiphyseal dysplasia congenita, spondyloepiphyseal dysplasia tarda, and pseudoachondroplastic spondyloepiphyseal dysplasia.

Spondylolisthesis: From "spondy" meaning spine and "listhesis" meaning to slip. This is a "slipped spine" or a spinal segment which has slipped onto another. This movement can be caused by a fracture in the pars interarticularis, degenerated facet joints which override one another (degenerative spondylolisthesis), or by an elongated pars. This condition can also be due to a congenital pars "fracture." Spondylolisthesis is graded type 1 through type 4 with type 1 being the least severe and type 4 being the most severe. Type 1 is usually treated nonoperatively. However, failure of conservative management may require surgical fusion. This diagnosis is not uncommon in children and adolescents as a congenital variant where there is an intrinsic weakness in the pars interarticularis or a dysplastic pars. The most common location is L5 (90%).

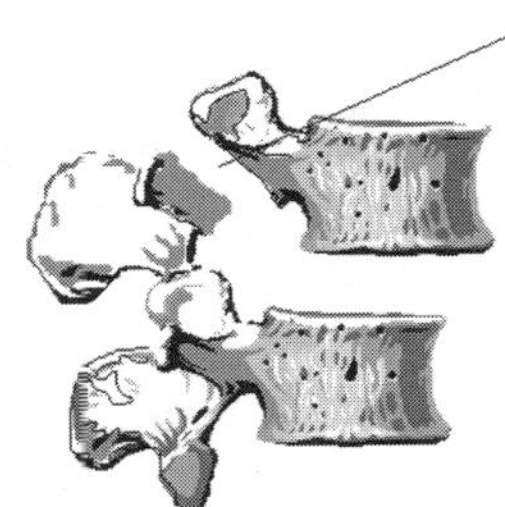

SPONDYLOLISTHESIS—A CRACK IN THE PARS INTERARTICULARIS ALLOWS THE TOP VERTEBRA TO SLIP FORWARD ON THE BOTTOM VERTEBRA.

Spondylolisthesis Acquisita: A stress fracture of the pars interarticularis one level above or below a spinal fusion. This likely occurs due to shunting of biomechanical forces to the pars above and/or below the fused segment. See Postsurgical Spondylolisthesis.

Spondylolisthesis Dysplasia: A congenital spondylolisthesis which occurs in the upper portion of the sacrum or neural arch of L5. There is slippage of L5 anteriorly on S1.

Spondylolisthesis—Isthmic: Spondylolisthesis due to fracture or elongation of the pars interarticularis. See Type II Spondylolisthesis, Isthmic Spondylolisthesis.

Spondylolysis: A defect in the pars interarticularis without slippage of the involved segment. This is similar to some types of spondylolisthesis without the "slip." See Pars Interarticularis Defect, Prespondylolisthesis.

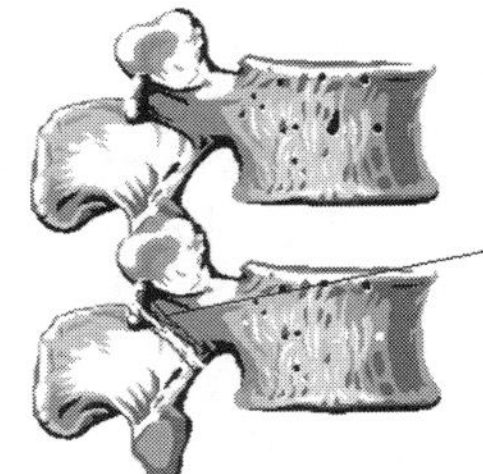

SPONDYLOLYSIS—A CRACKED PARS INTERARTICULARIS WITHOUT SLIPPAGE

Spondylolytis: Another term for ankylosing spondylitis. This is the ICD-9 diagnosis. See Ankylosing Spondylitis.

Spondylopathy: Referring to any disease or condition of the vertebrae.

Spondylophyte: A degenerative spurring (osteophyte) that arises from the vertebral end plate and usually projects somewhat horizontally.

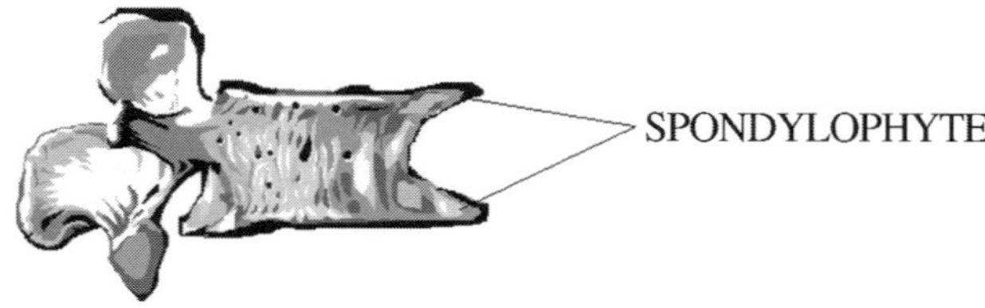

Spondyloptosis: A spondylolisthesis in which the vertebral body of L5 has slipped completely beyond the sacral promontory. This is a grade IV+ spondylolisthesis.

Spondylosis: A degenerative disease of the spine which is usually equated with the normal aging process. Bone spurs are seen on x-ray (osteophytes). On MRI, there is decreased disc height, as well as decreased hydration (loss of water) of the intervertebral discs. It is thought that disc degeneration with microtrauma occurring to the intervertebral disc also occurs. See Degenerative Disc Disease, Osteoarthritis, Senile Kyphosis.

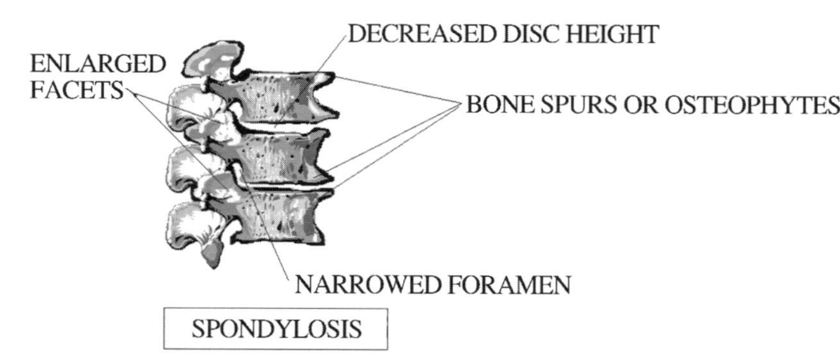

SPONDYLOSIS

Spondylosis—Cervical: A progressive degeneration of the intervertebral discs leading to bony spurring. See Cervical Spondylosis.

Spondylosis Deformans: A defect in the pars interarticularis. See Spondylosis.

Spondylotherapy: A chiropractic technique which involves the therapeutic application of percussion or concussion over the vertebrae to elicit reflex responses at the levels of "neuromeric" innervation.

Spondylotic: Pertaining to spondylosis.

Spondylotic Myelopathy: A compressive myelopathy caused by bony spurring and spondylosis. See Myelopathy, Spondylosis.

Sponge Test: A physical examination maneuver that tests for inflammation. With the patient lying in the prone position, a hot sponge is placed at the superior aspect of the thoracic spine. The sponge is then passed down the spinal column to the lumbosacral area; this is repeated several times. It is reported that pain is felt in locally inflamed areas as the hot sponge passes over that area. It is thought that this pain indicates local acute inflammation.

Spontaneous Potentials: A finding during an EMG exam which denotes denervation. When a muscle loses its nerve supply, the muscle membrane becomes electrically unstable and fires without being prompted. This can be picked up on an EMG screen as fibrillation potentials, fasciculations, or sharp waves (all examples of spontaneous potentials).

Sport Cord: A brand name for rubber surgical tubing which is used as resistance in an exercise program. The cords are color-coded with different colors representing different resistance levels. See Theraband.

SP PL: A chiropractic listing which refers to a spinous process that is found to be posterior and left of center. See PL, Spinous PL.

SP PLI: A chiropractic listing which refers to a spinous process that is found to be posterior, left of midline, and inferior. See PLI, Spinous PLI.

SP PLS: A chiropractic listing which refers to a spinous process that is found to be posterior, left of midline, and superior. See PLS, Spinous PLS.

SP PR: A chiropractic listing which refers to a spinous process that is found to be posterior and right of center. See PR, Spinous PR.

SP PRI: A chiropractic listing which refers to a spinous process that is found to be posterior, right of midline, and inferior. See PRI, Spinous PRI.

SP PRS: A chiropractic listing which refers to a spinous process that is found to be posterior, right of midline, and superior. See PRS, Spinous PRS.

Spr: An abbreviation for *sprain.*

Spray and Stretch: A technique described by Travell and Simons for the treatment of trigger points and tender points within muscle. Fluori-Methane spray (cold) is directed over a trigger point and its referral area while a stretch is applied. This is performed to deactivate the trigger point. See Trigger Point, Fluori-Methane Spray.

Springing: Assessing the mobility of a vertebral segment by PA mobilization. See Spring Test.

Spring Test: A physical exam maneuver used to assess mobility of the joint capsule. Direct pressure is placed over the spinous process or other structure in an anterior direction. The quality and quantity of motion is palpated. These are graded 0 through 6 with 0 being no movement and 6 being unstable.

Spring Testing: Assessing the mobility of a vertebral segment by PA mobilization.

Springy Block: A type of end feel which, according to Cyriax, points to internal derangement of a joint. See End Feel.

Sprung Pelvis: A complete separation of the symphysis pubis and disruption of one or both SI joints. There is usually severe damage to the internal organs of the pelvis such as the bladder. See Open Book Pelvis, Open Book Fracture.

Spurling's Sign: A physical exam maneuver which is used to screen for cervical radiculopathy or foraminal stenosis. The patient's head is traditionally turned to the side of symptoms with extension added to "close off" the foramina. The patient's head is tapped forcefully in the direction of the symptoms (force placed on the vertex of the head) to close off the foramina further. A positive test is electric shock-like pain or numbness that occurs in a dermatomal distribution (in the shoulder or hand). See Jackson Compression Test.

Squaring of the Vertebral Body: A radiographic sign in ankylosing spondylitis. The vertebral bodies appear to be square due to the loss of their normal anterior concavity.

Squats: A physical therapy exercise used to strengthen the quadriceps and gluteal muscles. The patient stands with the knees slightly bent. The knees are then bent slowly to an angle between 30° and 90°. The patient then re-extends the knees while contracting the quadriceps and moves back to an upright position. Proper pelvic positioning during this exercise should be emphasized. See Minisquats, Partial Squats.

Squish Test: A physical exam maneuver which involves placing slow, downward pressure on the anterior ilium on both sides with the patient lying supine. Mobility is assessed side to side. The superior, middle, and lower transverse axes can be accessed. The superior axis tests craniosacral motion, the middle axis tests sacroiliac motion, and the inferior axis tests iliosacral motion. The patient can complain of SI joint pain with this maneuver.

SSEP: A diagnostic technique used commonly to detect a sensory radiculopathy or significant myelopathy. This is also used to monitor the integrity of the dorsal columns during spinal surgery (to let the surgeon know if spinal cord or nerve root damage is occurring). This test is commonly performed in conjunction with EMG/nerve conduction studies. Sensory nerves and mixed nerves, such as the saphenous, superficial peroneal, and sural nerves, are studied in the lower extremities and are thought to reflect L4, L5, and S1 radiculopathies, respectively. These nerves are stimulated and the potentials are picked up as cortical evoked responses. As a control, a sensory nerve action potential is also taken at a site more proximally along the nerve to rule out poor electrode placement. See Dermatomal Somatosensory Evoked Potential, Somatosensory Evoked Potentials.

SSI: Spinal implants. See Segmental Spinal Instrumentation.

SSI: Social Security Insurance. This term is often used to refer to Social Security Disability Insurance.

SSDI: Social Security Disability Insurance.

St: An abbreviation for *strong*.

Stabilization Activities: One of many rehabilitation programs such as pelvic stabilization, lumbar stabilization, and core stabilization. See Dynamic Lumbar Stabilization.

Standing Flexion Test: A physical exam maneuver which screens for SI joint hypomobility. The patient is standing and both PSISs are palpated. The patient is then asked to flex forward while the PSIS motion is monitored bilaterally with the thumbs. If one PSIS rises more than the other, that side is considered to be hypomobile. This test can also be used to determine if a leg length discrepancy is exerting influence on the SI joint.

Standing Posture: The position of the spine while standing. Many different standing postures have been described for different areas of the spine. The most common in the cervical spine would be a forward head position with rounded shoulders implying overload of the cervical extensors and impingement of the lower cervical region. The most common in the thoracic spine would be a kyphotic deformity. In the lumbar spine, many different postural aberrations have been described. These include a swayback, decreased lordosis, increased lordosis, list, and others.

Star Sign: A radiographic sign in ankylosing spondylitis. Calcification of the superior SI ligaments creates a triangular-shaped radiodensity which looks like a three-point star.

Static Intersegmental Subluxation: A chiropractic term which refers to a malposition detected on static testing. This can be either in flexion, extension, lateral flexion, rotation, anterolisthesis, retrolisthesis, lateralisthesis, with altered interosseous spacing, or interosseous foraminal encroachment. See Malposition.

Static Listing: A chiropractic term describing the spatial orientation of one vertebra in relation to its adjacent segments. See Listing—Static.

Static Strength Evaluation: The measurement of strength by isometric means. No motion of the extremities or muscle groups is allowed during the measurement of force.

Static Traction: A steady traction force applied and maintained for a specific time interval. See Traction—Static.

Static Vertebral Malposition: A chiropractic term denoting abnormal or anomalous vertebral position. See Malposition.

Steel's Rule of Thirds: An anatomical rule pertaining to the atlantoaxial articulation between C1 and C2. The first anterior third of available space is for the dens, the second third of space is occupied by the cord, the posterior third of the available space is empty.

Steffee Plates: A transpedicular screw and plate system used for posterior spinal fusion in which the screws are rigidly attached perpendicular to the plating system. There are some potential problems. For instance, if the screw is not initially perpendicular to the plate, the shaft tends to get bent as the nut is tightened. Also, this system may impinge on the facet joint at the level above the instrumented segment. See Pedicle Screw Fixation.

Steindler's Test: A physical exam maneuver used to differentiate HNP from a low back strain. A local anesthetic agent is injected into the tender area. Low back strain is suspected if the needle aggravates the local pain or radiating pain, abolishes the local pain or radiating pain, or if there is normal straight-leg raising after the injection.

Stellate Block: The injection of a local anesthetic into the region surrounding the stellate ganglion in the cervical spine. See Stellate Ganglion Block.

Stellate Ganglion: A star-shaped collection of sympathetic cell bodies (ganglion) in the cervical spine. From there, sympathetic nerve fibers are distributed to the face, neck, upper extremities, and organs of the thorax. The stellate ganglion is composed of the inferior cervical and first thoracic sympathetic ganglia and is located between the base of the transverse process of C7 and the origin of the first rib. See Cervicothoracic Ganglion.

Stellate Ganglion Block: The injection of a local anesthetic into the region surrounding the stellate ganglion in the cervical spine. This is often performed as a diagnostic test for reflex sympathetic dystrophy (RSD). It is thought that a positive test will show decreased symptoms of RSD after the injection. See Cervicothoracic Block, Sympathetic Block.

Stenosis: This term most commonly refers to central canal stenosis. This is a narrowing of the canal for the spinal cord. This can be caused by bony enlargement due to degenerative disc disease. See Central Canal Stenosis, Foraminal Stenosis, Lateral Recess Stenosis.

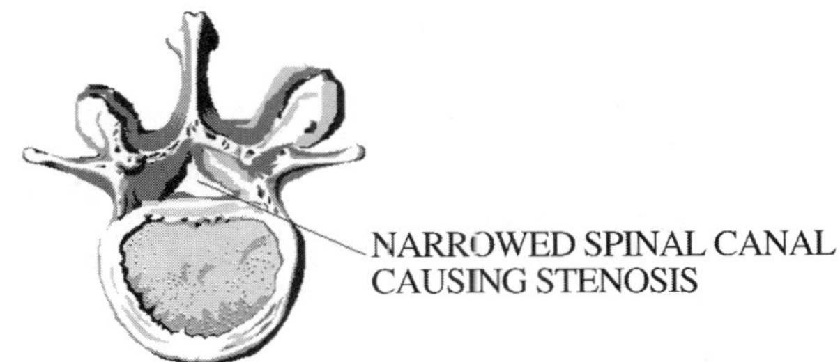

Step Defect: A radiographic sign of a vertebral compression fracture. This is seen on a lateral x-ray view as a sharp step-off of the anterior–superior vertebral margin along the otherwise smooth concave edge of the vertebral body.

Step Ladder Sign: A radiographic sign seen in spondylolisthesis. On an oblique x-ray, the alignment of the facet joints changes abruptly at the level of the slippage.

Steppage Gait: A high-stepping gait which resembles that of a Lipizzan stallion. This is usually due to paralysis of the tibialis anterior. The leg must be lifted abnormally high to clear the foot from the ground. See Drop Foot, Equine Gait.

Sternal Angle: The angle formed between the manubrium and the body of the sternum. See Angle of Louis.

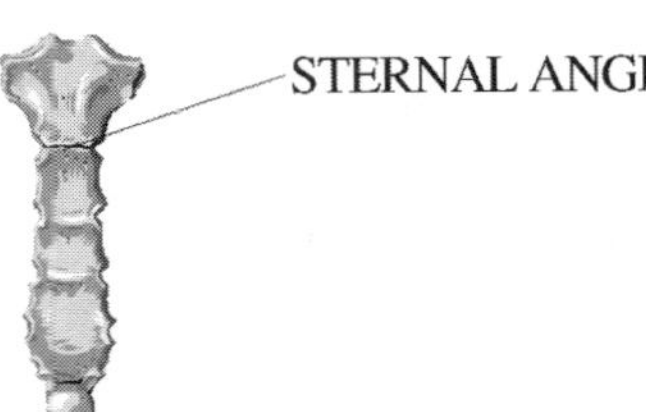

Sternal Compression Test: A physical exam maneuver which attempts to identify rib fractures. The patient is in a supine position with arms at the sides or crossed over the abdomen. The examiner places the pisiform of one hand in the vertical axis of the sternum. The examiner exerts a downward pressure on the sternum, and localized pain in the ribs is reported to indicate a fracture.

Sternal Occipital Mandibular Immobilizer: A type of hard cervical–thoracic orthosis commonly used for rigid cervical immobilization. See SOMI Collar.

Sternoclavicular Joint: The joint between the upper lateral portion of the sternum (breast bone) and the clavicle (collar bone). This acts as the anterior supporting strut of the shoulder girdle. The joint contains an articular disc and is surrounded by a joint capsule. In elevation of the shoulder, the clavicle depresses and "rolls into" the joint. On protraction of the shoulder, the clavicle also depresses and "rolls into" the joint. The spine participates in sternoclavicular motion. For example, thoracic extension is accompanied by shoulder retraction and the anterior fulcrum for this movement is the sternoclavicular joint. Also, in the opposite direction, thoracic flexion is accompanied by shoulder protraction and again the sternoclavicular joint is the anterior fulcrum for this movement. Also, in chronic thoracic flexion due to poor posture, the sternoclavicular joints can become overloaded. See SC Joint.

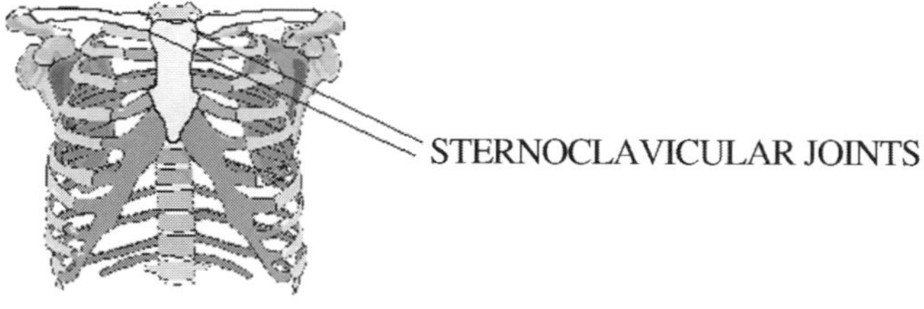

Sternocleidomastoid Muscle: An anterior neck muscle which originates from the sternum and clavicle (two heads) and inserts on the mastoid process of the skull. The muscle plays a major role in head and neck proprioception and is commonly injured in whiplash injuries. It has trigger points which refer to the head and can cause dizziness. The actions are to flex the neck when contracted bilaterally, turn the head to the opposite side, and side bend to the same side when contracted unilaterally. See SCM.

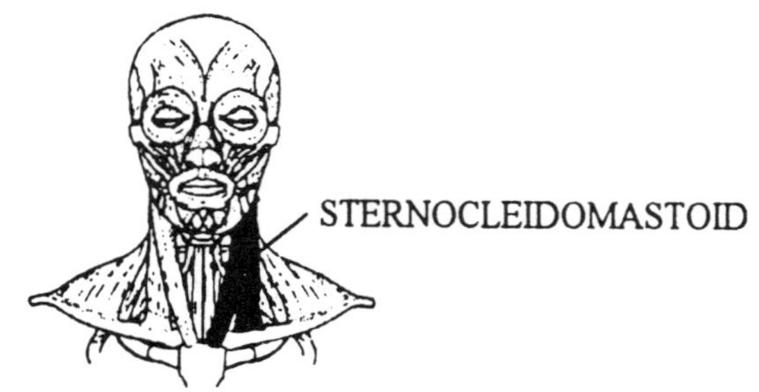

Sternum: The breast bone. This is a flat, long, rectangular-shaped bone which acts as the keystone of the rib cage. The sternum articulates with the clavicles and costal cartillage of the first through seventh ribs. From top to bottom, the three portions are the manubrium, the body, and the xiphoid process.

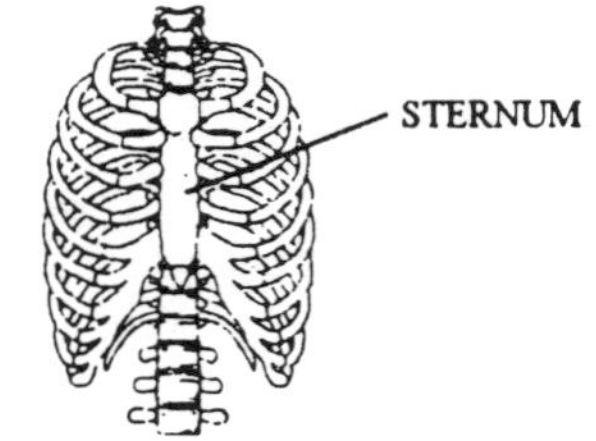

Steroid: A potent anti-inflammatory which can be administered in tablet form, IV, IM, into a joint capsule, or into a tendon sheath. In the spine, these are commonly used in such inflammatory conditions as radiculopathy and ankylosing spondylitis. Dosages vary depending on the type of glucocorticoid and condition. Injectable steroids are usually not recommended in the same location more than two to three times per year. This is due to steroid atrophy (fat atrophy, muscle necrosis, and weakening of collagen). Steroids are also used epidurally. Drug-induced secondary adrenal cortical insufficiency is possible. This is usually minimized by tapering the drug. There is an enhanced effect of corticosteroids on patients with hypothyroidism and in those with cirrhosis. Corticosteroids should also be used cautiously in patients with ocular herpes simplex. The lowest possible dose should be used to control the condition. Euphoria, insomnia, mood swings, personality changes, severe depression, and psychotic manifestations are possible. Steroids should also be used with caution in patients with ulcerative colitis, diverticulitis, peptic ulcer disease, renal insufficiency, hypertension, osteoporosis, and myasthenia gravis. There are drug interactions with cyclosporine, phenobarbital, phenytoin, rifampin, ketoconazole, high-dose aspirin, and oral anticoagulants.

Steroid Taper: Decreasing doses of steroid medication given over days to weeks to avoid the side effects of steroid withdrawal. A steroid burst is given to decrease inflammation in such disorders as radiculopathy.

stim: An abbreviation for *stimulate* or *stimulation*.

Stinger: A neuropraxic lesion of the brachial plexus which is self-limited. There is numbness and weakness in the upper extremity after a traumatic blow. See Burner.

STIR Image: An imaging technique that exploits the difference between the T1 relaxation time of fat and other tissues. Water has a very high signal intensity. See Short Tau Inversion Recovery.

STM: An abbreviation for *soft tissue manipulation* and *soft tissue massage.*

Stooping: Flexing the lumbar spine at the waist. Also known as bending.

Stoop Test: A technique used to detect lumbar central canal stenosis. The patient is asked to walk in an upright erect position. This should cause pain in the buttock and in the limbs and will intensify as the patient continues to walk in this position. The patient is then asked to stoop forward while continuing to walk in a standing position. This will decrease symptoms. The patient is then asked to stand upright again, and this increases symptoms, again.

Stork Test: A common physical exam test used to detect SI joint dysfunction. See Gillet's Test.

str: An abbreviation for *strain.*

Straddle Fracture: A comminuted fracture of the pubic arch which is the most common type of unstable fracture seen in the pelvis. This is a double vertical fracture which involves both superior pubic rami and the ischiopubic junctions bilaterally. The unstable segment places pressure on the bladder and a full 20% of these patients have a bladder rupture or urethral tear.

Straight Cervical Spine: The loss of the normal neck curvature usually seen after whiplash. It is thought that this is due to spasm in the longus colli musculature.

Straight-Leg Raise: A physical exam maneuver traditionally used to detect a lumbar radiculopathy (pinched nerve in the back, herniated disc). The patient is in the supine position, and the hip is brought into flexion with the knee extended. This places a stretch on the sciatic nerve which causes tension on the spinal nerves through the intervertebral foramina. A positive straight-leg test is usually considered reproduction of the patient's dermatomal pain pattern or numbness (numbness in the region of the foot or leg that corresponds to specific nerve root that might be pinched) past the knee. However, many physicians and therapists report a positive straight-leg test as an increase in back pain thought secondary to dural irritation. It is believed that the tibial nerve above the knee moves superior during this maneuver while below the knee it moves inferior. It is believed that the common peroneal nerve has the same type of movement with the attachment to the fibular head being the anchor point. This maneuver is sometimes also performed to check for hamstring length. See Nerve Root Tension Sign, Straight-Leg Raising, Straight-Leg Raising Manuever, SLR.

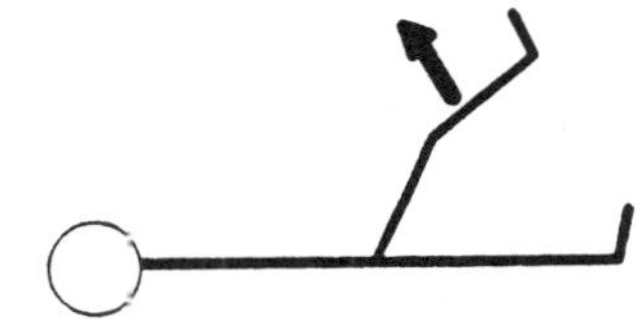

STRAIGHT-LEG RAISE

Straight-Leg Raising: A physical exam maneuver traditionally used to detect a lumbar radiculopathy (pinched nerve in the back, herniated disc). See Straight-Leg Raise, SLR, Stretch Root Sign.

Straight-Leg Raising Maneuver: A physical exam maneuver traditionally used to detect a lumbar radiculopathy (pinched nerve in the back, herniated disc). See Straight-Leg Raise.

Strain–Counterstrain: A technique which is advocated for the treatment of acute and subacute muscular strain. The concept is that there is injury to the muscle spindle complex. This technique involves shortening the muscle to "shut down" the overactive muscle spindles. A Jones point is identified in the muscle (a tender point in a specific area of the muscle which is used for monitoring). See Jones Strain–Counterstrain, Jones Point, Fold and Hold, Indirect Technique.

Strained Sacroiliac Joint: See SI Joint Syndrome, SI Dysfunction.

Strap Muscles: Long, ribbon-like muscles in the anterior neck which connect to the hyoid bone and then to the mandible. These include the thyrohyoid, the omohyoid, the sternohyoid, and sternothyroid muscles. These can be tender in patients who are using the otherwise phasic strap musculature as tonic supporters of the head and neck. This is commonly seen in TMJ syndrome and whiplash.

Stress Evaluation: X-rays taken in the extremes of flexion and extension to detect abnormal segmental movement. See Flexion–Extension Views.

Stretch Root Sign: A physical exam maneuver traditionally used to detect a lumbar radiculopathy. See Straight-Leg Raising.

Stretch Weakness: The weakening of muscles that are kept in a stretched position beyond their normal resting length. This can be detected with postural problems and may be a perpetuating factor of myofascial pain.

Stringiness: A palpable texture abnormality similar to a "taut band" in a muscle. It is used to denote a string-like area palpated in the muscle fibers.

Structural: Medical slang for a spinal curve which is caused by bony changes and not just soft tissue changes.

Structural Curve: (1) A fixed lateral curvature due to bony changes in the spine. This is usually seen on AP radiographs. If the curve does not correct on supine, lateral, or side bending films it is thought to be a "structural curve." See Scoliosis. (2) An irreversible curvature of the spine with bony changes and a fixed rotation of the vertebrae. See Structural Scoliosis.

Structural Integration: A body work system created by Ida Rolf used to correct posture or to integrate structure. See Rolfing.

Structural Leg Length: The functional length of a lower extremity measured from the umbilicus to the medial malleolus. See Apparent Leg Length.

Structural Leg Length Discrepancy: A short leg due to a difference in length of the femur or tibia. There is usually a small, subtle change in length.

Structural Scoliosis: An irreversible curvature of the spine with bony changes and a fixed rotation of the vertebrae. This is due to congenital bony structure with uneven growth or long-standing neuromuscular disease. Forward bending of the trunk usually produces a rib hump posteriorly on the convex side of the curve because of rotation of the vertebrae and rib cage. See Scoliosis—Structural, Scoliosis, Structural Curve.

Strumming: A very deep, often painful release technique for the fascial tissues. This can be done to break up long-standing hypomobility of one or more vertebra.

STT: A physical therapy abbreviation for *soft tissue techniques.*

Subacromial Bursitis: Compression of the supraspinatus and subacromial bursa underneath the coracoacromial arch. See Impingement Syndrome.

Subacute: In between acute and chronic.

Subarachnoid Space: The space below the arachnoid membrane which is filled with cerebrospinal fluid.

Subarticular Stenosis: A subcategory of lateral recess stenosis in which the superior articular facet compresses the nerve root just below the disc in patients with short pedicles. There is indentation of the recess by the subarticular portion of the lamina.

Subaxial: Referring to the C3–C7 region.

Subaxial Subluxation: A subluxation below the second cervical vertebra which occurs in 7–29% of patients with rheumatoid arthritis. This is most commonly seen at the C2–3 or C3–4 levels. The characteristic sign on x-ray is of a "staircase" produced by serial subluxations. It is thought that these lesions develop due to laxity in the ALL, PLL, or facet joint. Myelopathy is uncommon.

Subcapsular Pocket: Recesses in the capsule of the facet joints located in the superior and inferior poles of the joint. These recesses are filled with fat and communicate with the fat outside the joint through foramina in the superior and inferior capsules.

Subchondral Cyst: A focal region of bone loss within subarticular bone seen with signs of joint degeneration. There is an ovoid area of decreased bone density between 2 and 20 mm in diameter, often with a sclerotic margin. There is usually a decreased joint space. These cysts are due to increased biomechanical stress on bone due to cartilage loss. See Geode.

Subchondral Sclerosis: A thickening in the trabecula just below cartilage. There is a thinning in the cartilage which transmits increased mechanical forces to the subchondral bone. This causes a compensatory increase in bone mass just below the surface. The joint space is decreased due to the loss of cartilage. See Eburnation.

Subdural Space: The space below the dura.

Subjective: A finding on any exam that is reported by the patient and is dependent on patient report for its reliability.

Subjective Discography: A term which applies to the pain response reported by the patient during a discogram. The patient will report that the dye injected into the disc exactly reproduces their symptoms. This is the same as a P2 response or a concordant pain response. This is usually considered as a sign that the patient's pain complaints are being generated by the disc. See P2 Response, Concordant Pain Response.

Subligamentous Disc Herniation: A disc herniation that is contained by the posterior longitudinal ligament. It has been postulated that, because this ligament is innervated, this can be a source of pain. A sequestered fragment can migrate superiorly or inferiorly.

Subluxation: From an orthopedic standpoint, abnormal joint movement beyond normal range of motion (an incomplete dislocation). From a chiropractic standpoint, subluxations are much smaller in amplitude and represent abnormal positions of the vertebral segments that cause alternations in central nervous system function. See Fixation, Subluxation Complex, Hypermobile Subluxation, Interosseous Disc Relationship, Luxated Joint, Luxation.

Subluxation Complex: A chiropractic term used to denote a vertebral segment that does not move freely in all directions. See Subluxation, Fixation.

Subluxed Vertebra: A chiropractic term used to denote a vertebral segment that does not move freely in all directions. See Fixation.

Submental Triangle: An anatomic triangle located beneath the central portion of the mandible.

Suboccipital Stretch: A physical therapy stretch designed to stretch the suboccipital musculature. See Chin Tuck.

Subtotal Vertebral Vertebrectomy: Removal of the entire vertebral body and discs for severe compressive myelopathy due to degenerative arthritis, cancer, or trauma. A bone graft or metal cage is substituted for the body of the vertebra. Frequently, instrumentation fusion is required for stability.

Subtotal Vertebrectomy: Removal of the entire vertebral body and discs for severe compressive myelopathy. See Subtotal Vertebral Vertebrectomy.

Sudeck's Atrophy: Severe, regional osteoporosis which is detected on x-ray and can be associated with RSD. See Reflex Sympathetic Dystrophy.

Suicide Jumper's Fracture: A horizontal fracture of the upper sacrum at the S1–S2 level which can occur from a serious fall. It is usually associated with suicide attempts, thus its descriptive name. See Horizontal Sacral Fracture, Transverse Sacral Fracture.

Sulindac: A nonsteroidal anti-inflammatory drug in the indole class. See Clinoril.

Summation Effect: A radiographic term which refers to a decrease in the length of the neck due to decreased disc height, osteolysis, and an upward migration of the dens. This can be seen in advanced rheumatoid arthritis.

sup: An abbreviation for *supine*.

Superficial Posterior Sacrococcygeal Ligament: A superficial ligament on the posterior portion of the inferior sacrum covering the sacral hiatus.

Superior Articular Process: A specialized mass of bone projecting from the junction of the lamina and pedicle upward which articulates at the facet joint with the inferior articular process of the vertebra above. When viewed from the side, the vertebrae are said to look like a dog with the spinous process being the nose and the superior articular process representing the ear. The inferior articular process would then represent the front paw. The medial portion of this area is smooth and covered with cartilage and makes up a portion of the facet joint. See Facet Joint.

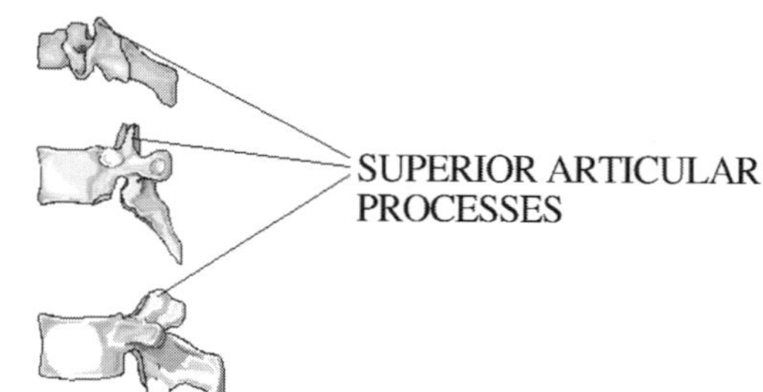

Superior Ilium: An osteopathic or manual physical therapy term used to refer to an SI joint dysfunction. See Up-slip.

Superior Innominate Shear: An osteopathic or manual physical therapy term used to refer to an SI joint dysfunction. See Up-slip.

Superior Nutation: See Counternutation.

Superior Pube: When one pubic symphysis is noted to be higher than the other. See Superior Pubic Shear.

Superior Pubic Bone: When one pubic symphysis is noted to be higher than the other. See Superior Pubic Shear.

Superior Pubic Ligament: One of the ligamentous structures that supports the pubic symphysis superiorly.

Superior Pubic Shear: When one pubic symphysis is noted to be higher than the other due to a shear force in the sagittal plane. There is greater mobility in the superior direction than in the inferior direction. See Superior Pube, Superior Pubic Bone, Superior Shear, Superior Pubis.

Superior Pubis: When one pubic symphysis is noted to be higher than the other. See Superior Pubic Shear.

Superior Sacral Notch: The notch between the sacral facet of S1 and the sacral ala. The dorsal ramus of the fifth lumbar nerve root passes through this notch.

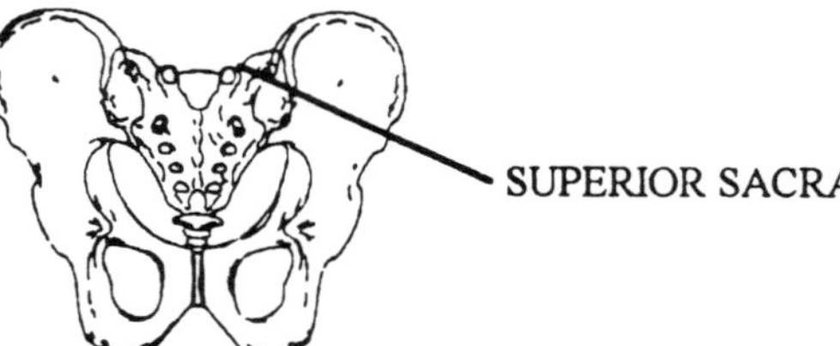

Superior Sacral Shear: An osteopathic or manual physical therapy term which refers to an abnormality in sacral positioning. See Unilateral Sacral Extension, Posterior Sacrum, Unilaterally Extended Sacrum.

Superior Shear: When one pubic symphysis is noted to be higher than the other. See Superior Pubic Shear.

Superior Subluxation: A chiropractic term which refers to increased space between a vertebral segment relative to the spacing of the segments above and segments below. The spinous process is noted to be a greater distance from the spinous process below when compared with the distance from the spinous process above. See Increased Interosseous Spacing.

Supervised Reconditioning: Instructing a patient in body mechanics, exercise to increase strength or range of motion, and general conditioning and flexibility. See Therapeutic Exercise.

Sup. Glut.: An abbreviation for *superior gluteal.*

Supinator Reflex: A physical exam maneuver that tests the integrity of the C6 nerve root. See Brachioradialis Reflex.

Supine Hamstring Stretch: A physical therapy stretch in which the patient lies supine with one leg raised and the other leg on the floor. The elevated leg is held behind the knee, and the patient slowly extends the knee until a stretch is felt in the hamstring area.

Supraligamentous Disc Herniation: A disc herniation which has broken through the constraints of the posterior longitudinal ligament and become "supraligamentous." See Supraligamentous Herniation.

Supraligamentous Herniation: A disc herniation which has broken through the constraints of the posterior longitudinal ligament and become "supraligamentous." See Disc Extrusion, Supraligamentous Disc Herniation.

Suprapubic: Above the symphysis pubis.

Suprascap.: An abbreviation for *suprascapular.*

Supraspin.: An abbreviation for *supraspinatus.*

Supraspinatus Tendinitis: Compression of the supraspinatus and subacromial bursa underneath the coracoacromial arch. See Impingement Syndrome.

Supraspinous Ligament: A ligament which attaches to and travels over the spinous processes. This is one of the ligaments that the lumbar spine "hangs" on when in a fully flexed position.

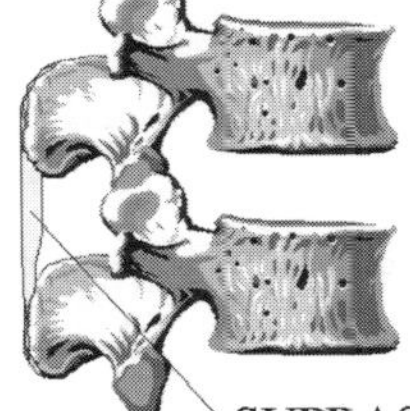

SUPRASPINOUS LIGAMENT

Supratentorial: Referring to a psychological problem. The problem is "above" the tentorium or in the brain (not in the body). An example would be a somatoform pain disorder.

Surgical Lesion: A term often used by surgeons to describe a problem that requires surgical intervention.

Sustained Activity Tolerance: A portion of a functional capacity evaluation which focuses on endurance for work or a specific activity.

Sustained Joint Mobilization: A mobilization technique applied to painful joints during which a constant force, intermittent distraction is used for 10 seconds with a few seconds of rest for several cycles. See Mobilization—Sustained.

Swayback: An anterior shift in the entire pelvis with hip extension and a posterior shift of the thoracic spine resulting in flexion of the thorax on the upper lumbar spine. This results in an increased lordosis of the lower lumbar region and usually a forward head. This is seen when the postural back muscles are unable to provide muscular support. The patient gives in fully to the effects of gravity, and all the passive structures are at their end range of motion.

Sweat Technique: A chiropractic cervical adjusting technique which uses an instrument for adjusting. This technique is controversial within the chiropractic community.

Swedish Massage: Traditional massage therapy that uses direct contact and light to deep pressure to relax muscles and stimulate blood flow.

Swimmer's Lateral: An x-ray view which demonstrates the lower cervical and upper thoracic vertebrae. The patient is positioned with one arm above the head and with that side obliquely against the x-ray cartridge.

Swiss Ball: A large, brightly colored rubber ball used in many lumbar stabilization programs. The balls come in various sizes and are large enough to sit on. The general idea is that it is difficult to stabilize on an unstable ball. The patient is asked to do various exercises while trying to stabilize the spine. See Gymnastic Ball, Gymnic Ball, Swiss Gym Ball.

Swiss Ball Exercises: An exercise program similar to a lumbar stabilization program. Patients are asked to stabilize their spine while on an unstable Swiss ball. Many different positions and techniques have been advocated. Because some of these exercises are difficult, this can also be an appropriate program for more advanced spinal stabilization patients.

Swiss Gym Ball: A large, brightly colored rubber ball used in many lumbar stabilization programs. See Swiss Ball.

Sx: An abbreviation for *symptoms*.

Symbols: All symbols are located in the front of this book.

Sympathetically Maintained Pain: Pain that is caused by an "overdrive" of the autonomic nervous system. Symptoms such as burning, hypersensitivity, sweating, and coldness are indicative of sympathetically maintained pain. See Reflex Sympathetic Dystrophy, Sympathetically Mediated Pain.

Sympathetically Mediated Pain: Pain that is caused by an "overdrive" of the autonomic nervous system. See Sympathetically Maintained Pain.

Sympathetic Block: The injection of anesthetic or another substance for the purpose of shutting down the sympathetic nervous system. The most common sympathetic block is a stellate ganglion block. Sympathetic blocks are also performed along the lumbar sympathetic chain. In both instances, this is performed diagnostically to rule out reflex sympathetic dystrophy (RSD). For instance, if the burning hyperpathic pain resolves with a sympathetic block, it is thought that RSD is the cause of the pain. Also, sympathetic blocks are performed therapeutically to try to decrease the sympathetic overdrive that occurs in RSD. See Stellate Ganglion Block.

Sympathetic Block—Lumbar: A block commonly used in patients with lower extremity reflex sympathetic dystrophy. See Lumbar Sympathetic Block.

Sympathetic Cervical Arthritis: A relatively uncommon syndrome characterized by dizziness, lightheadedness, vertigo, vasomotor face disturbances, retro-orbital pain, disturbances of vision, and other symptoms. See Syndrome of Barre-Lieou.

Sympathetic Chain: A portion of the autonomic nervous system that consists of a chain of ganglia that lies on either side of the vertebral column. See Sympathetic Trunk.

Sympathetic Dystrophy: A clinical syndrome characterized by the presence of pain out of proportion to the severity of the injury. See Reflex Sympathetic Dystrophy.

Sympathetic Ganglia: A portion of the autonomic nervous system that consists of a chain of ganglia that lies on either side of the vertebral column. See Sympathetic Chain, Paravertebral Sympathetic Ganglia.

Sympathetic Nervous System: One of the two divisions of the autonomic nervous system which is the opposite of the parasympathetic nervous system. When the sympathetic nervous system is activated, there is an increase in heart rate, blood pressure, and blood flow to the skeletal muscles, decreased blood flow to digestive organs and skin, bronchodilatation, dilation of the pupils, sweating, and other anticholinergic responses. See Sympathetic Trunk.

Sympathetic Posterior Cervical Arthritis: An uncommon syndrome characterized by dizziness, lightheadedness, vertigo, vasomotor face disturbances, retro-orbital pain, disturbances of vision, and other symptoms. See Syndrome of Barre-Lieou.

Sympathetic Trunk: A portion of the autonomic nervous system that consists of a chain of ganglia that lies on either side of the vertebral column. This system extends from the base of the skull to the coccyx and consists of between 21 and 25 ganglia. The gray rami communicantes connect the spinal nerves and portions of the chain by forming communicating pathways. See Sympathetic Chain, Sympathetic Nervous System.

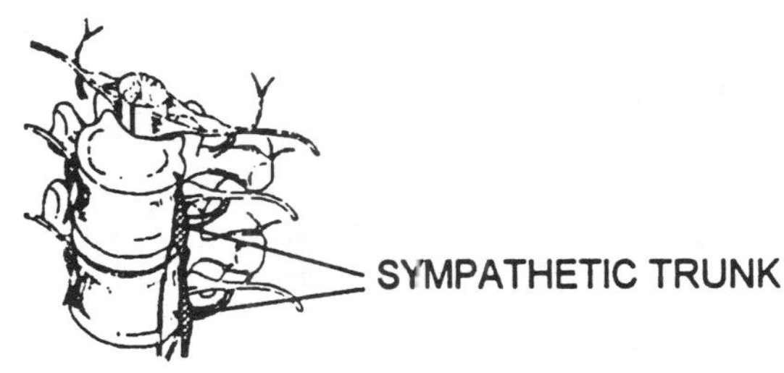

Symphyseal Shear: When the symphysis pubis is found to be displaced along a plane parallel to that of joint contact. This usually occurs in a superior–inferior direction but also occurs in an anterior–posterior direction.

Symphysis Pubis: The place in the anterior pelvis where the two halves of the pelvis articulate. See Pubic Symphysis.

Symphysis Pubis Avulsion Fracture: An avulsion of the superior or inferior pubic rami near the pubic symphysis caused by the adductor major. This injury is commonly seen in soccer players. See Avulsion Fracture of the Symphysis Pubis.

Symphysis Pubis Shotgun Method: A nonspecific treatment for SI joint dysfunction where the pubic tubercles are noted to be uneven. The patient lies in the hook-lying position and maximally abducts the hips against unyielding resistance applied by the therapist for 10 seconds. The patient then relaxes and reverses hand position so that resistance is applied to the medial thigh. Abduction is then maximally performed against the therapist's unyielding resistance for 10 seconds. This procedure is repeated three times. See Shotgun SI Treatment, Shotgun Treatment, SI Shotgun, Shotgun SI Treatment.

Symptom Magnification Syndrome: A nonspecific term implying unconscious magnification of symptomatology out of proportion to pathology. See Magnified Illness Behavior, Somatoform Pain Disorder.

Syndesmophyte: A vertically oriented calcification adjacent to the intervertebral disc or vertebra. These structures can bridge across vertebrae and are thought to be associated with the "degenerative cascade" as described by Kirkaldy-Willis. This is the concept that hypermobility occurs at a segment due to degenerative changes and that this bony "bridging" is the body's attempt to stabilize that segment.

Syndrome of Barre-Lieou: An uncommon syndrome characterized by dizziness, light-headedness, vertigo, vasomotor face disturbances, retro-orbital pain, disturbances of vision, and other symptoms. Rarely are all of these symptoms present concurrently. Theories as to the etiology include alternations in the flow of the vertebral artery caused by degenerative changes in the superior articular facet or uncovertebral joint, single-level cervical hypermobility due to degenerative disease or trauma or both, interference with the periarterial nerve plexus, irritation of the posterior cervical sympathetics, alar or transverse ligament laxity, C4 root sleeve defects, upper cervical ligamentous hypomobility, and myofascial pain. Specific vertebral artery maneuvers can be performed on exam which usually involve cervical rotation, extension, and lateral bending to the opposite side reproducing the patient's dizziness. ENG/AEBR may be helpful in ruling out vestibular disturbances. Vertebral artery angiography and MRA have been used to determine the location of the kinking; however, this can be extremely difficult to demonstrate on an imaging study. See Barre-Lieou Syndrome, Foramen Arcuale, Vertebral Basilar Insufficiency, Vertebral Artery Insufficiency, Bartschi-Rochain's, Sympathetic Posterior Cervical Arthritis, Posterior Cervical Sympathetic Syndrome, Sympathetic Cervical Arthritis, Vertebrogenic Dizziness, Cervical Dizziness.

Synovitis: Inflammation of the synovial membrane or an excess of normal synovial fluid within a joint. This inflammatory condition can occur in multiple locations in the spine including within the facet joints or within the SI joint.

Syracuse Plates: Instrumentation used for anterior interbody spinal fusion which consists of a steel plate in the shape of an "I" that is attached to the vertebral body with four screws. As with any plating system, there is a concern that screw "backout" can occur even once solid arthrodesis has been achieved. However, in this plating system the proximal part of the screw completely fills the plate hole producing a "press cold weld" fit.

Syringes: The plural of syrinx. See Syrinx.

Syringobulbia: A syrinx or fluid-filled cavity found within the brain stem. A cystic dilatation of the fourth ventricle in the brain stem. Nystagmus, atrophy of the tongue, and impaired facial sensation may result. See Syringomyelia.

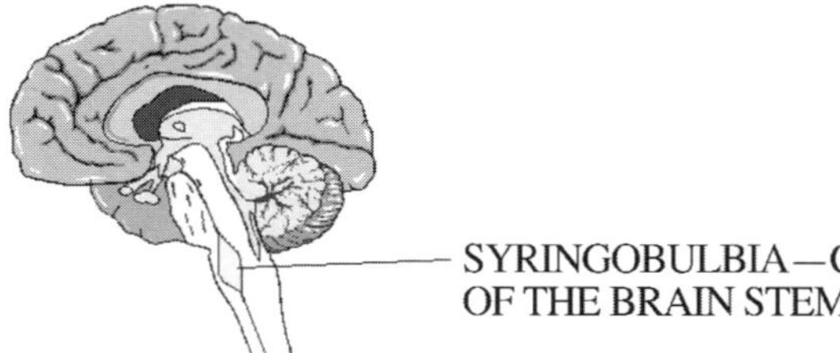

Syringohydromyelia: A cystic dilatation of the lower one-third of the spinal cord frequently associated with occult spinal dysraphism.

Syringomyelia: A cyst, or "syrinx," which occurs in the center of the spinal cord. This can affect pain and temperature sensation due to its location. There is greater motor loss in the upper extremities due to the position of the motor tracts in relation to the syrinx. This is a chronic, slowly progressive disease often seen in patients with previous spinal cord injury. See Syrinx, Syringobulbia.

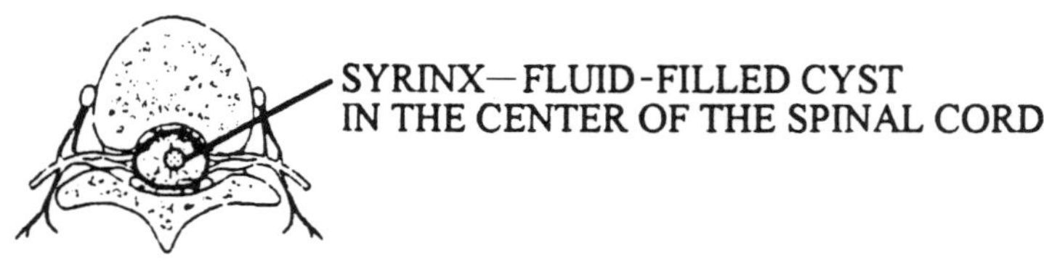

Syrinx: A cyst which occurs in the center of the spinal cord. See Syringomyelia, Syringes.

Systemic Hypermobility: Excessive mobility found in multiple areas of the body. The disease process associated with this condition is Ehlers-Danlos syndrome. However, many individuals are born with excess mobility. Many physical therapists believe that this excess mobility predisposes these patients to further hypermobility through ligamentous injury. See Congenital Hypermobility.

T

T: An abbreviation for *thoracic.*

t: A chiropractic abbreviation for *transverse process.*

T1–T12: Referring to the entire thoracic spine.

T1 Weighted Image: An MRI sequence which is designed to show fat as a bright signal. This is particularly helpful in the lumbar spine, as many of the structures are outlined by fatty tissue and show up dark against the bright fat signal. This is part of the standard MRI sequence in the lumbar spine which also includes a proton density sequence and a T2 weighted sequence. A T1 weighted sequence has a short TR and a short TE.

T2 Weighted Image: An MRI sequence that is designed to show water or fluid as bright. This is particularly helpful in the spine, because young healthy discs contain a significant amount of water. Thus, the nucleus pulposus of the discs shows up as bright on a T2 weighted sequence. Degenerated discs show up as darker because they contain less water. A T2 weighted image has a long TR and a long TE. It is one of the standard lumbar sequences for MRI which also includes T1 weighted images and proton density images.

Tabes Dorsalis: A now relatively rare, progressive form of neurosyphilis seen in approximately 5% of patients with untreated disease. Due to the advent of antibiotics, this has become rare and is seen today in third world countries or in the homeless. There is selective degeneration of the posterior columns. Symptoms often take 5–20 years to develop. Due to the selective nature of the spinal cord and spinal nerve root destruction, disturbances of sensation and proprioception are the most common complaints.

Talwin: An analgesic containing pentazocine (roughly equivalent, milligram to milligram, to the analgesic effect of codeine). This is used for the relief of moderate pain. Physical dependence is possible. The usual dosage is two caplets three or four times a day. Talwin also comes in a compound formulation that contains 650 mg of aspirin.

Tandem Gait: Normal walking. The act of literally putting one foot in front of the other.

Tapotement: A tapping or percussing movement in massage that includes clapping, beating, and punctation.

TART: An osteopathic abbreviation for *tissue texture abnormality, asymmetry, restriction of motion, and tenderness*. These are the elements that define the osteopathic somatic dysfunstion.

Taut Band: A palpable band of muscle fibers usually associated with a trigger point. See Palpable Band.

Taylor Brace: A thoracolumbosacral orthosis (TLSO) brace used to stabilize the thoracic and thoracolumbar spine. See Taylor Spinal Brace.

Taylor Brace with Lateral Uprights: A type of TLSO used to stabilize the thoracic and thoracolumbar spine. Unlike the Taylor brace without lateral uprights, this restricts all three axes of movement in the thoracic spine. It provides overall intermediate control over thoracic mobility.

Taylor Spinal Brace: A TLSO. See Taylor Brace.

TD: An abbreviation for *temperature differential.* This has been proposed by some chiropractors as a way to measure the vertebral subluxation complex. A temperature analysis of the spine is undertaken with an electronic thermocouple. This is thought to be directly proportional to the amount of neurophysiologic involvement caused by the vertebral subluxation complex. There is some controversy even among chiropractors as to the reliability of these measurements.

TE: Echo time in an MR image. The time at which data is acquired.

Teardrop Fracture: A fracture of the cervical spine seen on lateral x-rays. This resembles an anterior fracture of the vertebral body with a fragment adjacent to the end plate anteriorly and inferiorly. This has been said to resemble a drop of water dripping from the vertebral body on x-ray. The mechanism of injury is usually hyperflexion or flexion with an axial load. This fracture can be associated with neurologic signs. A teardrop fracture has also been associated with a fracture plane oriented in the sagittal plane. This often splits the vertebral body into left and right halves which may rotate backward and cause encroachment of the spinal canal and cord. This can occur in up to half of all teardrop fractures.

Tectorial Membrane: A continuation of the posterior longitudinal ligament in the cervical spine that runs superiorly from the body of C2 and up and over the posterior portion of the dens. It then runs toward the foramen magnum and becomes the tectorial membrane of the brain.

Tegretol: An anticonvulsant sometimes used in chronic intractable neuropathic pain. It is contraindicated in patients with a history of previous bone marrow depression or sensitivity to tricyclic compounds. Aplastic anemia and agranulocytosis have been reported in association with the use of Tegretol. The common dosage for the relief of pain is 100 mg twice a day to start, gradually increasing by 100-mg increments every 12 hours, until pain is relieved. The dosage to relieve pain may range from 200–1200 mg and should not exceed 1200 mg daily. After pain is relieved, a maintenance dosage of 400–800 mg is usually adequate. See Carbamazepine.

Temperature Differential: See TD

Temporal: Toward the temples. This also refers to a type of headache with pain on the sides of the head.

Temporalis Muscle: A muscle used in chewing which is often associated with TMJ syndrome and has trigger points which can cause temporal or frontal headache. This muscle is also likely associated with upper cervical biomechanics. It originates from the side of the skull and inserts on the coronoid process of the mandible. It is responsible for closing the jaw and moving it from side to side to facilitate grinding (along with the masseter and medial pterygoid). Innervation is through the mandibular branch of trigeminal nerve (cranial nerve 5).

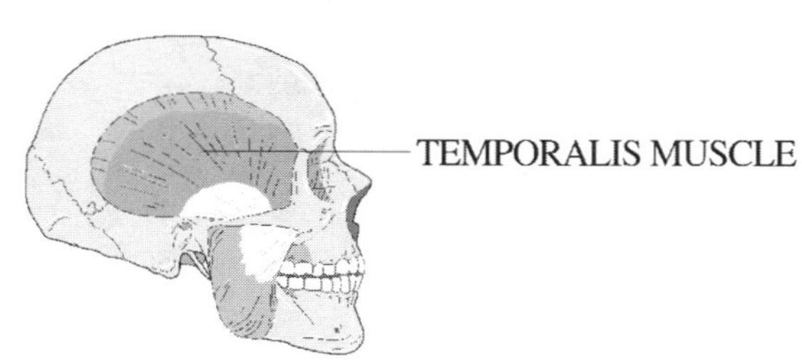

Temporary Partial Disability: The inability of a worker to return to his full work capacity. The worker is employable in a different job full duty with fewer hours. Benefits are paid to supplement the worker's income. An example is a worker who was returned to light duty work or part time.

Temporary Total Disability: When a worker is unable to earn wages and return to work as expected, and the medical condition has not yet stabilized. This is when the patient's medical condition prevents return to work and benefits are paid. See TTD.

Temporomandibular Dysfunction: Pain emanating from the temporomandibular joint. See TMJ Dysfunction, Arthrosis Temporomandibularis, TMJ Myofascial Pain, Temporomandibular Joint Arthrosis, Mandibular Pain Dysfunction Syndrome.

Temporomandibular Joint: The jaw joint between the mandible and the articular surface of the temporal bone. This joint allows opening and closing of the jaw, as well as numerous other movements including lateral deviation and protrusion. The joint contains an articular disc. It is surrounded by the articular capsule, the temporomandibular ligament, the stylomandibular ligament, and the sphenomandibular ligament. It is also surrounded by the temporalis, masseter (superficial and

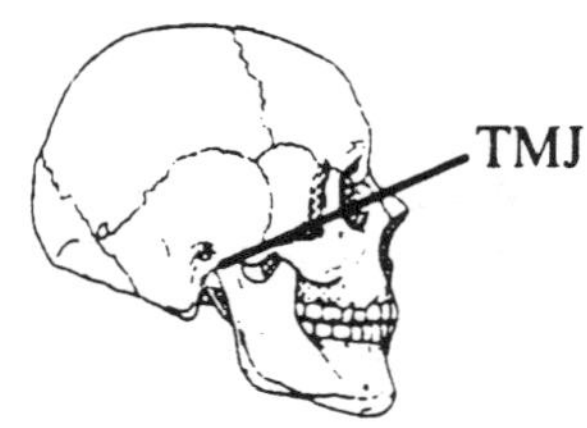

deep), lateral pterygoid, stylohyoid, posterior belly of the digastric, thyrohyoid, omohyoid, sternohyoid, mylohyoid, geniohyoid, and other muscles. See TMJ.

Temporomandibular Joint Arthrosis: Pain emanating from the temporomandibular joint. See TMJ Dysfunction, Arthrosis Temporomandibularis, TMJ Myofascial Pain, Temporomandibular Dysfunction, Mandibular Pain Dysfunction Syndrome.

Temporomandibular Joint Capsulitis: An inflammatory reaction within the TMJ joint. See TMJ Dysfunction, TMJ Joint Capsulitis, TMJ Capsulitis.

Tender Point: A circumscribed (discrete) area of tenderness within a muscle. This term is used generally to sometimes refer to a trigger point (area within a muscle which can be palpated, is tender, and refers pain to another area). Also, it is used to refer to a Jones tender point. See Jones Tender Point.

Tendinitis Calcarea: The deposition of hydroxyapatite crystals in multiple locations. See Hydroxyapatite Deposition Disease.

Tendon Jerk: A physical exam maneuver that checks the integrity of the neurologic "wiring" of the muscle being tested. See Deep Tendon Reflex, Tendon Reflex.

Tendon Reflex: A physical exam maneuver that checks the integrity of the neurologic "wiring" of the muscle being tested. See Deep Tendon Reflex, Tendon Jerk.

TENS: Transcutaneous electrical nerve stimulation, a form of electrical anesthesia used to block pain perception. It is based on Melzack and Wall's "gate theory" that pain can be blocked in the CNS at the spinal level before being transmitted to the brain and being perceived as pain. Cells in the substantia gelatinosa act as the "gate." However, the gate theory does not explain all the effects of TENS. TENS units are simple devices in the form of portable battery-powered units. Currents vary between 0 and 100 milliamps and pulse rates between 1 and 200 hertz. The width of the electrical pulse can be modulated, and the shape of wave form can be chosen. Asymmetric wave forms are usually chosen because they are more comfortable. Stimulus intensity can also be modulated. Electrodes are placed over a variety of spots including peripheral nerves, acupuncture meridians, and trigger points. TENS has been shown to be effective in acute and chronic pain. However, effectiveness with chronic pain varies widely depending on study. See Transcutaneous Electrical Nerve Stimulation, MENS, Interferential E-stim.

Tension Band: A resistive band used for progressive resistance exercises. See Theraband.

Tension Cephalgia: A headache caused by cervical myofascial pain. See Tension Headache.

Tension Headache: A headache caused by cervical myofascial pain. Trigger points in the suboccipitals, sternocleidomastoids, upper trapezius, semispinalis capitis, and other associated musculature can cause headaches. This condition is usually worsened by stress, thus the term "tension." This problem can also be caused by biomechanical overload of the cervical musculature and weakness in the deep cervical musculature following whiplash injury. It is currently thought that tension headaches may lead to migraine headaches. See Muscle Contraction Headache, Migraine Headache, Headache.

Tension Myalgia: Pain emanating from the muscles which often radiates to other areas of the body. See Myofascial Pain.

Tension Test: Stressing specific nerves through maneuvers of the extremities or spine. See Adverse Neural Tension Test.

Tensor Fasciae Latae Stretch: A stretch for the tensor fasciae latae and iliotibial band. See Tensor Stretch.

Tensor Stretch: A stretch for the tensor fasciae latae and iliotibial band. The patient stands and places one leg behind the other while crossing the legs. The patient then leans in the direction opposite the crossed side. See TFL Stretch, Tensor Fasciae Latae Stretch.

Terminal Point Adjustive Thrust: A chiropractic technique using a mechanical drop mechanism with an adjusting table. See Thompson Technique.

Tethered Cord Syndrome: A progressive neurologic deficit seen in patients with spina bifida and myelomeningocele. The spinal cord or filum terminale is anchored to bony structures and is put under traction as the patient grows. The progressive tethering results in progressive neurologic deficits in the legs, bladder, and bowel. MRI shows the conus medularis to be low riding, usually below L2. Surgical release may be necessary. See Filum Terminale Syndrome, Cord Traction Syndrome.

Texas Scottish-Rite Hospital Instrumentation: A rodding system used in the correction of idiopathic scoliosis. It was designed to provide a better interface fit of the rods to newly designed hooks. This system apparently allows for greater ease of removal and adjustment during revision surgeries. This system maintains the normal sagittal contours of the spine when in use.

TFL Stretch: A stretch for the tensor fasciae latae and iliotibial band. See Tensor Stretch.

Thecal Sac: Another name for the dural sac. This is the sac-like covering of the spinal cord.

Theraband: A brand name of resistive bands used for progressive resistance exercises. They are color-coded so that yellow has the least resistance and black the most resistance. Any length can be cut and given to the patient to use in a home program. See Sport Cord.

Therapeutic Exercise: Instructing a patient in body mechanics, exercise to increase strength or range of motion, and general conditioning and flexibility. See Supervised Reconditioning.

Therapeutic Massage: Deep or light pressure applied to muscles and or fascia for the purpose of muscle relaxation, fascial release, or increasing local blood flow. See Massage.

Ther Ex: An abbreviation for *therapeutic exercise.*

Therex: An abbreviation for *therapeutic exercise.*

Thermal Treatment: The application of heat or cold in order to decrease spasm, decrease inflammation, or promote circulation.

Thomas Collar: A hard cervical collar with intermediate effectiveness in limiting cervical range of motion, specifically flexion/extension and lateral rotation.

Thomas Test: A physical exam maneuver which detects tightness in the hip flexors. It is often positive in patients with facet syndrome or long-standing SI syndromes. One leg is brought to the chest while the other is observed as it hangs off the end of a table. If the non-test leg is found to be in significant flexion (compared side to side), this is a positive modified Thomas test. The full Thomas test looks to find other areas of tightness around the hip. If there is greater hip extension when the hip is allowed to abduct and/or internally rotate, TFL-ITB tightness is thought to be the cause. If there is greater hip extension when the knee is passively extended, then the rectus femoris is thought to be the cause. See Modified Thomas Test.

Thompson Technique: A chiropractic technique using a mechanical drop mechanism with an adjusting table, which reduces the spinal adjusting force. This technique is also thought to reduce the patient's sensitivity and pain during spinal adjustments. A specific technique has been developed to be used in conjunction with a Thompson table. Some consider this a nonforce technique. This technique is used by just over 40% of the U.S. chiropractors. See Terminal Point Adjustive Thrust.

thor: An abbreviation for *thoracic.*

Thoracic: Of or pertaining to the upper back. The thoracic spine contains 12 vertebrae that are connected to the rib cage.

Thoracic Curve: A lateral curvature of the spine in which the apex is between T2 and T11.

Thoracic Disc Disorder with Myelopathy: An ICD-9 diagnosis code for a thoracic HNP causing compression of the spinal cord. Large, central thoracic HNPs are rare, but when they do occur, they often produce myelopathy.

Thoracic Inlet Release: A myofascial release technique for the anterior chest wall musculature. This is a superficial release over the anterior chest wall musculature, and it is commonly used in preparation for other release techniques in this area.

Thoracic Outlet Syndrome: Compression of the neurovascular bundle (usually irritation of nerves) in the shoulder girdle area between the first rib and clavicle, by a cervical rib, at the second and third ribs, between the anterior and middle scalenes, or underneath the pectoralis minor and clavipectoral fascia. Symptoms include paresthesia, numbness, pain in the arm and hand, and weakness in the hand. There are many physical exam maneuvers. One such test involves having the patient bring the shoulders into retraction and down and then applying overpressure to this position. Common treatments include postural exercises, mobilization of the cervical spine, increasing the strength of the upper back musculature and scapular stabilizers, first rib mobilizations, clavicular mobilizations, adverse neural tension work, deep tissue work on the surrounding musculature, spray and stretch to the surrounding musculature, muscle energy techniques, Jones strain–counterstrain, and others. True neurovascular thoracic outlet syndrome is rare. This is defined as decreased vascular flow detected first on physical exam by an Adson's test. This is more commonly seen in young athletes and can involve loss of arterial flow to the hand or loss of venous return. Axonal loss secondary to frank brachial plexus compression is also rare. EMG–nerve conduction study is notoriously nonsensitive for this diagnosis. It is thought that neurogenic thoracic outlet syndrome does have a characteristic constellation of the EMG findings. An arteriogram or venogram can be helpful when diagnosing true vascular TOS. However, the diagnosis of brachial plexus irritation is a clinical diagnosis. See TOS, Myogenic TOS, Anterior Scalene Syndrome, Scalene Anticus Syndrome, Cervicobrachial Syndrome, Claviculocostal Syndrome, Clavipectoral Syndrome, Pectoralis Minor Syndrome, Femoral Nerve Stretch Test.

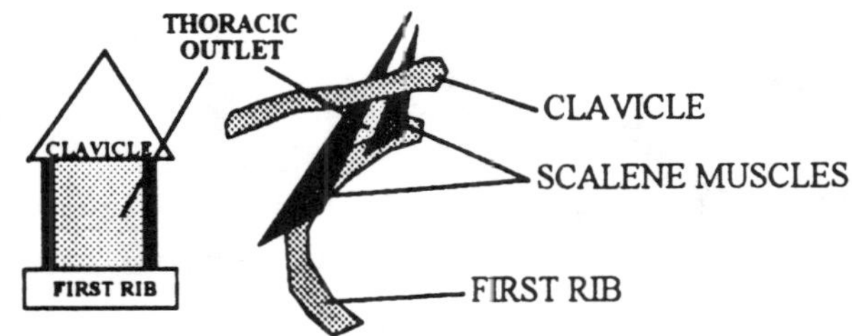

THE THORACIC OUTLET REPRESENTED BY A HOUSE, WITH THE CLAVICLE AS THE ROOF, THE FIRST RIB AS THE FLOOR, AND THE SCALENE MUSCLES AS THE WALLS.

Thoracic Scoliosis: A scoliosis where the apex of the curve is within the thoracic spine.

Thoracic Spine Pain: An ICD-9 diagnosis which is extremely nonspecific. This can be caused by numerous factors, such as biomechanical dysfunction within the thoracic segments, pain emanating from overload of the scapular stabilizers, myofascial pain of the scapular stabilizers or thoracic erector spinae, rib pain, pain emanating from the rib facet, and diaphragmatic pain.

Thoracodorsal Fascia: A thick sheet of connective tissue that covers the superficial musculature of the lumbar spine. It is connected to the latissimus dorsi and gluteus maximus and, consequently, is a link in the kinetic chain that connects the upper and lower extremities. The obliques connect into the fascia laterally and form a muscular corset. The two structures help to off-load the weight of the trunk onto the abdominal contents by allowing the trunk to float on the abdominal cavity. The thoracodorsal fascia connects to the spinous processes in the midline and, as such, helps pull the lumbar spine into extension. See Lumbodorsal Fascia, Thoracolumbar Fascia.

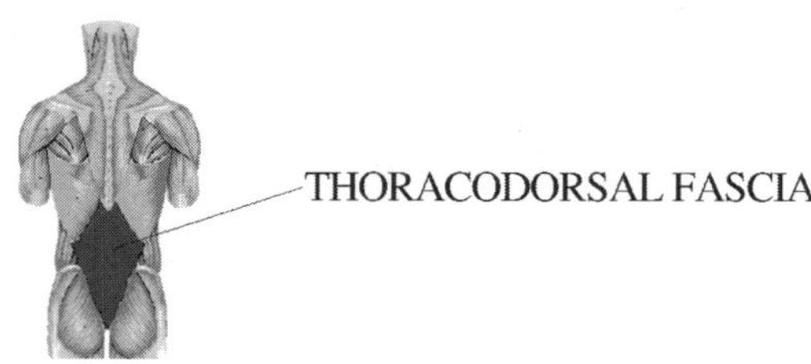

Thoracolumbar Burst Fracture: A collapse of the vertebral body posteriorly with widening of the pedicles. Bony fragments are retropulsed into the spinal canal with 50% of these patients presenting with neurologic deficits. There is a high incidence of instability. See Burst Fracture.

Thoracolumbar Curve: A scoliosis with its apex at T12 or L1.

Thoracolumbar Fascia: A thick sheet of connective tissue that covers the superficial musculature of the lumbar spine. See Thoracodorsal Fascia.

Thoracolumbar Junction: The T12–L1 area. This is the region where the relatively immobile thoracic spine (due to the rib cage) joins with the more mobile lumbar spine.

Thoracolumbosacral Orthosis: A hard shell brace which extends from just below the shoulders to just below the hips. See TLSO.

Thoracolumbosacral Thigh Orthosis: A hard shell brace which extends from just below the shoulders to just below the hips. There is an additional portion which extends down to one thigh. See TLSOT.

Three-Point Brace: A three-point brace with two pads anteriorly over the sternum and pubis and one pad posteriorly over the thoracolumbar area. See Jewett Brace.

Thrombotic Myelopathy: Myelopathy caused by a thrombotic event with ensuing spinal cord ischemia. A dural AV fistula or juvenile AVM can be the etiology.

THSPS: An instrumentation system. See Titanium Hollow Screw Plate System.

t.i.d.: An abbreviation for *three times a day* (from the Latin *ter in die*).

Tietze's Syndrome: Inflammation of the costal cartilage (area between the ribs) which can be due to trauma but more likely is idiopathic. See Costochondritis.

ting: An abbreviation for *tingling*.

Tinnitus: A ringing in the ears or in the head. This can represent any auditory sensation and can be continuous, intermittent, or pulse-like. Tinnitus can also be heard by the examiner if it is caused by intravascular turbulence, fluid within the eustachian tube, or sounds emanating from the TMJ.

Tissue Texture Abnormality: An osteopathic term describing a palpable change in the tissues that is associated with somatic dysfunction. See TTA.

Titanium Hollow Screw Plate System: An instrumentation system designed for anterior cervical fusion which attempts to prevent the migration and loosening of screws by using a cross-split screw head that can be locked into place. This also eliminates the requirements for posterior cortex purchase and decreases the risk of spinal cord injury. This is often used for tumor resection, fracture, and correction of kyphotic deformities. See THSPS.

T-L: An abbreviation for *thoracolumbar*.

TLSO: A hard shell brace which extends from just under the shoulders to just above the hips. This type of immobilization commonly is used after a lumbar fusion or with a vertebral compression fracture. See Thoracolumbosacral Orthosis.

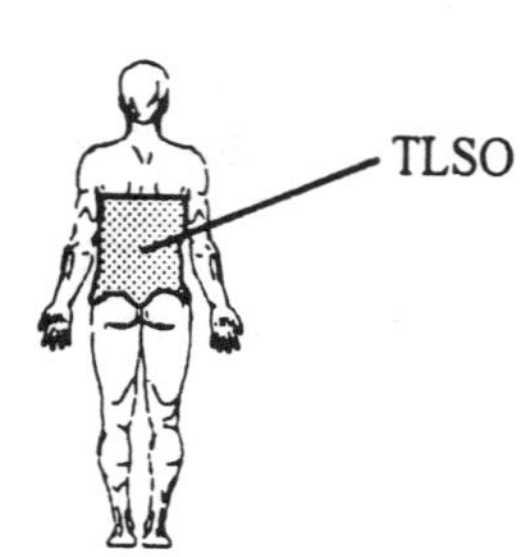

TLSOT: A hard shell brace which extends from just below the shoulders to just below the hips. There is an additional portion which extends down to one thigh. It is thought that this type of orthosis better immobilizes L5–S1 and L4–L5. This is more restricting than a TLSO. See Body Cast with a Leg In, Thoracolumbosacral Thigh Orthosis, TLSO with a Leg In.

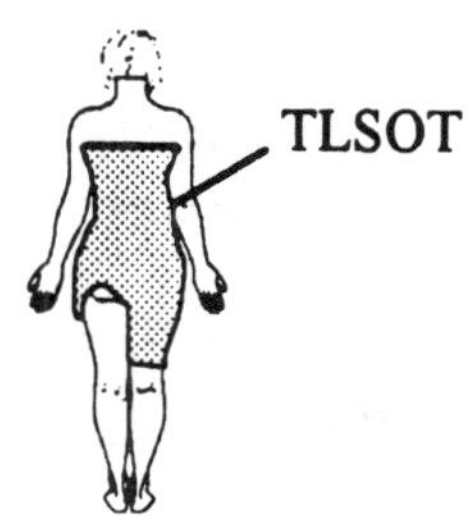

TLSO with a Leg In: A hard shell brace which extends from just below the shoulders to just below the hips. There is an additional portion which extends down to one thigh. See TLSOT.

TMJ: The articulation between the mandible (jaw bone) and the skull. See Temporomandibular Joint.

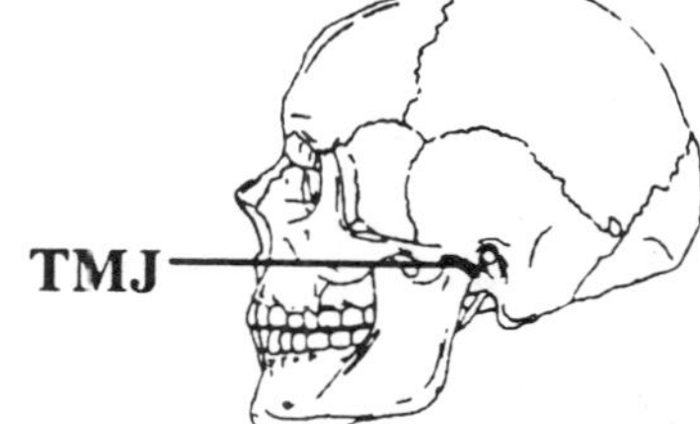

TMJ Capsulitis: An inflammatory reaction within the TMJ joint. See TMJ Dysfunction, TMJ Joint Capsulitis, Temporomandibular Joint Capsulitis.

TMJ Dysfunction: Pain emanating from the temporomandibular joint usually due to direct trauma to the joint. This most commonly occurs in patients between the ages of 20 and 40 and is more frequently found in women. Early symptoms include clicking, subluxation, and recurrent dislocation. The syndrome first manifests itself in the form of decreased coordination of the mandibular muscles. There is hypermobility of the joint and tendency to protrude with initial opening movement. There is often pain on palpation of the joint or movement of the joint. The pain is also common during mastication (chewing). Gradually, as the pain becomes worse, there is decreased mobility within the joint. It is thought that in unilateral conditions the joint deviates toward the side of dysfunction. Catching and locking can occur in certain positions. See Mandibular Pain Dysfunction Syndrome, Arthrosis Temporomandibularis, Temporomandibular Joint Arthrosis, TMJ Myofascial Pain, Temporomandibular Dysfunction.

TMJ Joint Capsulitis: An inflammatory reaction within the TMJ joint. See TMJ Dysfunction, TMJ Capsulitis, Temporomandibular Joint Capsulitis.

TMJ Myofascial Pain: Pain emanating from the temporomandibular joint, usually due to direct trauma to the joint. See TMJ Dysfunction.

TMJ Syndrome: Pain due to TMJ dysfunction but not necessarily directly from the TMJ. This appears to be directly related to head and neck position. For instance, the otherwise phasic strap musculature can become tonic head and neck supporters in a forward head position. This can cause overload of the musculature and can lead to problems within the joint. Myofascial trigger points can be found in numerous locations including the temporalis, masseter, sternocleidomastoid, and medial or lateral pterygoid. Many manual therapists believe that this syndrome is intimately associated with upper cervical dysfunction. The cause can be whiplash or neck trauma.

TMT: An abbreviation for *treatment.*

TNS: A variation of TENS. See TENS.

Tofranil: A tricyclic antidepressant used for chronic pain. See Imipramine.

Toftness Technique: A chiropractic technique that uses a tube-shaped instrument with a series of lenses to help detect areas of subluxations and neurologic disturbances. This instrument is reported to detect minute radiation and electromagnetic disturbances that exist with spinal subluxation. There is a very light nonforce adjustment technique used in conjunction with this instrument to make spinal corrections. This is not an accepted technique in most chiropractic associations and is used by only 3% of U.S. chiropractors. See Nonforce Technique.

Toggle Recoil: A chiropractic adjusting technique in which a high-velocity (high-acceleration), low-amplitude thrust is applied to the upper cervical spine. See Recoil Adjustment.

tol: An abbreviation for *tolerated.*

Tolectin: A nonsteroidal anti-inflammatory drug in the pyrrole class. It is thought, as with all NSAIDs, that the mechanism of action is through inhibition of prostaglandin synthesis. As with all NSAIDs, GI, renal, and hepatic side effects are possible. There are drug interactions with oral anticoagulants and methotrexate. Unlike other NSAIDs, no interactions have been found with oral hypoglycemic agents. The recommended starting dosage is 400 mg three times a day. The normal adult dosage range is 600–1800 mg daily in divided doses. The therapeutic response may take a few days to a week. This drug is supplied in 200-, 400-, and 600-mg capsules. See Tolmetin Sodium.

Tolmetin Sodium: A nonsteroidal anti-inflammatory drug in the pyrrole class. See Tolectin.

Tomography: An x-ray technique usually used to examine thin sections of bony structures. The x-ray tube is moved while the rest of the body remains stationary. Only a thin slice of the bony structure in question remains in focus while the surrounding structures are blurred.

Tonus Receptor Technique: The technique used to resolve Nimmo points or trigger points. See Nimmo Technique.

Torticollis: An abnormal twisting posture of the head and cervical spine. See Focal Cervical Dystonia, BOTOX.

TOS: Compression of the neurovascular bundle (usually irritation of nerves) in the shoulder girdle area between the first rib and clavicle, by a cervical rib, at the second and third ribs, between the anterior and middle scalenes, or underneath the pectoralis minor and clavipectoral fascia. See Thoracic Outlet Syndrome.

Total Gym: A piece of exercise equipment which utilizes a rolling platform on steel rails. Pulleys connect to this platform so that the patient can pull against varying degrees of resistance depending on the inclination of the platform. This is commonly used in spinal rehabilitation with a "medical exercise therapy" approach. For instance, a patient with severe lumbar pain who cannot tolerate full-gravity quadriceps strengthening can lie down on the inclined rolling platform and perform half squats while giving assist to the quadriceps through the upper extremity pulleys.

Total Laminectomy: A surgical technique. See Laminotomy.

tp: An abbreviation for *treatment plan.*

TP: An abbreviation for *transverse process.*

TP: An abbreviation for *trigger point.* See Trigger Point.

TPI: An injection of usually procaine, lidocaine, xylocaine, or marcaine into a trigger point in an effort to deactivate the trigger point. See Trigger Point Injection.

TPL: A chiropractic x-ray marking technique in which dots are placed at the lateral mass-transverse process intersection in the upper cervical spine.

TPT: An abbreviation for *trigger point therapy.* See Trigger Point.

TR: Repetition time in an MR image. This is the time between subsequent radio frequency pulses and is a crucial factor for image contrast.

Trabeculae: Small connective tissue extensions (thin rods of bone oriented in vertical and transverse planes making up the struts and cross beams of the vertebra) between the arachnoid membrane and the pia mater. These form a delicate, sponge-like network and appear very similar to the trabeculae of bone. These act as the internal architecture of the bones and provide strength. The spaces between the trabeculae are used as channels for blood supply and venous drainage and further act as a system for transmitting the loads of weight bearing and absorbing force. See Arachnoid Trabeculae.

Traction: An axial distraction that is applied by manual means (i.e., hands). See Manual Traction, Pelvic Traction.

Traction—Intermittent: Traction that is alternatively applied and then released at short intervals. See Intermittent Traction.

Traction Spur: A type of spinal osteophyte (bone spur) which projects horizontally from the corner of the vertebral body and is located 5 mm or more from the vertebral margin. These are thought to be the direct result of degenerative disc disease. Abnormal motion between the vertebral segments places unusual and pathologic stresses on the outermost fibers of the annulus and causes traction spurs. This type of osteophyte is thought to be associated with segmental instability.

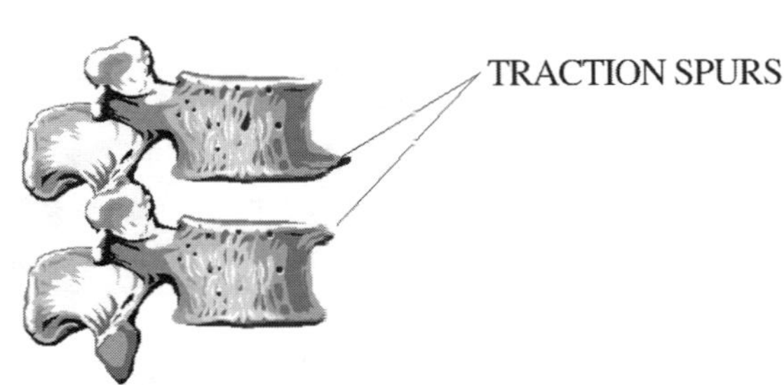

Traction—Static: A steady traction force applied and maintained for a specific time interval. See Static Traction.

Trager: A mechanical soft tissue technique involving neuromuscular re-education developed by Milton Trager, M.D. There are no rigid protocols, and the nervous system is used to make changes, rather than making mechanical changes in the connective tissues themselves. Trager practitioners believe that "for every physical non-yielding condition there is a psychic counterpart in the unconscious mind." The system uses general passive motions that emphasize mobilization concentrating on traction and rotation. There is also a system of active movements called mentastics. This is used to alter the neuromuscular balance to establish more normal movement patterns. See Trager Psychophysical Integration.

Trager Psychophysical Integration: A mechanical soft tissue technique. See Trager.

Transcranial Electrical Stimulation: An electrical stimulation device used to treat headaches.

Transcranial Magnetic Stimulation: A method of monitoring the integrity of the corticospinal tract and motor pathways during spinal surgery. See Motor Evoked Potential.

Transcutaneous Electrical Nerve Stimulation: A form of electrical anesthesia used to block pain perception and based on Melzack and Wall's "gate theory." See TENS.

Transderm-Scōp: A trademark name for a transdermal patch delivery system which is designed for continuous release of scopolamine. This has been used in patients with chronic dizziness. Scopolamine is a belladonna alkaloid with anticholinergic side effects. It is believed that scopolamine inhibits the vestibular input to the CNS. This drug is contraindicated in patients with glaucoma. Also, some drowsiness or disorientation may be associated with this drug, so it is to be avoided in combination with activities that require mental alertness. It should also be used only rarely in patients with pyloric obstruction or urinary bladder neck obstruction. Also, patients with impaired metabolic, liver, or kidney functions (e.g., the elderly) should use this drug with caution. Alcohol may potentiate some of the CNS side effects. Dosage is one

Transderm-Scōp disc (0.5 mg of scopolamine over three days) applied to the hairless area behind one ear at least four hours before the drug is required. If the disc becomes displaced, another disc can be applied. The drug is supplied as a 2.5 cm^2 containing 1.5 mg of scopolamine programmed to deliver 0.5 mg of scopolamine over three days. Packages of four discs are available. See Scopolamine Patch.

Transforaminal Ligament: An anomalous ligament that spans a lumbar foramen. It may have implications for additional sites of nerve root entrapment.

Transient Quadriplegia: Numbness and weakness in the bilateral upper extremities and lower extremities seen in patients with cervical central canal stenosis. These symptoms are usually dependent on head position, such as flexion or extension. There is usually no permanent neurologic deficit involved.

Transitional: A vertebra that adjoins another spinal region with some characteristics of that spinal region. See Transitional Segment, Transitional Vertebra.

Transitional Segment: A vertebra that adjoins another spinal region with some characteristics of that spinal region. Transitional Vertebra, Transitional.

Transitional Vertebra: A vertebra that adjoins another spinal region with some characteristics of that spinal region. An example is a first lumbar vertebra with rudimentary ribs. Another example would be a sacralized L5 or a lumbarized S1. The most common level is L5–S1. See Transitional Segment, Transitional.

Transitional Vertebrae: A term used in describing the neutral vertebrae in patients with scoliosis. These are the vertebrae that make the transition from one curve to the next.

Translaminar Facet Screw Fixation: A form of spinal fusion which involves inserting a screw at the base of the spinous process, through the opposite lamina, transversing the facet joint, and ending in the base of the transverse process. This provides a very solid fusion by immobilizing the facet joints. See Translaminar Fixation.

Translaminar Fixation: A form of spinal fusion. See Translaminar Facet Screw Fixation.

Translated Sacrum: An osteopathic term which refers to a sacrum that has moved forward or backward relative to the ilia. This is not just movement of the sacral base but also of the sacral apex such that the entire sacrum has moved either forward or backward between the ilia.

Translated Sacrum—Anterior: An osteopathic term which refers to a sacrum that has moved forward relative to the ilia. The entire sacrum has moved forward between the ilia, not just the base or the apex. There is increased movement in an anterior direction relative to the posterior direction. See Anterior Translated Sacrum.

Translated Sacrum—Posterior: An osteopathic term which refers to a sacrum that has moved backward relative to the ilia. The entire sacrum has moved backward, not just the base or the apex. There is increased movement in a posterior direction relative to the anterior direction. See Posterior Translated Sacrum.

Translatory Gliding Motion: A lateral translation of the spine. See Side Glide.

Transpedicular Fixation: The use of pedicle screws for anterior fusion. Because the failure rate of anterior fixation systems that drill into the vertebral body can be significant, this technique has been proposed. A special guide is used to drill the pedicle screw into the anterior vertebral body and into the pedicle from an anterior approach. It is thought that this allows for anterior immobilization of shorter segments with fewer screws due to the better purchase in bone. See Anterior Fusion.

Transpedicular Screws: Screws which are placed into the pedicle and used in many different types of spinal fixation.

Transverse Axes of the Sacrum: In osteopathic literature, it is postulated that there are three transverse axes of sacral movement: inferior, middle, and superior. The inferior axis is for iliosacral motion, the middle axis (passes through S2) for postural motion (movement of the sacrum while standing), and the superior axis for respiratory motion (movement that occurs with respiration and with craniosacral movements). See Iliosacral Motion.

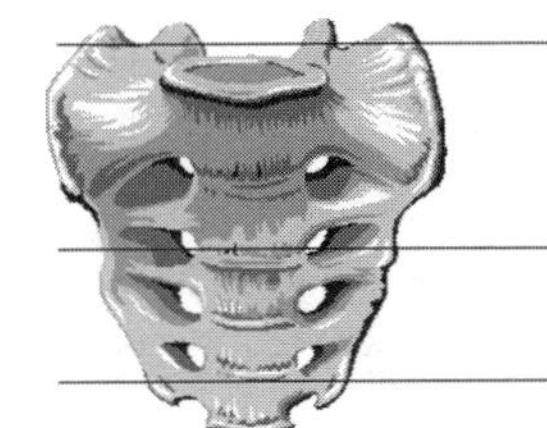

Transverse Foramen: The hole through the transverse processes of C1– C6 through which the vertebral artery passes.

Transverse Foramen of the Axis: The hole in the axis through which the vertebral artery passes.

Transverse Fracture of the Sacrum: The most common type of sacral fracture, usually seen at the level of the third and fourth sacral segments near the lower end of the SI joint. See Horizontal Fracture of the Sacrum.

Transverse Friction Massage: A muscle goading technique in which deep pressure is applied in a perpendicular direction to the muscle fibers.

Transverse Ligament of the Atlas: The ligament which holds the dens against the anterior arch of the atlas. It is continous with the overlying cruciform ligament. Biomechanically, it allows rotation of C2 on C1 through holding the dens in its pivot point. There is a bursa between the dens and the transverse ligament. Isolated traumatic rupture of this ligament is not well studied. Traditionally, it has been thought that rupture of this ligament without fracture is rare. In rheumatiod arthritis, the ligament can be eroded through causing atlantoaxial instability. In Down syndrome, there can be significant ligamentous laxity. See ADI.

Transverse Ligament Rupture: Rupture of the ligament that can occur in association with a Jefferson's fracture, inflammatory arthritis, and Down syndrome. See Rupture of the Transverse Ligament.

Transverse Ligament Test: A test for the integrity of the transverse ligament. The patient is in the supine position with the examiner at the head of the table and the occiput supported in the palms with the upper cervical spine slightly extended. With the fingertips, posterior-anterior pressure is applied against the posterior arch of C1 (the posterior arch of C1 can be found just superior and lateral on each side of the spinous process of C2). A negative test should have a ligamentous or firm end feel with approximately 1–3 mm of motion. A positive test is suspected if the patient reports cord signs or nausea or if there is excess movement.

Transverse Process: A projection of bone which takes its origin from the junction of the pedicle and lamina. When the vertebral body is viewed from the front or from behind, the transverse processes look like arms extending outward on either side. On the posterior surface there is an irregular bony prominence called the accessory process.

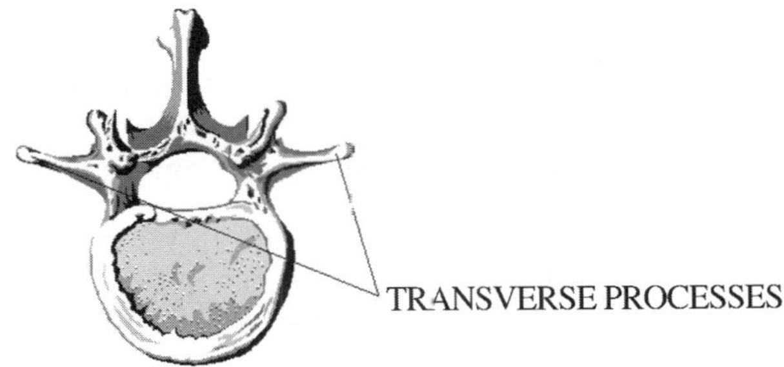

Transverse Process Fracture: A fracture of the lateral bony projection of the vertebra. This is the second most common fracture of the lumbar spine (vertebral compression fracture is the first). They usually occur secondary to a severe hyperextension/lateral flexion injury of the lumbar spine. The most common levels fractured are L2 and L3 with multiple fractures being more common. There may be loss of the psoas shadow due to hemorrhage. Fractures of the L5 transverse process are commonly found in association with pelvic fractures (fractures of the ala or SI joint disruption). Because damage to the kidneys can be seen after these fractures, urinalysis is mandatory to rule out hematuria.

Transverse Sacral Fracture: The most common type of sacral fracture, usually seen at the level of the third and fourth sacral segments near the lower end of the SI joint. See Horizontal Fracture of the Sacrum, Suicide Jumper's Fracture.

Trap: An abbreviation for *trapezius.*

Trapezius: An upper back muscle which is responsible for such diverse actions as retracting the shoulders, aiding in abducting the shoulder, and turning the head. The upper fibers attach to the nuchal ligament and to the spinous processes of C1–C5 and then attach distally to the outer third of the clavicle. This portion of the trapezius elevates the shoulder, laterally bends the neck to the same side, and aids in extreme rotation of the head to the opposite side. Acting bilaterally, the upper fibers extend the head and neck. The upper trapezius plays a postural role. The levator scapulae, upper serratus anterior, and the upper trapezius are part of a force couple that rotates the scapula upward. There are two trigger points, one anteriorly, which refers up the neck laterally and to the temporal area, and one posterolaterally, which refers to the occiput. The upper trapezius may be a source of "tension headaches." The middle fibers of the trapezius attach medially to the spinous processes and interspinous ligaments of C6–T3 and distally to the acromion and spine of the scapula. These fibers retract the scapula and assist in flexion and abduction of the shoulder by tilting the scapula upward. There are three trigger point areas in the middle trapezius. The first is located just medial to the medial border of the scapula and refers burning pain toward the spinous processes. The second is found near the acromion and refers an aching pain to the superior shoulder or AC joint area. The last is in the middle portion above the superior-medial border of the scapula and refers pilomotor activity to the lateral arm. The fibers of the lower trapezius attach to the spinous processes and interspinous ligaments of T4–T12 medially and insert on the spine of the scapula. These fibers retract the scapula and rotate it upward while assisting in flexion and abduction of the arm. There are two trigger points. The first is located in the middle portion of the muscle laterally and refers to the high cervical region. This is usually referred to as "soreness" by the patient. The second trigger point is located laterally near the fiber attachment to the spine of the scapula. This refers a steady burning pain to the medial border of the scapula. Innervation of the trapezius is through the spinal accessory nerve (cranial nerve XI).

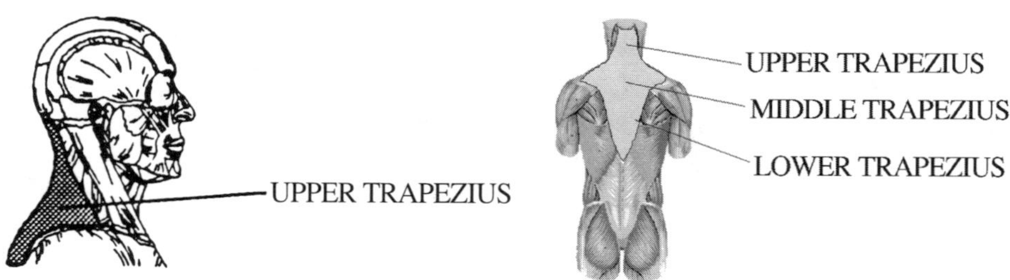

Traumatic Atlanto-occipital Dislocation: A traumatic injury of the upper cervical spine that occurs as a result of a high-speed MVA or auto–pedestrian accident. This is a traumatic dislocation of the atlanto-occipital joint.

Traumatic Scoliosis: A structural scoliosis that is caused by a traumatic vertebral body fracture.

Traumatic Spondylolisthesis: A fracture of the neural arch other than the pars interarticularis. See Type IV Spondylolisthesis.

Trendelenburg Gait: Weakness in the gluteal musculature that causes a tilting of the pelvis and trunk toward that side during the stance phase of walking. This is known as a compensated Trendelenburg gait. An uncompensated gait is when the opposite pelvis drops during the stance phase due to severe gluteal weakness. See Coxalgic Gait, Gluteus Medius Gait, Gluteus Medius Lurch, Gluteal Gait.

Tri: An abbreviation for *triceps.*

Triad of Dejerine: A test for dural irritation or compression. See Dejerine's Sign.

Triazolam: A benzodiazepine used to induce sleep in insomnia. See Halcion.

Tric: An abbreviation for *triceps.*

Trigger Point: Classically, a taut palpable band in muscle that is painful to touch and refers pain in a characteristic distribution to another (often adjacent) body area. However, it may be confused to mean any tender spot within a muscle (not the classical definition). One theory is that a trigger point is a hyperirritable focus within a muscle or its surrounding fascia associated with a taut band on palpation. The trigger point may be the downstream consequence of a biomechanical imbalance. There are both active and latent trigger points. Common treatments include myotherapy, acupressure, ischemic compression, spray and stretch, or trigger point injections. See Active Trigger Point, Myofascial Trigger Point, Myofascial Pain Syndrome, Myofascial Pain, Massage, Nimmo Technique, Nonforce Technique.

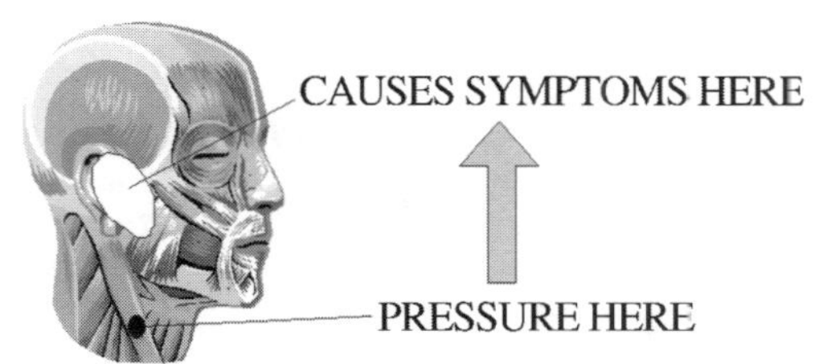

AN EXAMPLE OF A TRIGGER POINT—PRESSURE OVER AN AREA OF THE STERNOCLEIDOMASTOID MUSCLE CAUSES SYMPTOMS IN THE EAR.

Trigger Point Injection: An injection of usually procaine, lidocaine, xylocaine, or marcaine into a trigger point in an effort to deactivate the trigger point. It is usually followed by stretching techniques. Steroids can also be added, but in anything greater than small amounts there may be evidence of muscle necrosis. See TPI.

Trigger Point Myotherapy: The application of progressively stronger pressure on a trigger point. This pressure causes ischemia within that portion of the muscle followed by a hyperemic response on the release of pressure. This is thought to "release" the trigger point. See Myotherapy.

Trochanteric Bursitis: Inflammation of the trochanteric bursa. This can be caused by a tight iliotibial band impinging the trochanteric bursa (over the greater trochanter). This may be associated with an SI joint syndrome. Common treatments: iliotibial band stretching, treating the SI joint syndrome, or injection into the trochanteric bursa of corticosteroids. Iontophoresis can also be helpful in thin patients. Pain here may be confused with a Jones point at the posterior lateral trochanter. See Iontophoresis, Iliotibial Band Syndrome.

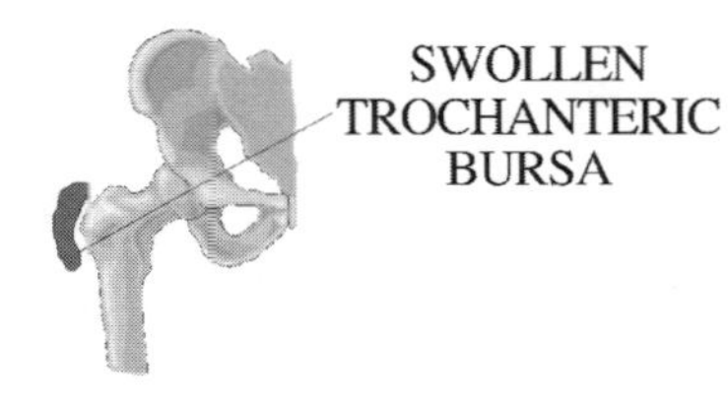

Trolley Track Sign: A radiographic sign seen in ankylosing spondylitis. This is caused by ossification of the joint capsule, ligamentum flavum, and interspinous ligaments. Parallel linear densities are seen on AP film that resemble a train track.

Tropism: Facet joints that are asymmetrical with respect to the plane of articulation. See Facet Tropism.

Trough Graft: A bony graft that is placed into troughs cut into the vertebral body above and the vertebral body below. The graft is placed in the disc space and used for immediate postoperative stability in problems like instability or spondylolisthesis. The troughs prevent movement of the vertebral body above on the vertebral body below. Usually a large piece of iliac bone is used for this type of fusion.

True Hypomobility: Severe limitation of movement in a joint which requires more effort to mobilize or is unchangeable. An excellent example of this is ankylosing spondylitis causing a fused SI joint.

Trunk Curl: A form of sit-ups used to increase the strength of the upper abdominals. This also gives an indication of overall trunk flexibility. In this abdominal strengthening exercise, most of the movement comes from the thoracic spine. Some would advocate having the patient in a hook-lying position, while others would advocate having the patient perform this maneuver with a straight leg.

Trx: An abbreviation for *traction.*

TSRH: Texas Scottish-Rite Hospital Instrumentation.

TTA: An osteopathic term. See Tissue Texture Abnormality.

TTD: When a worker is unable to earn wages and return to work as expected and the medical condition has not yet stabilized. See Temporary Total Disability.

TTF: An abbreviation for *taut tender fibers*.

Tuberculous Spondylitis: A tuberculosis infection involving the spine which can cause collapse of the vertebral bodies. See Pott's Disease.

Tuohy Needle: A needle commonly used for epidural steroid injection that has a curved end with either a sharp or blunt tip. The blunt tip is thought to cause less potential injury to the dura.

Twitch Response: A sudden contraction of muscle seen as a twitch in response to stimulation of a trigger point. The twitch usually occurs within the trigger point being stimulated. Stimulation is by snapping, palpation, or needling. See Local Twitch Response, Jump Sign.

Two-Point Discrimination: A test of sensation involving mechanoreceptors usually tested on the hand or on the feet. The patient should be able to distinguish two separate points 3 mm apart on the pads of the fingers or 2–3 cm apart on the sole of the foot. This test can be used to define sensation loss.

Tx: An abbreviation for *treatment*.

Tylenol: An analgesic and antipyretic (reduces fever). See Acetaminophen.

Tylenol No. 2: A narcotic pain reliever which contains 300 mg of acetaminophen and 15 mg of codeine phosphate. See Codeine.

Tylenol No. 3: A narcotic pain reliever which contains 300 mg of acetaminophen and 30 mg of codeine phosphate. Codeine is an addictive narcotic. Common adult dosage is one to two tablets every 4 hours. See Codeine, Acetaminophen and Codeine Phosphate.

Tylenol No. 4: A narcotic pain reliever which contains 60 mg of codeine and 300 mg of acetaminophen. See Tylenol No. 3, Codeine.

Tylox: A narcotic pain reliever containing 5 mg of oxycodone and 500 mg of acetaminophen. The drug is contraindicated in patients taking other CNS depressant medications (i.e., alcohol). There is a significant abuse potential. The usual dosage is one Tylox every 6 hours as needed for pain. Note that the drugs Percocet, Percodan, and Roxicet also contain oxycodone.

Type 1 AVM: A type of arteriovenous malformation which is commonly located on the dorsal spinal cord surface. See AVM—Type 1, Single-Coiled Vessel AVM, Dural AV Fistula.

Type 1 Dysfunction: A system used in evaluating lateral bending movements with stress radiography. See Type 1 Lateral Flexion.

Type 1 Dysfunction Based on Fryette's First Law: An osteopathic or physical therapy term which signifies a group of dysfunctions usually involving three or more vertebral segments. The barrier to movement is found with the spine in a neutral position. Because this is based on Fryette's first law, these vertebral segments will be restricted in side bending in one direction and in rotation to the other. These dysfunctions usually occur as compensatory "fixes" because of a type 2 dysfunction. These dysfunctions must be treated after the type 2 dysfunction.

Type 1 End Plate Changes: Changes in the bone marrow of the vertebral bodies near the intervertebral disc. See End Plate Changes—Type 1.

Type 1 Lateral Flexion: A system used in evaluating lateral bending movements with stress radiography. As the spine is laterally flexed, the spinous process of each lumbar segment rotates toward the same side. See Coupling, Type 1 Motion, Type 1 Dysfunction.

Type 1 Marrow Changes: Changes in the bone marrow of the vertebral bodies near the intervertebral disc. See End Plate Changes—Type 1.

Type 1 Mechanoreceptors: Mechanoreceptors which are found within the joint capsule and around the joint. See Ruffini End Organs.

Type 1 Motion: A system used in evaluating lateral bending movements with stress radiography. See Type 1 Lateral Flexion.

Type 1 Nerve Root Anomaly: A nerve root anomaly with an aberrant course, e.g., two pairs of nerve roots that arise from a single dural sleeve. See Nerve Root Anomaly—Type 1, Anomaly—Type 1.

Type 2 AVM: A glomus type, intradural, arteriovenous malformation which, together with Type 3 AVMs, comprise approximately 15–20% of all spinal AVMs. See AVM—Type 2, Glomus AVM.

Type 2 Dysfunction: A system used in evaluating lateral bending movements with stress radiography. See Type 2 Lateral Flexion, Nonneutral Dysfunction.

Type 2 Dysfunction Based on Fryette's Second Law: An osteopathic or manual physical therapy term referring to a vertebral segment which is hypomobile (not moving as much as it should) because of a restriction to its movement. Because this is based on Fryette's second law, the segment is most restricted in the flexion or extension test positions. This usually occurs secondary to trauma. The segment is restricted in side bending and rotation to the same side.

Type 2 End Plate Changes: The bone marrow becomes replaced with fat. See End Plate Changes—Type 2.

Type 2 Lateral Flexion: A system used in evaluating lateral bending movements with stress radiography. A lateral bending film is taken, and normal coupling behavior is seen. As the spine is laterally flexed, the spinous process of each lumbar segment rotates toward the same side. Type 2 refers to a spine that laterally bends but does not axially rotate. See Type 1 Lateral Flexion, Type 2 Motion, Type 2 Dysfunction.

Type 2 Marrow Changes: The marrow becomes replaced with fat. See End Plate Changes—Type 2.

Type 2 Motion: A system used in evaluating lateral bending movements with stress radiography. See Type 2 Lateral Flexion.

Type 2 Nerve Root Anomaly: A nerve root anomaly where the number of roots in an intervertebral foramen is variable, e.g., if a foramen is empty and the foramen above or below contains two sets of roots. See Nerve Root Anomaly—Type 2, Anomaly—Type 2.

Type 3 AVM: An intradural arteriovenous malformation which is considered "juvenile." See AVM—Type 3.

Type 3 Dysfunction: Type 3 motion describes a spine that does not laterally flex. See Type 3 Lateral Flexion.

Type 3 End Plate Changes: Instead of replacement by fibrous vascular tissue or fat, there is replacement with sclerotic bone. See End Plate Changes—Type 3.

Type 3 Lateral Flexion: A system used in evaluating lateral bending movements with stress radiography. A lateral bending film is taken, and normal coupling behavior is seen. As the spine is laterally flexed, the spinous process of each lumbar segment rotates toward the same side. Type 3 motion describes a spine that does not laterally flex but has the normal coupling motion of axial rotation. See Type 1 Lateral Flexion, Type 3 Motion, Type 3 Dysfunction.

Type 3 Marrow Changes: Replacement with sclerotic bone. See End Plate Changes—Type 3.

Type 3 Motion: A spine that does not laterally flex. See Type 3 Lateral Flexion.

Type 3 Nerve Root Anomaly: A nerve root anomaly in which there are extra dural connections between roots, and a bundle of nerve fibers leaves one dural sleeve to enter an adjacent root. This is also known as a conjoined nerve root. See Nerve Root Anomaly—Type 3, Anomaly—Type 3, Conjoined Nerve Root.

Type 4 Dysfunction: A system used in evaluating lateral bending movements with stress radiography. See Type 4 Lateral Flexion.

Type 4 Lateral Flexion: A system used in evaluating lateral bending movements with stress radiography. A lateral bending film is taken, and normal coupling behavior is seen. As the spine is laterally flexed, the spinous process of each lumbar segment rotates toward the same side. Type 4 motion is a segment that is not laterally bending or rotating. See Type 1 Lateral Flexion, Type 4 Motion, Type 4 Dysfunction.

Type 4 Motion: A system used in evaluating lateral bending movements with stress radiography. See Type 4 Lateral Flexion.

Type I Mechanoreceptor: A classification of mechanoreceptors which is defined as postural and located in joint capsules. According to Paris, these mechanoreceptors are activated by graded or progressive oscillatory type mobilizations.

Type I Spondylolisthesis: A congenital malformation of the upper sacrum or neural arch of the L5 vertebra which results in an anterior displacement of the L5 vertebral body on the sacrum. This is commonly associated with a large spina bifida occulta. Unlike other types of spondylolisthesis, this is not associated with a pars interarticularis defect. This type of spondylolisthesis does not usually progress to more severe stages. It occurs with about 25% of the frequency of isthmic spondylolisthesis. See Dysplastic Spondylolisthesis.

Type II Mechanoreceptor: A classification of mechanoreceptors that are considered dynamic and located in joint capsules. According to Paris, these are activated by graded or progressive oscillatory mobilizations.

Type II Spondylolisthesis: Spondylolisthesis due to fracture or elongation of the pars interarticularis. There are three types: A, B, and C. Type A is caused by biomechanical stress or a fatigue fracture of the pars interarticularis. This is the most common type of spondylolisthesis found in patients under the age of 50. Type B is an elongation of the pars interarticularis without actual fracture or separation. This is thought similar to type A in that repeated stresses cause elongation of the pars without actual fracture. Type C is spondylolisthesis from an acute pars fracture following severe trauma. This is usually caused by a hyperextension injury to the lower lumbar spine. See Isthmic Spondylolisthesis.

Type III Mechanoreceptor: A classification of mechanoreceptors which is considered inhibitive. They are located in joint capsules and ligaments. According to Paris, they are activated by stretching or sustained pressure. They are also activated by manipulative thrusts.

Type III Spondylolisthesis: A spondylolisthesis caused by severe degeneration of the facet joint. The neural arch is intact, and, for this reason, this is sometimes referred to as pseudospondylolisthesis. Unlike isthmic spondylolisthesis, this occurs most commonly at L4 and is most common in females over the age of 60. This type of disorder is rare in patients younger than 50 years. It is more common in blacks than whites and is four times more likely to be found in association with a sacralized L5. See Degenerative Spondylolisthesis, Pseudospondylolisthesis.

Type IV Spondylolisthesis: A fracture of the neural arch other than the pars interarticularis. This is common at C2. See Hangman's Fracture, Traumatic Spondylolisthesis.

Type V Spondylolisthesis: Slippage of one vertebra onto another due to a fracture of the neural arch as a result of a systemic or cancerous process. Examples include metastatic carcinoma, Paget's disease, and osteoporosis. See Pathological Spondylolisthesis.

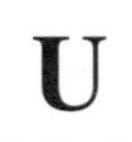

U: An abbreviation for *upper.*

UC: An abbreviation for *upper cervical.*

UID: A cervical spine injury involving dislocation of one facet as a result of a flexion and rotation injury. See Unilateral Facet Dislocation, Unilateral Interfacetal Dislocation.

Ullmann's Line: A radiographic line for determining if there is anterolisthesis of L5 on S1 (spondylolisthesis). A line is drawn parallel to the sacral base and a second line perpendicularly through the anterior margin of the sacral base. If the anterior/inferior corner of L5 is beyond the perpendicular line, then an anterolisthesis is suspected. This can be helpful when there is poor visualization of the pars interarticularis. See Right Angle Test Line, Garland-Thomas Line.

Ullmann's Sign: An x-ray finding in spondylolisthesis. A line is drawn perpendicular to the anterior surface of the sacrum on a lateral radiograph. This line is extended up toward L5. In normal studies, the anteroinferior angle of L5 lies slightly behind this line. In spondylolisthesis, the L5 vertebral body intersects with this line.

Ulnar Neuropathy: An isolated lesion of the ulnar nerve which can cause numbness in the fourth and fifth fingers or paresthesias in the same sensory area. A varying amount of motor dysfunction can also be present including weakness of the intrinsics of the hand and weakness in the ulnar innervated forearm musculature (FCU). The most common site of entrapment is at the cubital tunnel (elbow). The ulnar nerve can also be entrapped as it passes through the two heads of the flexor carpi ulnaris and in Guyon's canal at the wrist. However, thoracic outlet syndrome is much more common than ulnar neuropathy at the elbow. Also, a C8 radiculopathy can also be confused with this diagnosis.

Ultrasound: High-frequency sound that is applied as a therapeutic treatment in rehabilitation. Continuous or pulsed versions can be used. Continuous ultrasound is used for deep heating. Pulsed ultrasound is used for its "nonthermal effects" such as "cavitation." As frequency increases, tissue penetration decreases. Ultrasound increases temperature most effectively at tissue interfaces. This treatment modality is used for a variety of musculoskeletal diagnoses including bursitis, tenosynovitis, trigger points, and tissue stretching. See U/S.

ULTT: A series of maneuvers to elicit adverse neural tension in the upper extremities. Often, passive neck flexion or extension is added to intensify or sensitize these tests. This is considered the straight-leg raise of the upper extremity. See Adverse Neural Tension, Upper Limb Tension Test, BPTT.

UMN: An abbreviation for *upper motor neuron.*

Uncinate Process: The joints which occur in the lower cervical spine from C2–C7. See Uncovertebral Joint.

Uncompensated Scoliosis: A scoliotic condition of the spine which results in an unlevel pelvis or shoulder girdle.

Uncovertebral Joint: The joints which occur in the lower cervical spine from C2–C7. These are formed by the lateral projections on the rim of the vertebral bodies. They are independent of the disc and facet joints. Clinically, degenerative changes are commonly seen with spondylosis. Osteophyte formation at this joint can impinge on the neuroforamina and cause foraminal stenosis. See Luschka's Joint, Joint of Von Luschka, Von Luschka's Joint, Uncinate Process.

Uncovertebral Joint Hypertrophy: An "overgrowth" of the uncovertebral joints which can lead to stenosis of cervical foramina. See Von Luschka Joint Arthrosis, Uncovertebral Joint.

Underburg's Test: A physical exam test that is very similar to a Romberg test or a pronator drift test. The patient stands with the eyes open and arms resting at his or her sides. The feet are placed together, and the examiner observes for any difficulty with equilibrium. The patient then closes the eyes and both arms are elevated with forearms supinated and palms towards the ceiling. The examiner observes for any pronator drift or loss of equilibrium with this maneuver. The patient then is asked to rotate the head and neck to one side while maintaining a narrow postural base (reportedly to detect vertebrobasilar insufficiency). This part of the test is very similar to Hautant's test.

Unilateral Anterior Nutation of the Sacrum: An osteopathic abnormality of sacral motion. See Unilateral Sacral Flexion.

Unilateral Anterior Sacral Nutation: An osteopathic abnormality of sacral motion. See Unilateral Sacral Flexion.

Unilateral Bar: A type of congenital scoliosis in which failure of segmentation of the posterior elements causes a unilateral congenital fusion of two or more vertebral segments. Without surgical correction, scoliosis will progress.

Unilateral Facet Dislocation: A cervical spine injury involving dislocation of one facet which occurs as a result of a flexion and rotation injury. This can occur with or without fracture. Fracture is usually to the superior facet joint and sometimes extends into the lamina. Unilateral facet dislocation without fracture is usually painful, but the spine is clinically stable. When there is disruption of the anulus fibrosus and fracture, neurologic complications are more common. See Facet Dislocation—Unilateral, Unilateral Interfacetal Dislocation.

Unilateral Inferior Nutation of the Sacrum: An osteopathic term which denotes an abnormality of sacral motion. See Unilateral Sacral Flexion.

Unilateral Inferior Sacral Nutation: An osteopathic term which denotes an abnormality of sacral motion. See Unilateral Sacral Flexion.

Unilateral Inferior Sacral Shear: An osteopathic abnormality of sacral motion. See Unilateral Sacral Flexion.

Unilateral Interfacetal Dislocation: A cervical spine injury involving dislocation of one facet which occurs as a result of a flexion and rotation injury. See Unilateral Facet Dislocation, UID.

Unilateral Isometric Hip Flexion: A lumbar stabilization exercise. The patient lies in the supine position with knees bent and feet on the floor. The patient is asked to tighten the stomach and raise one knee to meet the outstretched arm. The arm is kept straight while pushing against the knee and keeping the spine stabilized. This is repeated on the opposite side. See Hip Flexion—Unilateral Isometric.

Unilaterally Extended Sacrum: An osteopathic or manual physical therapy term which refers to an abnormality in sacral positioning. See Unilateral Sacral Extension, Posterior Sacrum.

Unilaterally Flexed Sacrum: An osteopathic or manual physical therapy term which refers to a sacrum with the sacral base anterior relative to the ilium on one side. See Anterior Sacrum.

Unilateral Posterior Nutation of the Sacrum: An osteopathic or manual physical therapy term which refers to an abnormality in sacral positioning. See Unilateral Sacral Extension.

Unilateral Posterior Sacral Nutation: An osteopathic or manual physical therapy term which refers to an abnormality in sacral positioning. See Unilateral Sacral Extension.

Unilateral Sacral Extension: An osteopathic or manual physical therapy term which refers to an abnormality in sacral positioning. The sacrum (which follows type I mechanics) is extended, side bent to the same side, and rotated to the opposite side. Usually the left side is involved, and the sacral base is more prominent on the dysfunctional side with the patient seated or in the prone position. The ILA on that side is elevated and there does not appear to be any symmetry in ILAs side to side. A pelvic obliquity is present, and, in the prone position, the sacral base will not flex forward with lumbar backward bending. This can be differentiated from a forward or backward sacral torsion by the fact that one ILA stays fixed in both forward and backward bending on a seated flexion test. See Unilaterally Extended Sacrum, Posterior Sacrum, Superior Sacral Shear.

Unilateral Sacral Extension—Right: An osteopathic or manual physical therapy term which refers to a sacrum in which the right sacral base is restricted in flexion. There is a positive forward bending test on the right in sitting and a positive stork test on the right. The left ILA is inferior and posterior, the right sacral base is posterior, and the right leg is short in prone lying due to a lumbar spine that is concave to the right. The right sacral base remains fixed throughout testing in flexion or extension. See Right Unilateral Sacral Extension, Right Superior Sacral Shear, Right Anterior Sacrum.

Unilateral Sacral Flexion: An osteopathic abnormality of sacral motion defined by a postive standing flexion test on the side of dysfunction, a deep sacral sulcus on the side of dysfunction, and an inferior ILA on the side of dysfunction. See Sacral Shear, Unilateral Anterior Nutation of the Sacrum, Unilateral Anterior Sacral Nutation, Unilateral Inferior Nutation of the Sacrum, Unilateral Inferior Sacral Nutation, Unilateral Inferior Sacral Shear, Unilateral Sacral Flexion—Left, Unilateral Sacral Flexion—Right.

Unilteral Sacral Flexion—Left: An osteopathic or manual physical therapy term which refers to a sacrum in which the left sacral base is found in flexion. There is a positive forward bending test on the left in sitting and a positive stork test on the left. The right ILA is inferior and posterior, the left sacral base is posterior, and the left leg is short in prone lying due to a lumbar spine that is concave to the left. The left sacral base remains fixed throughout a testing in flexion or extension. See Left Unilateral Sacral Flexion, Left Superior Sacral Shear, Left Anterior Sacrum.

Unilateral Sacral Flexion—Right: An osteopathic or manual physical therapy term which refers to a sacrum in which the right sacral base is found in flexion. There is a positive forward bending test on the right in sitting and a positive stork test on the right. The left ILA is inferior and posterior, the right sacral base is posterior, and the right leg is short in prone lying due to a lumbar spine that is concave to the right. The right sacral base remains fixed in flexion on flexion or extension of the lumbar spine. See Right Unilateral Sacral Flexion, Right Superior Sacral Shear, Right Anterior Sacrum.

Unilateral Spondylolysis: A fracture of the pars interarticularis that involves only one side. This may allow a 5–10% slippage. This can cause sclerotic changes and hypertrophy in the opposite pedicle, which can be seen on an AP radiograph.

Unilateral Superior Nutation of the Sacrum: An osteopathic or manual physical therapy term which refers to an abnormality in sacral positioning. See Unilateral Sacral Extension.

Unilateral Superior Sacral Nutation: An osteopathic or manual physical therapy term which refers to an abnormality in sacral positioning. See Unilateral Sacral Extension.

Unilateral Superior Sacral Shear: An osteopathic or manual physical therapy term which refers to an abnormality in sacral positioning. See Unilateral Sacral Extension.

Unisegmental Mobility: The mobility of one spinal segment. This can be evaluated either through mobilization or through passive or active range of motion testing.

Universal Reformer: One of the more common pieces of Pilates equipment used by physical therapists, athletic trainers, and Pilates instructors. This is a bench with a moveable platform and resistance. Many different exercises can be performed, including quadriceps strengthening, lateral stability work for SI joint patients, and general spine stability for spinal stabilization work. See Pilates, Reformer.

University Plate: A proprietary name for an anterior spinal fusion system used between T10 and L5. This may be used to stabilize fractures or instability secondary to tumors.

Unlevel Pelvic Base: A proprietary name for an obliquity within the pelvis due to a functional or structural short leg or an SI joint dysfunction. This causes an unlevel base of support for the spine.

Unloading Therapy: A rehabilitation technique used in patients unable to tolerate exercises in normal gravity without pain. See Gravity Unloading, Medical Exercise Therapy, SOMA.

Up-going Toe: A physical exam maneuver performed to detect an upper motor neuron dysfunction. See Babinski Sign.

Upledger: The name of an osteopathic craniosacral technique.

Upper Back Pain: Pain in the upper back musculature. See Upper Dorsal Pain.

Upper Cervical Dysfunction: A restriction in movement of the atlanto-occipital or atlantoaxial joints following a cervical injury. This usually causes pain in the upper cervical region as well as radiating pain experienced as headaches in the posterior occipital region or radiating to just behind the eyes. This headache pain can be either unilateral or bilateral. Common etiology is MVA whiplash injury. Common treatments include upper cervical mobilization or manipulation, cervical traction, nonsteroidals, immobilization if hypermobility is suspected, TENS or MENS to block the headache pain, muscle energy techniques, Jones strain–counterstrain, strengthening, specific stretches, or passive modalities to reduce spasm or inflammation. Patients with pre-existing degenerative arthritis at C1 or C2 may be more prone to upper cervical dysfunction. Some believe that if there is a significant arthritic component, more of the headache pain is experienced in the posterior occipital region.

Upper Dorsal Pain: Pain in the upper back musculature, such as the trapezius, rhomboids, serratus posterior superior, or thoracic spine. See Upper Back Pain.

Upper Limb Tension Test: A series of maneuvers designed to elicit adverse neural tension in the upper extremities. This is the upper extremity equivalent of the straight-leg raise. Often, passive neck flexion or extension is added to intensify or sensitize these tests. See Adverse Neural Tension, BPTT, ULTT.

Up-slip: An osteopathic or manual physical therapy term used to refer to an SI joint dysfunction. The ilium in this condition has "slipped up" relative to the sacrum. Both the PSIS and pubic tubercle are noted to be more superior on exam. This is commonly seen after a sudden impact to one lower extremity, such as stepping into a hole. There is usually tenderness in the quadratus lumborum. The ipsilateral sacrotuberous ligament is slack. See Superior Innominate Shear, Superior Ilium, Up-slipped Innominate, Vertical Ilium.

Up-slipped Innominate: An osteopathic or manual physical therapy term used to refer to an SI joint dysfunction. See Up-slip.

URSA: An osteopathic foundation which promotes osteopathic treatment techniques. URSA is a major force in educating physical therapists in osteopathic manual techniques.

U/S: Abbreviation for *ultrasound*.

UT: An abbreviation for *upper thoracic* and *upper trapezius.*

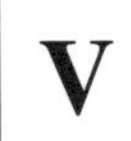

Vacuum Cleft Sign: A radiographic sign which can be seen after whiplash injury. On lateral cervical extension views, a radiolucent linear shadow is seen in the anterior disc space. This is a focal accumulation of nitrogen within an annular tear of the disc. See Lucent Cleft Sign.

Vacuum Phenomenon: Gas noted to be within the disc space on radiographs. This gas appears as a radiolucent (dark) spot within the disc space and is usually thought to denote disc degeneration and possibly segmental instability. The prevalence of vacuum phenomenon increases with the age of the individual and is apparently poorly correlated with present or historic back complaints. Ninety percent of the gas is thought to be nitrogen which has accumulated in the small clefts of the nucleus pulposus. See Vacuum Sign, Gas in Nucleus Pulposus.

Vacuum Sign: Gas noted to be within the disc space on radiographs. See Vacuum Phenomenon.

Valium: A benzodiazepine, which is a central nervous system depressant and a muscle relaxant, that acts directly on skeletal muscle. It is used most commonly for the short-term management of anxiety disorders. It is also used with central nervous system spasticity. There is significant abuse potential. This drug is contraindicated in patients with acute narrow-angle glaucoma. Phenothiazines, narcotics, barbiturates, MAO inhibitors, and antidepressants potentiate the action of this drug. The clearance of Valium can be delayed in association with cimetidine (Tagamet). It is available in 2-mg, 5-mg, and 10-mg tablets. The usual adult dosage is 2–10 mg two times a day to four times a day. See Diazepam.

Vallois Lumbar Index: A numeric rating system which relates the height of the posterior border of the vertebral body to its anterior body. This index is found to be lower in spondylolysis and spondylolisthesis.

Valsalva Maneuver: A forced expiration against a closed glottis which increases venous and cerebral spinal fluid pressure. This is the "bearing down" maneuver. If there is irritation in the covering surrounding the spinal cord (dura) this *may* reproduce the patient's low back pain.

Van Akkerveeken's Measurement of Lumbar Instability: A radiographic evaluation for lumbar instability due to trauma or degenerative disease. A lateral lumbar spine x-ray is taken in neutral, flexion, and extension. Two lines are drawn through and parallel to the opposing end plates. These are allowed to intersect posteriorly. The distance from the posterior body margins to the point of intersection is measured. A distance greater than 1.5–3 mm likely represents clinical instability. See Lumbar Instability, Spinal Instability, Clinical Instability.

Variable Resistance Exercise: Exercise where the weight varies during the range of motion. An example would be a Nautilus system where the weight is varied through the range of motion by the use of cams. A Cybex Eagle system is a similar strength-training device.

Variable Screw Placement System: A type of Steffee plate in which transpedicular screws are used in variable slots. Each plate has a series of "nests" into which the tapered portion of the nut can be securely fixed. The position of the screw can vary along the entire length of the plate for adjustment of fit. See VSP.

VAS: A pain scale in which the patient records pain from 1, which is very mild, to 10, which is excruciating. This is often used to help quantify pain complaints or to follow-up pain complaints during treatment. See Visual Analog Scale.

Vasa Nervorum: The blood supply to the peripheral nervous system which consists of extrinsic vessels which supply feeder arteries to the nerve. There is also an intrinsic system of blood supply within the nerve itself. Blood supply from the nerve roots is from two distinct afferent vessels. In the proximal radicular artery, blood circulates from the longitudinal spinal artery and flows distally. The distal radicular artery arises segmentally and supplies blood to the proximal nerve root. There is a complex intraneural blood supply within the nerve root. The blood supply intraneurally allows for movement of the nerve root by way of arterial coils which allow stretch. In the spinal cord, the anterior spinal artery supplies about 75% of the cord. There are approximately eight medullary feeder arteries that make up this longitudinal system of functioning independent vascular supplies. Posteriorly, there are two small posterior spinal arteries. It should be noted that the nervous system consumes approximately 20% of the available oxygen in the circulating blood yet consists of only 2% of body mass.

Vascular Headache: A headache caused by excessive dilatation of the arteries in the brain. This is considered a vascular headache, and the etiology is unknown. See Migraine Headache.

VATER: An acronym for *v*ertebral defects, imperforate *a*nus, *t*racheo*e*sophageal fistula, and radial and renal dysplasia. This syndrome of congenital vertebral malformations is associated with visceral abnormalities.

Ventral Osteophyte: A bone spur which occurs on the anterior surface of the spine. Large cervical ventral osteophytes can compress the esophagus and cause dysphagia.

Ventral Ramus: The portion of the exiting nerve root which is directed ventrally or toward the anterior aspect of the body. The ventral rami innervate the musculature of the trunk and extremities.

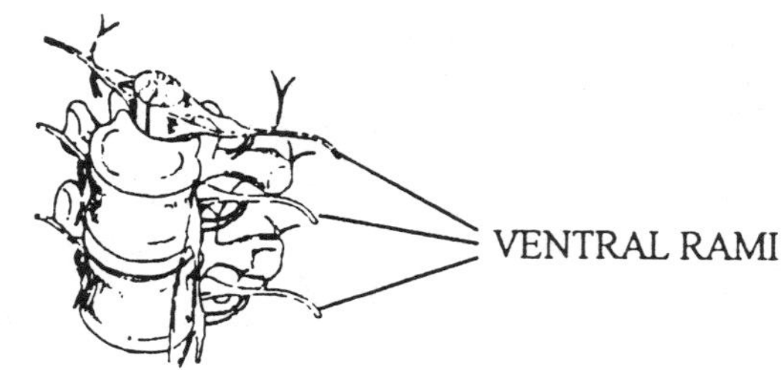

Ventral Root: The anterior motor nerve fibers that exit the anterior horn of the spinal cord and join with the dorsal root and dorsal root ganglion to become the spinal nerve.

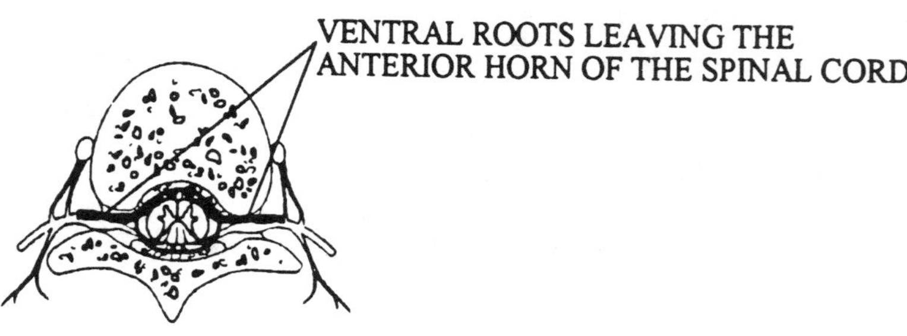

Ventral Sacroiliac Ligament: The relatively thin ligament that lies across the front of the SI joint. It has been demonstrated recently on SI arthrography that this ligament is prone to rupture in traumatic injuries to the joint.

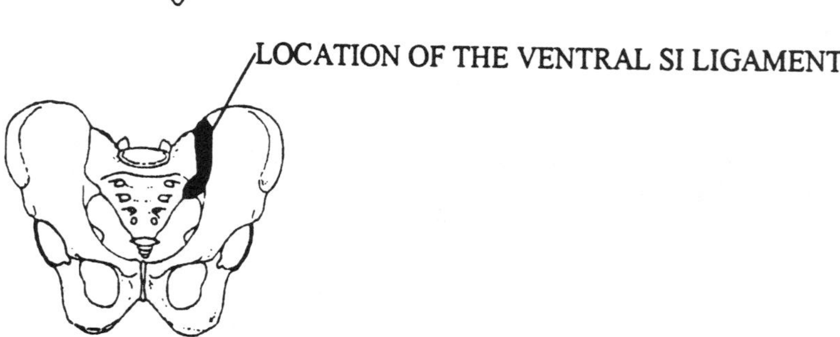

Vermont Spinal Fixator: A proprietary name for instrumentation used for posterior spinal fusion which attaches with pedicle screws. This is a highly adjustable system with two attachment points separated by a rod. A locking bolt clamps the system into place once the appropriate spinal alignment has been attained. See Krag Fixator, VSF.

vert: Abbreviation for *vertebral.*

Vertebra: One of the 24 bones that make up the spine. There are three types: cervical, thoracic, and lumbar. The plural of *vertebra* is *vertebrae*.

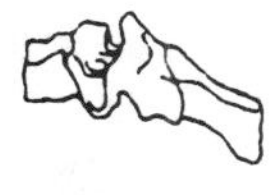

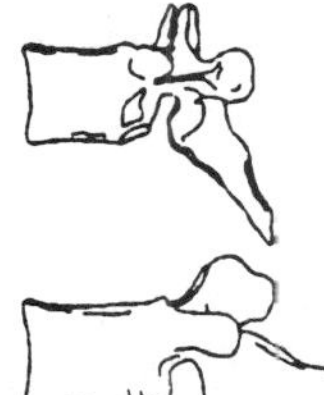

Vertebral Artery: A posterior artery of the neck supplying blood (along with the basilar) to the cerebellum, medulla, spinal cord, and pons. See Vertebrobasilar Artery.

Vertebral Artery Aneurysm: An uncommon ballooning out of the vertebral artery. The most frequent site is C1–C2. The dilatation of the artery may result in erosion adjacent to the C2 pedicle and transverse foramen. Age-related tortuousity of the artery has shown to cause resorption of the pedicle in the mid-cervical spine. The patient may present with suboccipital headaches or features of the syndrome of Barre-Lieou. See Syndrome of Barre-Lieou.

Vertebral Artery Compression Syndrome: An uncommon syndrome characterized by dizziness, light-headedness, vertigo, vasomotor face disturbances, retro-orbital pain, disturbances of vision, and other symptoms. See Vertebral Basilar Syndrome, Syndrome of Barre-Lieou.

Vertebral Artery Insufficiency: An uncommon syndrome characterized by dizziness, light-headedness, vertigo, vasomotor face disturbances, retro-orbital pain, disturbances of vision, and other symptoms. See Syndrome of Barre-Lieou.

Vertebral Artery Syndrome: Spondylitic compromise of the vertebral artery, also known as foramen arcuale. See Syndrome of Barre-Lieou.

Vertebral Basilar Insufficiency: An uncommon syndrome characterized by dizziness, light-headedness, vertigo, vasomotor face disturbances, retro-orbital pain, disturbances of vision, and other symptoms. See Syndrome of Barre-Lieou.

Vertebral Basilar Syndrome: An uncommon syndrome characterized by dizziness, light-headedness, vertigo, vasomotor face disturbances, retro-orbital pain, disturbances of vision, and other symptoms. See Syndrome of Barre-Lieou.

Vertebral Body: The anterior portion of the vertebra which forms the vertebral column when stacked on another vertebra. The circumference of the vertebral bodies increases from the cervical to lumbar areas.

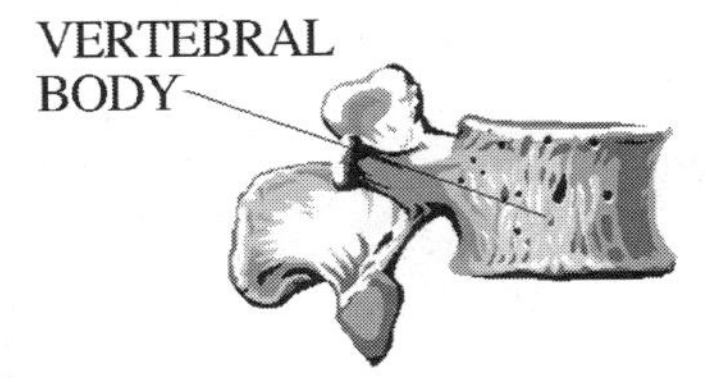

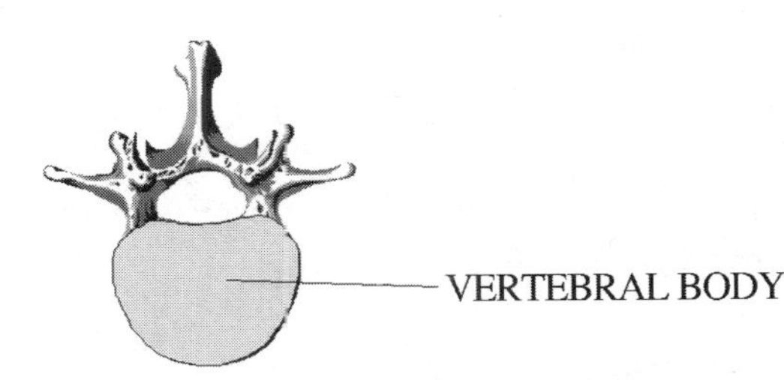

Vertebral Body Instability: Excessive vertebral motion that is beyond normal physiologic motion. This can be due to a traumatic disruption of the ligamentous supporting structures, degenerative disc disease, or fracture. See Instability.

Vertebral Body Sclerosis: Increased density within the vertebral body adjacent to the site of disc narrowing. This can be confused with neoplasm. See Sclerosis—Vertebral Body.

Vertebral Canal: The canal that runs the length of the spine formed by the vertebral foramina. If one stands in the vertebral canal and faces anteriorly, the posterior surfaces of the lumbar vertebrae, the disc, and the posterior longitudinal ligament would be directly ahead. Behind would be the lamina and the ligamentum flavum. To either side would be the pedicles. The intervertebral foramina would be the "windows" to either side.

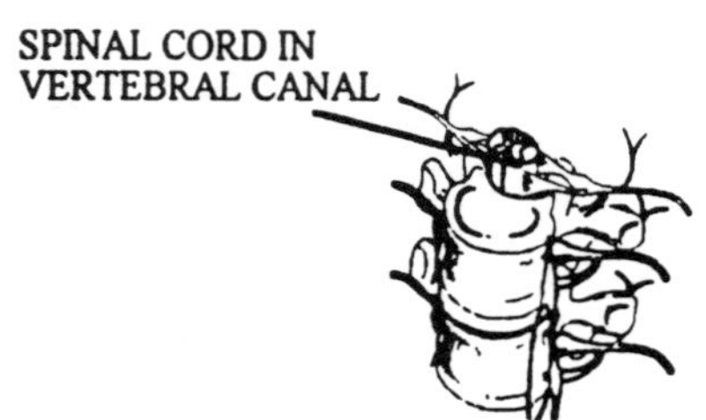

Vertebral Compression Fracture: A collapse of the vertebral body usually seen in elderly patients with osteoporosis. See Compression Fracture.

Vertebral End Plate: A layer of cartilage approximately 1 mm thick which is located on the top and bottom of the vertebral bodies and encircled by the ring apophysis. This consists of hyaline cartilage and fibrocartilage. In older individuals, the end plates are almost entirely fibrocartilage. In younger individuals, the end plate is more extensive and extends out to Sharpey's fibers as the outermost annulus inserts into the intervertebral disc. As the ring apophysis ossifies, the end plate becomes less extensive. It is thought that the end plate has a shock-absorbing function. It has been reported that with axial loads, the end plates will fracture before the nucleus pulposus herniates through the annulus. See End Plate.

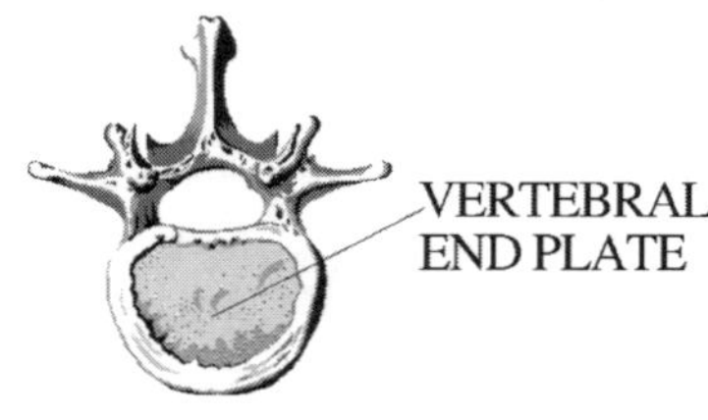

Vertebral End Plate Fracture: A fracture of the end plate. There are three types: a central portion fracture, a peripheral portion fracture, or fractures that are transverse across the entire end plate. See End Plate Fracture.

Vertebral Foramen: A notch above and below each pedicle that is seen when the vertebra is viewed from the side. The superior notch is smaller, and its boundaries include its base at the top of the pedicle; posteriorly, the superior articular process; and, anteriorly, the upper-most posterior edge of the vertebral body. The inferior notch is much deeper. The lower portion of the vertebral body is anterior, and the inferior articular process is posterior. When two vertebral bodies are stacked on top of each other, an intervertebral foramen is formed from the notch above and notch below. This acts as the "window" for the exiting nerve root. See Intervertebral Foramen, Foramen.

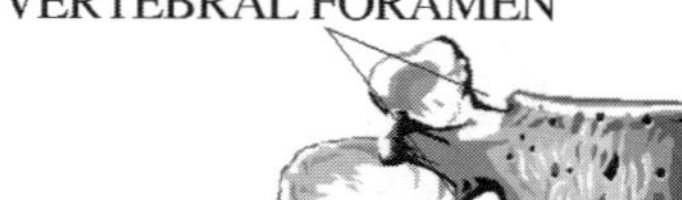

Vertebral Growth Plate: A cartilaginous covering of the superior and inferior aspects of the vertebral body that is responsible for linear growth in the immature skeleton.

Vertebral Hemangioma: A common benign tumor of the spine. See Hemangioma.

Vertebral Lamina: The upper portion of the neural arch which projects from the pedicles toward the midline. See Lamina.

Vertebral Notching: An x-ray finding seen in the preadolescent vertebral body that represents the epiphyseal ring. These notches are seen both superiorly and inferiorly along the vertebral margins.

Vertebral Pedicle: Pillars of bone which project from the back of the vertebral body. See Pedicle.

Vertebral Ring Apophysis: The narrow rim of smoother, less perforated bone which is on the superior and inferior surfaces of each vertebral body. See Ring Apophysis.

Vertebral Subluxation Complex: A chiropractic term which refers to an abnormality of spinal biomechanics involving a loss of normal movement of a vertebral motion segment. See Abnormal Spinal Segmental Motion, Osteopathic Lesion, Joint Blockage, Somatic Dysfunction, Articular Dysfunction.

Vertebral Vein System: The network of venous plexus surrounding the vertebral column that is just anterior to the posterior longitudinal ligament. See Batson's Plexus.

Vertebral Venous Plexus: A system of venous drainage for the spinal cord which exists in the spinal canal. Intermedullary veins drain into a series of longitudinal veins in the epidural space. The venous plexus takes up much of the nonneural space in the spinal canal and also apparently offers some protection from trauma. The veins in this venous plexus do not have valves and thus allow for flow reversibility to accommodate a sudden intake of blood that might occur with such physiologic movements as coughing or straining. Together with the CSF pressure, a balance of intraspinal canal pressure is maintained.

Vertebra Plana: An extremely flat vertebral body associated with vertebral collapse. While this has been associated with osteoporosis, it is uncommon and should arouse suspicion of malignant bone disease or eosinophilic granuloma. See Pancake Vertebra.

Vertebrobasilar Artery: A posterior artery of the neck that supplies blood (along with the basilar) to the cerebellum, medulla, spinal cord, and pons. The arteries (one on each side) pass through the transverse foramina (holes in the cervical transverse processes) and pierce the posterior atlanto-occipital membrane to enter the vertebral canal. They then pass into the foramen magnum where they join with the basilar artery on the anterior surface of the medulla. The basilar artery goes on to unite with the circle of Willis through the posterior cerebral artery. Vertebrobasilar insufficiency can cause posterior circulation symptoms such as dizziness, light-headedness, ocular headache, and loss of consciousness. It has been long postulated that the artery can be compressed secondary to whiplash injuries or spondylosis. See Syndrome of Barre-Lieou, Vertebral Artery.

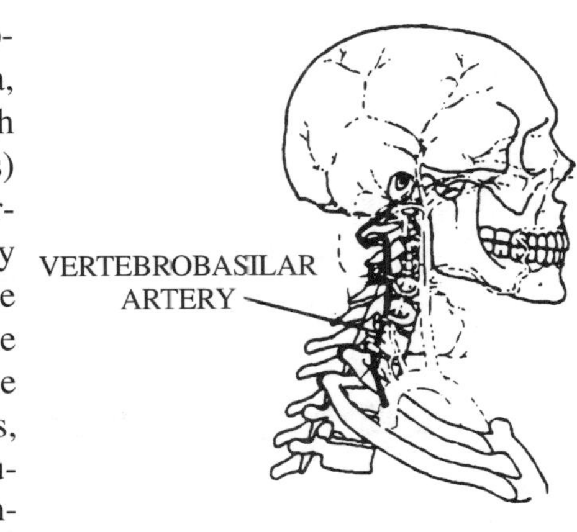

Vertebrogenic Dizziness: An uncommon syndrome characterized by dizziness, light-headedness, vertigo, vasomotor face disturbances, retro-orbital pain, disturbances of vision, and other symptoms. See Syndrome of Barre-Lieou.

Vertex Headache: Headache at the top of the head.

Vertical Cervical Compression Test: The application of vertical, downward pressure on the spine. See Axial Loading Test.

Vertical Fracture of the Sacrum: A fracture of the sacrum which usually occurs due to indirect trauma to the pelvis. These fractures are seen on AP pelvis or outlet views. The fracture line usually runs the entire length of the sacrum and is, of course, vertical. Because an isolated fracture of the sacrum is uncommon, other fractures associated with the pelvic ring or symphysis pubis should be ruled out. See Vertical Sacral Fracture, Sacral Fracture—Vertical, Fracture Sacral—Vertical.

Vertical Ilium: An osteopathic or manual physical therapy term used to refer to an SI joint dysfunction. See Up-slip.

Vertical Sacral Fracture: A fracture of the sacrum which usually occurs due to indirect trauma to the pelvis. See Vertical Fracture of the Sacrum, Sacral Fracture—Vertical, Fracture Sacral—Vertical.

Vertical Settling: An abnormality of a skull base. See Basilar Invagination, Vertical Subluxation.

Vertical Subluxation: Vertical subluxation of the odontoid into the foramen magnum due to erosion of the occipital condyles, lateral masses of the atlas, or lateral facet joints of C1–C2. This is a severe complication of advanced rheumatoid arthritis. The odontoid can compress the medulla oblongata causing myelopathy and possible death from brain stem compression. See Atlantoaxial Impaction, Vertical Settling, Cranial Settling.

Vertigo: Dizziness with a sensation of spinning. The patient usually describes the room spinning around, and this is significantly disabling. There are many different causes including labyrinthitis, Menière's disease, a perilymph fistula due to traumatic causes, a tumor within the semicircular canals or inner ear, myofascial pain of the sternocleidomastoid musculature, and Barre-Lieou syndrome. See Benign Positional Vertigo.

Very Heavy Work: An NIOSH work category which corresponds to lifting more than 100 pounds frequently. This would also include frequently carrying objects weighing greater than 100 pounds.

Vestibulitis: Inflammation of the semicircular canals (labyrinth) in the inner ear. See Labyrinthitis.

Vestibulo-occular Reflex: A centrally mediated reflex which adjusts the eyes to compensate for body movement so that the visual field remains stable. See VOR.

Vestibulospinal Reflex: A centrally mediated reflex which keeps the visual field level by making postural adjustments to the spine. It is also responsible for providing proprioceptive input to the vestibular system. It is thought that this reflex may be the cause of adaptive changes within the spine. See V Sp R, VSR.

vib: An abbreviation for *vibration.*

Vibratory Therapy: A chiropractic technique that uses the fingers or a mechanical device to produce oscillations in body tissues to stimulate proprioceptors.

Vicodin: A powerful narcotic pain reliever containing 5 mg of hydrocodone and 500 mg of acetaminophen. Addiction is possible. The usual dosage is one to two tablets every 4–6 hours as needed for pain. This formulation is very similar to Lortab 5.0.

Vicodin ES: An extra-strength form of the narcotic pain reliever Vicodin. This contains 7.5 mg of hydrocodone with 750 mg of acetaminophen. Physical addiction is possible. The usual dosage is one tablet every 4–6 hours as needed for pain. The total 24-hour dose should not exceed five tablets. This is a very similar formulation to Lortab 7.5, except that Vicodin ES contains 250 mg more acetaminophen.

Vig: An abbreviation for *vigorous high voltage.*

vis: An abbreviation for *visible.*

Viscoelastic: Joint play is usually taken to mean the viscoelastic properties, or "give," of a joint. See Somatic Dysfunction, Loss of Joint Play.

Visual Analog Scale: A pain scale. See VAS.

Voltaren: The delayed-release (enteric-coated) form of diclofenac sodium, which is a nonsteroidal anti-inflammatory drug of the benzeneacetic acid group. It has anti-inflammatory, analgesic, and antipyretic activity. This drug should not be given to patients who have experienced asthma, urticaria, or other allergic reactions due to taking aspirin or other NSAIDs. There is risk of GI side effects, as well as hepatic side effects. There are drug interactions with aspirin, anticoagulants, digoxin, methotrexate, cyclosporine, oral hypoglycemics, diuretics, and other drugs. This drug does increase platelet aggregation time but does not affect bleeding time. Voltaren is supplied in 25-mg, 50-mg, and 75-mg delayed-release tablets, and the usual adult dosage is 50–75 gm taken twice a day. Cataflam is essentially the same drug in the potassium salt and is an immediate-release version. See Cataflam, Diclofenac Potassium.

Von Bechterew Disease: An inflammatory disease of the spine which greatly restricts spinal movement. It is often associated with morning pain and occurs primarily in young adults. It is also known as bamboo spine because of its bamboo shoot-like appearance on x-rays. See Marie-Strumpell Disease, AS, Ankylosing Spondylitis, Rheumatoid Spondylitis, Pelvospondylitis Ossificans.

Von Luschka Joint Arthrosis: An "overgrowth" of the uncovertebral joints which can led to stenosis of cervical foramina. See Uncovertebral Joint Hypertrophy, Uncovertebral Joint.

Von Luschka's Joint: The joints which occur in the lower cervical spine from C2–C7. See Uncovertebral Joint.

Von Luschka's Nerve: The sinuvertebral nerve that emerges from the dorsal root just distal to the dorsal root ganglion. See Sinuvertebral Nerve.

VOR: A centrally mediated reflex. See Vestibulo-occular Reflex.

VS: An abbreviation for *vital signs*.

VSF: Instrumentation used for posterior spinal fusion. See Vermont Spinal Fixator.

V Sign: A radiographic sign seen on a lateral x-ray view which may represent a ruptured or elongated transverse ligament. On a lateral radiograph, C1 is tilted in relation to the dens and a "V" is created by a line drawn on the posterior aspect of the anterior atlas and the anterior aspect of the dens. There is some disagreement as to whether this represents clinical instability. If neurologic signs are present, C1–C2 fusion is usually considered. See ADI.

VSP: A type of Steffee plates. See Variable Screw Placement System.

V Sp R: A centrally mediated reflex. See Vestibulospinal Reflex.

VSR: A centrally mediated reflex. See Vestibulospinal Reflex.

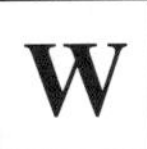

Waddell's Test: A series of five tests thought to be associated with nonorganic pain behavior. The first is light touch or rolling of the skin. This is positive if the patient complains of an exaggerated pain response. The second is a simulation test involving axial rotation of the pelvis and shoulders. A positive test causes back pain. The third is a distraction test. This is positive if distraction by the examiner causes pain behaviors during a maneuver to decrease. The fourth is nonanatomic numbness or nonanatomic weakness. The fifth is overreaction. This is scored positive when there is excessive body language, grimacing, verbalizations, groans, or tremors. It should be noted that Waddell's test can be positive in patients who are symptom magnifiers. It also should be noted that the literature consistently shows that true malingering is rare, occurring in approximately 2% of the population. See Nondermatomal Sensory Loss, Nonorganic Signs, Symptom Magnification Syndrome.

Wallerian Degeneration: Damage to a nerve fiber through trauma or prolonged compression which results in degeneration and disintegration of the fiber both distal to the point of injury and proximal (back toward the body). Regeneration is possible after the debris has been cleared. Regrowth occurs at about 1 mm per day.

Wall Lateral Glide: A physical therapy exercise used to increase side gliding. See Wall Lateral Shear.

Wall Lateral Shear: A physical therapy exercise used to increase side gliding. The patient stands sideways against a wall with the elbow or forearm resting on the wall with the hand against the wall on the rib cage. The other hand is on the lateral surface of the opposite hip. The patient pushes sideways to the point where range of motion ends. See Wall Lateral Glide.

Wall Slides: A physical therapy exercise to strengthen the quadriceps and promote dynamic stability of the pelvis while dependent on the quadriceps in a standing position. The patient is asked to lean the back against a wall and stabilize the pelvis. The knees are bent. The patient then slides along the wall increasing flexion at the knees and then pushes back up with the quadriceps. This is then repeated for quadriceps strengthening.

Warm and Form Back Brace: A soft low back brace. See Warm and Form Low Back Brace.

Warm and Form Low Back Brace: A soft, low back brace with a thermoplastic insert that can be custom molded to the lumbar spine and then placed within a special insert posteriorly. This obviously provides more support than a traditional soft low back brace. See Warm and Form Back Brace, Back Brace—Warm and Form.

WCE: A test of physical strength and stamina used to determine working restrictions and work tolerance. See Functional Capacity Evaluation, Work Capacity Evaluation.

Weaver's Bottom: An inflammation of the ischial bursa. See Ischial Bursitis.

Wedge Fracture: A compression fracture of the vertebra which is caused by anterior collapse of the vertebral body from a hyperflexion injury.

Wedge-shaped Vertebra: A vertebra with its anterior height much smaller than its posterior height. This is commonly seen in the thoracic spine and is due to compression fractures in osteoporotic patients. See Wedge Vertebra.

Wedge Vertebra: A vertebra with its anterior height much smaller than its posterior height. See Wedge-shaped Vertebra.

Weight-bearing Line of L3: The imaginary line that represents a plumb line dropped from the vertex of the head in a patient with perfect posture. See Gravitational Line.

Weizhong Acupont: An acupuncture point used to treat low back pain that is located in the popliteal fossa.

Well-Leg Raising: A physical exam maneuver in which one leg is raised with the patient in the supine postion. See Fajersztajn Sign.

Well-Leg Raising Test of Fajersztajn: A physical exam maneuver in which one leg is raised with the patient in the supine postion. See Crossed Straight-Leg Raising Test.

West Coast Method: An injection technique used for prolotherapy. See Ongley's Technique, Prolotherapy.

Westergren Sedimentation Rate: A nonspecific test that is an indicator of the overall level of inflammation. See Erythrocyte Sedimentation Rate, WSR.

West Tool Sort: A test of perceived disability commonly used during a functional capacity evaluation. The patient is asked to sort through 65 cards, which contain a picture and description of a tool and how it is most commonly used. The patient is asked to sort these cards into five different categories such as: I would have no change in the speed I work, I would be unable to work, I do not know whether or not I could use this tool. There are three pairs of duplicate tools in the 65 cards. These serve as a check for validity. If the patient does not place these cards into matching categories, there is suspicion of symptom magnification or malingering. The test also helps to determine the patient's perception of disability. See Loma Linda Activity Sort, Spinal Function Sort.

WFL: An abbreviation for w*ithin functional limits.*

Whiplash Injury: A sprain or strain syndrome of the cervical spine caused by a hyperextension–

hyperflexion injury. This most commonly occurs in motor vehicle accidents. In rear-end accidents, this can involve injury to the sternocleidomastoid musculature, the longus colli, anterior longitudinal ligament, or cervical discs. The poorest prognosis for recovery is for patients involved in rear-end accidents and patients with a previous whiplash injury, pre-existing degenerative disc disease, or neurologic symptoms soon after the accident. In one study, some patients who had experienced a rear-end MVA were still symptomatic at one year after the accident regardless of litigation or compensation issues. Common treatments include short course of immobilization, nonsteroidals, muscle relaxants, muscle energy techniques, cervicothoracic stabilization techniques, Jones strain–counterstrain, traction, deep tissue work such as massage or myotherapy, stretching, modalities to reduce inflammation and muscle spasm, strengthening of the cervical extensors, and mobilization or manipulation of individual restricted cervical segments. See Acceleration–Deceleration Injury, Flexion–Extension Injury.

Whiskering: A radiographic sign in ankylosing spondylitis. This is a calcification of the entheses (area where muscle and tendon attach to the bone). Spicules of bone extend away from the bone due to periostitis.

Wide Foraminotomy: A foraminotomy that is more extensive for additional nerve root decompression.

Wigraine: An ergotamine and caffeine tablet or a suppository that is used primarily as an abortive for vascular headaches, such as migraine. The use of Wigraine is contraindicated in pregnant patients and in patients with peripheral vascular disease, heart disease, hypertension, impaired hepatic or renal function, and sepsis. The average adult dose is two tablets at the start of a vascular headache, followed by one tablet every half hour if needed, up to six tablets per attack. Two Wigraine suppositories are given for each individual attack.

Williams Brace: A lumbar support brace that controls flexion, extension, and side bending but not lumbar rotation.

Williams Flexion Exercises: A series of exercises first developed by Paul Williams (an orthopedic surgeon) in 1934. It is based on the concept that controlling the pelvic angle will reduce overall stress forces on the lumbar spine. Exercises involve abdominal strengthening, pelvic tilts, gluteal strengthening, and iliopsoas stretches. Some components of this program have found their way into lumbar stabilization programs.

Willner Instrument for Spinal Stabilization: A lumbar support brace. See WISS.

Wiltse Fixator: A type of pedicle screw fixation used for a posterior spinal fusion.

Wiltse System: A proprietary name for a system of instrumentation for posterior spinal fusion which involves pedicle screws which are attached by cable with adjustable clamps. This allows for three-dimensional adjustability between the screws and longitudinal linking devices. See Pedicle Screw Fixation.

Wiltse Technique: One technique for posterior lateral fusion in which bilateral incisions are made off the midline, and the muscle and fascia are split to obtain access to the transverse processes. An intertransverse fusion is then performed.

Winking Owl Sign: A radiographic sign seen with lytic metastases of the spine. See One-eyed Pedicle Sign.

Winter Anterior Osteotomy: A technique for anterior spinal fusion to correct congenital kyphosis.

Wintrobe: A nonspecific test for the overall level of inflammation. See ESR, Westergren, Erythrocyte Sedimentation Rate.

Wisconsin Segmental Spine Instrumentation: A posterior spinal instrumentation system which is commonly used to correct scoliotic deformities. This is a combination of traditional Harrington rod instrumentation and Luque segmental fixation through the base of the spinous processes. This system is capable of correcting deformities in all planes See WSSI.

WISS: A lumbar support brace with adjustable side straps that provides adjustable lumbar support through a tightening knob in the back. A trial adjustable orthosis is worn, and the measurements are used to fabricate a final solid brace. See Willner Instrument for Spinal Stabilization.

WNL: An abbreviation for *within normal limits.*

Work Capacity Evaluation: A test of physical strength and stamina used to determine working restrictions and work tolerance. See Functional Capacity Evaluation.

Work Conditioning: A program designed to progress an injured worker from the acute stages of an injury to optimal recovery and return to work. Usually, strength, cardiovascular fitness, and flexibility are emphasized.

Work Conditioning Program: A rehabilitation program. See Work Hardening Program.

Work Hardening Program: A rehabilitation program involving gradually progressive work-related activities performed with good body mechanics in an attempt to prepare that person to return to work. This may involve a psychological component to prepare the worker mentally and emotionally for a safe return to work. See Work Conditioning Program.

Work Restriction: Limitations on lifting, positions, postures, and upper and lower extremity use that are specified after a work injury for the purposes of allowing the injured tissue to heal.

Work Simulation: A component of a work hardening program in which specific job tasks are simulated to replicate the work enviroment.

Work Tolerance: The ability to sustain a work effort at a specific frequency over a given period of time. Work tolerance can be measured sitting, reaching, kneeling, standing, stooping, crouching, pushing, pulling, walking, climbing, fingering, handling, feeling, listening, gripping, talking, and seeing.

Work Tolerance Screening: A test of physical strength and stamina used to determine working restrictions and work tolerance. See Functional Capacity Evaluation.

WR: An abbreviation for *work restriction.*

Wright's Hyperabduction Maneuver: A physical exam test used to evaluate thoracic outlet syndrome at the first rib. The patient is asked to protract the shoulders bilaterally. This narrows the space in the thoracic outlet between the clavicle and the first rib and should reproduce radiating symptoms in the upper extremity. However, having the patient inhale has also been described and possibly sensitizes the maneuver. This further narrows the space between the clavicle and the first rib by elevating the first rib. See Costoclavicular Maneuver, Hyperabduction Maneuver, Adson's Test.

Wryneck: A congenital condition which causes the head and neck to be side bent to the affected side and the chin to face the opposite direction. See Congenital Torticollis.

WSR: A nonspecific test that is an indicator of the overall level of inflammation. See ESR, Westergren Sedimentation Rate.

WSSI: A posterior spinal instrumentation system. See Wisconsin Segmental Spine Instrumentation.

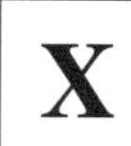

X

Xanax: A benzodiazepine with the chemical name of alprazolam. This is a central nervous system depressant indicated for use in patients with generalized anxiety, panic disorder, or acutely stressful situations which cannot be controlled without medications. The use of this medication is contraindicated in patients with acute narrow-angle glaucoma. There is a significant abuse potential. The usual dosage for patients with anxiety is 0.25–0.5 mg three times a day. The maximum daily dose is 4 mg, and the drug can usually be increased in three- to four-day intervals. In elderly patients, or in patients with advanced liver disease or debilitating disease, the usual starting dose is 0.25 mg two to three times a day. The elderly may be very sensitive to the effects of this drug and other drugs in the benzodiazepine class. Xanax is provided in 0.25-mg, 0.5-mg, 1-mg, and 2-mg tablets, which are all scored.

Xenograft: A graft used for spinal fusion that is from another animal species. See Heterograft.

Xylocaine: An amino amide which is commonly used for anesthetic infiltration. See Lidocaine.

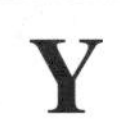

Y Ligament of Bigelow: One of the strongest ligaments of the body. It resembles an inverted Y. See Iliofemoral Ligament.

Yeoman's Sign: A test for SI joint dysfunction. The patient lies in the prone position, and pressure is placed over the SI joint on the affected side to fix the pelvis to the table. The leg is raised into hyperextension at the hip with the knee flexed. Increased pain in the SI joint is considered to be a positive sign.

yest: An abbreviation for *yesterday*.

Yuan Plates: Plates used for instrumentation of an anterior fusion in the thoracolumbar spine.

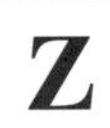

ZB: A system of musculoskeletal treatment. See Zero Balancing.

Zero Balancing: A system of musculoskeletal treatment developed by Fritz Frederick Smith. The concept of balancing body energy is combined with balancing body structure. There is an attempt to blend the traditional Western concepts of anatomy, physiology, and kinesiology with Eastern concepts such as energy channeling and chakras. See ZB.

Zielke Device: Instrumentation used for an anterior interbody spinal fusion which is a modification of the Dwyer cable system. A flexible rod is used in place of a cable and attached to screws implanted laterally into the vertebral bodies. A special outrigger device can be used to enhance the lordosis during curve correction, which is a benefit over the cable systems where this is not possible. During correction of the curve, the nuts in the compression side of the device are tightened, and the surgeon works away from the apex of the curve sequentially. This is considered one of the implants of choice for correction of thoracolumbar scoliosis.

Zielke Instrumentation: Instrumentation used for an anterior spinal fusion of long segments. It is often used in idiopathic scoliosis correction. See Zielke Screws, Zielke Device.

Zielke Screws: Instrumentation used for an anterior interbody spinal fusion. See Zielke Instrumentation.

Z-joint: An abbreviation for zygapophyseal joint. See Facet Joint, Zygapophyseal Joint.

Zoloft: An antidepressant in the selective serotonin reuptake inhibitor (SSRI) class. It is contraindicated for use in patients on MAO inhibitors. There are drug interactions with warfarin (Coumadin), digoxin, cimetidine, diazepam, lithium, and atenolol. The use of alcohol with this drug is not recommended, although it apparently does not potentiate any CNS side effects. All SSRIs are activating to some degree, and this is a common complaint. The initial dose is 50 mg once a day. The dosage range is 50–200 mg per day. In patients with hepatic or renal impairment, lower dosage should be given. Zoloft is supplied in 50- and 100-mg capsule-shaped scored tablets. See Sertraline Hydrochloride.

Zolpidem Tartrate: A nonbenzodiazepine sleeping medication. See Ambien.

Zone of Impaction: A radiopaque band which can sometimes be seen in the middle of a compression fracture. This is an area where the bone has been driven together following a forceful flexion injury.

Zone of Irritation: A direction of vertebral movement which irritates a spinal segment when mobilized.

Zone of Reference: The referred pain pattern of a trigger point or the region of the body that contains the referred pain pattern.

Zuni: A proprietary name for a gravity-unloading system. See SOMA, Gravity Unloading, Medical Exercise Therapy.

Zygapophyseal: Of or pertaining to the facet joints.

Zygapophyseal Blocks: Injection of local anesthetic and steroid into the facet joints (usually lumbar) under fluoroscopic guidance. See Facet Block.

Zygapophyseal Joint: The facet joint. This term is derived from the Greek *apophysis*, meaning "outgrowth," and *zygos*, meaning "bridge." This, therefore, translates to "a bridging outgrowth." This refers to how the superior and inferior articular processes form a bridge over the posterior portion of the foramen. See Facet Joint.